RESEARCH TRENDS IN NUTRITION FOR THE MIDDLE AGED AND ELDERLY

Johan P. Urster

Editor

Nova Science Publishers, Inc.
New York

Library of Congress Cataloging-in-Publication Data

Research trends in nutrition for the middle aged and elderly / Johan P. Urster (editor).
    p. ; cm.
 Includes bibliographical references and index.
 ISBN 978-1-60456-147-0 (hardcover)
 1. Middle-aged persons--Nutrition. 2. Older people--Nutrition. I. Urster, Johan P.
 [DNLM: 1. Nutrition Physiology. 2. Aged. 3. Aging--physiology. 4. Diabetes Mellitus--prevention & control. 5. Middle Aged. 6. Socioeconomic Factors. QU 145 R4323 2007]
TX361.M47R48 2007
613.2084'4--dc22
                            2007046682

Published by Nova Science Publishers, Inc. ✦ New York

Contents

Preface

The aging process changes body composition and thus nutritional status changes as one gets older. At the same time the body becomes more susceptible to diseases and diet becomes an even more significant or at least visibly significant than in earlier years. Moreover, there is frequently socio-economic downward drifting in this age group making nutritious foods more difficult to afford. This new book presents leading-edge research from around the world.

Short Communication - Aims: 1) Describe the characteristics of a typical adult with type 2 diabetes mellitus (DM) in a developing country; 2) develop interventions to overcome the barriers to effective self management of type 2 diabetes mellitus, based on evidence.

Method: Current literature regarding barriers, models of education and development of patients' self management skills with evidence based interventions were reviewed.

Successful interventions in Chile, Costa Rica, Israel, and USA were reviewed and useful elements extracted to inform an educational/ behavior change intervention strategy for the adult patient with DM in a developing country.

Results: The typical adult with type 2 DM is obese, poorly motivated, poorly equipped to manage his or her illness and confused by inconsistent information. Important elements of a successful intervention would include: assessment of the knowledge and practices of the health care providers, patients and patients' families; instruction and support in the regular and effective use of a portable glucose monitor; nutritional and exercise interventions to effect weight loss in overweight and obese patients; continuous monitoring and assessment of patients in their knowledge and self care practices, recognizing that knowledge does not necessarily relate to effective self care.

Conclusion: The most important element of any successful intervention is an effective plan based on evidence. Research is necessary to assess the barriers, including cultural and psychosocial barriers to effective self care in the target population. Guidance should be sought from recommended "standards of care" and input developed by a multidisciplinary team to develop a specific program. The material would be frequently evaluated, modified, and updated as required. Major components should include instruction and support in the regular use of a portable glucose monitor and input from nutritionists and dietitians in a weight loss program. The use of indigenous low glycemic foods should be encouraged. It is important to transmit information in a way that is consistent with the educational level of the target population. It is also important to motivate patients to learn about DM, and to empower them to set realistic goals and actively assume their roles in treatment and care.

Chapter 1 - The inflammatory bowel diseases (IBD) and colorectal cancer (CRC) share common global geographic distributions. Similarly in both, pathogenesis depends on host and environmental influences. In particular, genetic background and intestinal microflora both contribute to disease formation. While diet is strongly implicated in CRC, such a pathogenic role is less clear in IBD. This focused review discusses the role of vitamin D obtained either through geographic exposure to sunlight or diet in both diseases as a modefier of risk, It reviews the evidence that risk of both disease is also linked epidemiologically to national dairy food consumption and the population prevalence of lactase status. The potential effector contribution of calcium is discussed. Based on these similarities in the two diseases, it is hypothesized that the observed paradoxical reduction in risk with dairy foods observed for CRC may also apply to IBD. If hypotheses put forth are supported, future studies on the effects of dairy foods on some diseases may need to consider lactase status and the use of lactose free products or digestive aids should be markedly reduced.

Chapter 2 - Cardiovascular disease, a leading cause of mortality in most industrialized countries, is associated with non-modifiable and modifiable risk factors. For some of the modifiable risk factors (hypertension, dyslipidemia, obesity and type 2 diabetes mellitus) nutritional therapy is recommended. The prevalence of these diet-modifiable risk factors, as well as of CVD, increases in middle-aged and older people. A body of evidence is accumulating that gender has an impact on the presentation, management and outcomes of CVD. It also has an impact on the modifiable risk factors and on the way they affect CVD risk and outcomes in this population. Gender differences exist also in relation to nutrition and may affect the nutrition-CVD risk factors interrelation in several ways: The sexes differ in the effect of nutrients and diet patterns on CVD risk, in the establishment of dietary habits, in the outcome of nutritional interventions and in compliance with dietary modification. Understanding of the impact of gender on the influence of nutrition on CVD and on the contributing risk factors may improve nutritional interventions in the primary and secondary prevention of CVD.

This chapter will include a short overview of the CVD risk factors, modifiable by diet and their gender-related aspects. The authors will emphasize the rationale for the dietary recommendations for primary and secondary prevention of CVD.

Chapter 3 - Diabetes mellitus is a group of metabolic diseases characterized by hyperglycemia resulting from defects in insulin secretion, insulin action, or both. The chronic hyperglycemia is associated with long-term damage causing dysfunction and failure of various organs, especially the eyes, kidneys, nerves, heart, and blood vessels. The prevalence of type 2 diabetes is increasing dramatically across the globe and in some regions has reached almost epidemic proportions. An estimated 135 million people worldwide had diagnosed diabetes in 1995, and this number is expected to rise to at least 300 million by 2025. This increase in prevalence is primarily being driven by environmental factors: "western" type of diet and more sedentary lifestyle. In addition, the ageing of the world population, particularly the western population, will increase the number of type 2 diabetes over the next years, unless adequate preventative actions are undertaken. Indeed, there are strong evidences that diabetes may be preventable, even in high-risk groups. Therefore, this chapter is focused on dietary factors which are important in the type 2 diabetes prevention in the elderly. The paper has been written based on research and epidemiological data. Topics include epidemiology informations as well as nutrients and recommendation. Special attention is paid on energy, fats, carbohydrates supply in prevention of the disease. In this paper, each of these nutrients is discussed separately. The efficacy of selected vitamins and minerals as well as alcohol at preventing type 2 diabetes in elderly are also discussed.

Chapter 4 – Nutrition has been recognized as a major determinant of health for centuries. Many studies showed that both food overabundance and macronutrient deficiency in older people increase the risk of many metabolic diseases. The costs associated with hospitalization resulting from many chronic diseases are usually higher than the costs of their prevention. The role of nutrition in health promotion and prevention of non-communicable or diet related diseases has not been given proper consideration. Aging of population is related to an increasing risk of chronic diseases such as cardiovascular disease (CVD) because an age has been included in groups of independent heart disease risk factors. Therefore, the primary target of this chapter is focus on the CVD prevention in the elderly. The paper has been written based on research and epidemiological data. Topics include epidemiology as well as nutrients and recommendation. In this paper, each of important diet ingredients in the prevention of cardiovascular disease such as fats, saturated fatty acids, cholesterol, carbohydrates, fiber, protein and B-groups vitamins, antioxidants, minerals as well as flavonoids is discussed separately. In conclusion there is a diet for the elderly. This chapter gives practical dietary recommendation for older people. Nutritional education of people even above 60 years old might be effective and useful because it is never too late to change nutritional habits for healthy ageing.

Chapter 5 – Obesity in adults is an increasing health problem. The increasing prevalence of obesity in many developing countries can be due to adoption of Western-style diet. In some countries obesity has reached epidemic levels and obesity related complications are the most important problems globally. It seems that in current strategy to stop obesity escalation too little attention has been given to the prevention of this disease. In the prevention of obesity three components: total energy intake, diet composition and portion size play a crucial role. Management of older, obese patients is difficult, and it is not obvious whether weight reduction is associated with beneficial health effect. Therefore prevention in earlier ages, rather than intervention in late life, is the recommended, most cost-effective strategy for successful aging. General nutritional strategies for obesity prevention include promotion of fruit, vegetables and whole grain product intake, restriction of energy-dense (salty, fatty and sugary), micronutrients-poor foods intake, and reduction of consumption of sugars-sweetened beverages. These strategies can result in improving the quality of diet.

This chapter focuses on energy and nutrients intake as well as on portions sizes as possible causative factors for unhealthy weight gain. Topics include epidemiology information as well as nutrients and recommendations. Special attention is paid on energy intake and density of food in weight gain prevention. Dietary fat, carbohydrates and selected micronutrients intakes are also discussed. The paper has been written based on research and epidemiological data.

Chapter 6 – Adults age 60 and older will comprise two-thirds of the diabetic population by the year 2025. Nutritional needs and patterns change with age, especially in the presence of a chronic metabolic disease such as diabetes. More than any other factor, the process of aging defines the daily requirements of protein, fat, carbohydrate, vitamins, and trace elements. It is expected that the prevalence of overweight and obesity will increase in the elderly and be a significant contributory factor to insulin resistance, hyperglycemia, and comorbid health conditions like hypertension and dyslipidemia. The issue of attainment and maintenance of an optimal body weight in elderly diabetic persons may not be as straightforward as in other age groups, and the risk-benefit ratio may be different as well. On the other hand, older inhabitants of long-term care facilities who suffer from diabetes tend to be underweight, which may signify malnutrition and be a risk factor for increased morbidity and mortality. The attendant problems of appetite changes, palatability of food, dietary restrictions, loneliness, and depression may affect the type and quantity of food consumed by elderly persons. Any involuntary change of greater than 10 pounds or 10% of body weight within a short time-frame may be nutrition-related and warrants further investigation from this standpoint. Overall, there is a paucity of information on the nutritional aspects of older patients with diabetes. This area would benefit from ongoing research because of the enormous increase in diabetes underway in the elderly population.

Chapter 7 – Acute pancreatitis is an acute inflammatory process of the pancreas with variable involvement of peripancreatic tissues or remote organ systems, usually caused by gallstones or alcohol. Supportive care rather than specific therapy characterizes the current management of acute pancreatitis and the arsenal of valuable options is pretty scarce. Thereby, the role of artificial nutrition as a novel therapeutical modality in acute pancreatitis should be carefully explored.

While the concept of "pancreatic rest" and a nil-per-mouth regimen dominated throughout the 20th century, the latest studies demonstrate unequivocal benefits of enteral over parenteral nutrition in terms of better glucose tolerance as well as reduction in infectious complications and mortality in patients with severe acute pancreatitis. Now that the advantages of enteral feeding have become apparent, the next step would be to clarify the optimal timing of onset of nutritional support. Theoretically, enteral feeding can prevent mucosal barrier dysfunction, small bowel bacterial overgrowth, and bacterial translocation and, therefore, should be instituted as early as possible in the course of disease. However, this hypothesis should be tested in the randomized trial on early versus delayed enteral nutrition.

Furthermore, as two recent randomized controlled trials demonstrated no difference in morbidity and mortality between nasogastric and nasojejunal feeding, the potential cumbers with the positioning of feeding tube in the jejunum with the aid of endoscopy or interventional radiology might be solved. Apart from this, intermittent feeding may probably decrease the gastric retention in patients on nasogastric tube feeding. Thereby, the effect of intermittent versus continuous enteral tube feeding should be investigated in the setting of acute pancreatitis.

Another important aspect for the optimizing of management of acute pancreatitis is observed in the modification in composition of enteral formula. Such immune-enhanced supplementations as glutamine, arginine and ὡ-3 fatty acids are unlikely to be effective. At the same time, the use of enteral nutrition supplemented with pro- pre- and synbiotics may potentially bring benefits to the patients with acute pancreatitis. However, further adequately powered studies are warranted before implementing them in clinical practice.

To this end, enteral nutrition appears to be an indisputable tool in acute pancreatitis and further high-quality studies should focus on the ways to elaborate it.

In: Research Trends in Nutrition…
Editor: Johan P. Urster, pp. 1-6

ISBN: 978-1-60456-147-0
© 2008 Nova Science Publishers, Inc.

Short Communication

Barriers to Control of Diabetes Mellitus in a Developing Country: A Search for Effective Interventions.

E.M. Duff[1], N. McFarlane-Anderson[2] and R.A. Wright-Pascoe[3]

[1] The University of the West Indies School of Nursing,
[2] Biochemistry Section, Basic Medical Sciences, UWI,
[3] Department of Medicine,
The University of the West Indies (UWI), Kingston 7, Jamaica

Abstract

Aims: 1) Describe the characteristics of a typical adult with type 2 diabetes mellitus (DM) in a developing country; 2) develop interventions to overcome the barriers to effective self management of type 2 diabetes mellitus, based on evidence.

Method: Current literature regarding barriers, models of education and development of patients' self management skills with evidence based interventions were reviewed.

Successful interventions in Chile, Costa Rica, Israel, and USA were reviewed and useful elements extracted to inform an educational/ behavior change intervention strategy for the adult patient with DM in a developing country.

Results: The typical adult with type 2 DM is obese, poorly motivated, poorly equipped to manage his or her illness and confused by inconsistent information. Important elements of a successful intervention would include: assessment of the knowledge and practices of the health care providers, patients and patients' families; instruction and support in the regular and effective use of a portable glucose monitor; nutritional and exercise interventions to effect weight loss in overweight and obese patients; continuous monitoring and assessment of patients in their knowledge and self care practices, recognizing that knowledge does not necessarily relate to effective self care.

Conclusion: The most important element of any successful intervention is an effective plan based on evidence. Research is necessary to assess the barriers, including cultural and psychosocial barriers to effective self care in the target population. Guidance should be sought from recommended "standards of care" and input developed by a multidisciplinary team to develop a specific program. The material would be frequently evaluated, modified, and updated as required. Major components should include instruction and support in the regular use of a portable glucose monitor and input from nutritionists and dietitians in a weight loss program. The use of indigenous low glycemic foods should be encouraged. It is important to transmit information in a way that is consistent with the educational level of the target population. It is also important to motivate patients to learn about DM, and to empower them to set realistic goals and actively assume their roles in treatment and care.

Introduction

The prevalence of diabetes mellitus (DM) continues to increase in the developing world as a result of changes related to modern lifestyles, decreased physical activity, high calorie diets and escalating obesity. In the Americas the number of people with DM was estimated at 35 million in 2000 and this is expected to increase to 64 million by 2025 [1].

Characteristics of a Typical Adult with Type 2 Diabetes

In Jamaica, for example, where the prevalence of DM in adults is12.7 (9.1-17.4)% for males and 18.4 (14.9-22.8)% for females [1], the typical individual with type 2 DM attending a specialty clinic tends to be female, of African ethnicity, has a mean age of 55 years, has had diabetes for more than 12 years, has a low level of basic education, is likely to be married or in a common law union, be unemployed or employed in a low-paying job and be largely dependent on a spouse or other family members for financial and psychosocial support [2,3]. Her body mass index (BMI) is high with a mean of 30 kg/m^2, her waist circumference large at 100cm, her systolic blood pressure (SBP) elevated at a mean of 139mmHg and the diastolic (DBP) at 81mmHg. She exercises 1.5 hours per week, her HbA1c is 8.4%, sugar intake is high at 140 g/week and is mainly in the form of sweetened beverages [2]. Her mean total cholesterol is 5.4mmol/L, HDL cholesterol is 1.2mmol/L. Her mean LDL cholesterol is 3.6mmol/L, and triglycerides 1.5mmol/L. The mean microalbuminuria is 74 mg/L. The parameters for oxidative stress are elevated, further increasing the risk of target organ damage [4].

She relies mainly on her physician for information about her illness. She tries to follow the "doctors' orders" but her knowledge is not sufficient for her to manage her illness effectively. She lacks perception of the risks of the chronic complications of diabetes, therefore, she pays little attention to her diet, does not use a portable glucose monitor and is generally noncompliant with medication, including insulin. She is poorly motivated and poorly equipped to manage her illness and confused by the inconsistent information she receives on diabetes mellitus. Her obesity may be culturally acceptable [5]. Although her medication is funded by a government agency, and she may have some insurance, she has little spare cash for such items as diagnostic tests, hospitalization, transportation, diabetes education, and any special dietary requirements. She has been taught to take care of her feet and eyes and attends clinics regularly but neglects dental care. She has however, more knowledge than her male counterparts at the public clinic, who tend to be older, and although less knowledgeable, manage to score higher on their self care rating scales [2,3].

Interventions

A similar population in Brazil, demonstrated a low basic education and limited knowledge regarding DM, its causes, management and prevention of acute and chronic complications [6]. A study in Costa Rica, found that patients did not did not make the link between a family history of obesity and diabetes, and received inconsistent nutritional messages from health care providers. This qualitative study was done to determine the knowledge and practices of patients and health care providers, looking at diabetes prevention and control and the local availability of foods. Based on these results, an educational methodology was developed and courses for health care providers, patients and patients' families were implemented. The model was successfully incorporated into the El Guarco-area health centers [7].

A study in the USA used self reports and automated clinic data to identify gaps in diabetes management and linked clinical depression with less physical activity, unhealthy diet and decreased adherence to medication [8]. Another study, in Caucasian and African Americans found no consistent relationships between glycemic control, social support, and self efficacy [9].

Simmons (2001) in summarizing personal barriers to optimal diabetes care, classified these as "educational," "internal physical," "external physical (systems)," "psychosocial," and "psychological" barriers. He included poor knowledge of diabetes mellitus, personal finance issues, need for more helpful health professionals and inappropriate diabetes care as some of the problems. He stated that "A team approach seems most likely to succeed with patients, and where appropriate, caregivers and family members as part of the diabetes team" [10].

Risk factors for the chronic complications of diabetes mellitus may be reduced with good glycemic control, thus reducing short term and long term complications [11]. A change in individual lifestyles and behavior, so as to effect adequate self management are essential components for attaining euglycemia [12].

During an eight-year follow-up study conducted in Israel, patients with diabetes were provided with in depth information about their disease, motivated to actively pursue their therapeutic goals and given tools to modify their modifiable risk factors. This was achieved by individual teaching sessions and enabling contact between patients and consultants. During eight years of follow up, BMI, $HbA_{1c,}$ systolic and diastolic blood pressure and cardiovascular disease were significantly reduced in the intervention group. Success was attributed to the availability of contact with consultants over time, the reinforcement of education and motivation of the patients during repeated consultation sessions [13].

An intervention in Chile which included patient education, self-monitoring of blood glucose and determination of HbA_{1c} was conducted according to the standards of their Ministry of Health. Educators, nurses and nutritionists were involved and materials were approved by external consultants and by the multidisciplinary intervention committee. Strategies were developed for groups according to age, educational level, clinical manifestations, the duration of diabetes, treatment and hospitalization history. The final analysis included those patients who had attended at least seven of the nine educational sessions and the evaluation process. The researchers concluded that "educating patients improved metabolic control, a fact that can be attributed mainly to the intervention's positive impact on those persons' diet." [14]

In the USA, a study to assess the efficacy of a lifestyle intervention program for obese patients with type 2 DM, included individual and group education, support and referral by registered dietitians. Case management for 12 months resulted in greater weight loss, reduced waist circumference, reduced HbA_{1c}, less use of prescription medications and improved health related quality of life. This study demonstrated that a moderate-cost dietitian-led lifestyle case management could improve diverse health indicators in obese patients with type 2 DM [15]. Contrary to expectations, case management participants with less formal education achieved a greater risk reduction than the other better educated participants. However, those in the control group with less education gained significantly more weight than those with greater education [16].

Conclusion

The most important element of any successful intervention is an effective plan based on evidence. Research to assess barriers to effective self care, such as cultural and psychosocial barriers in the target population should be carried out. Guidance from standards of care should be sought [17]. Input from a multidisciplinary team to develop an effective educational program is also important. The program should start with educating all the health care providers. Frequent evaluation of such a program should result in modifications to make the program more efficacious. The patient should be sensitized and empowered as an equally important part of the team providing care. Information on the role and use of a portable glucose monitor and interpretation of results is essential as it empowers patients to take control of their diabetes [18]. However, consideration must be given to the most prudent and cost effective use of the monitor to keep costs affordable [19]. Major input from nutritionists and dietitians in weight loss and activity programs are also essential components of a successful program. The use for instance, of indigenous products which may be grown in back yard gardens is to be encouraged. Utilizing low glycemic root crops, bananas, breadfruit and legumes maximizes the patients' scarce food dollar in a culturally acceptable way [20].

In a developing country, the cost of education is frequently a factor. However, effective self-care is ultimately cost effective over time [15]. Often patients in the developing world are burdened with an education model developed for first world audiences. This adds to their confusion and defeats the purpose, especially when it is also not well understood by all members of the health care team. It is important to transmit information in a simple way, taking into consideration educational ability which in many third world nations may be low. Motivating patients to learn about their disease and empowering them to actively assume their roles in treatment and care is critical to the success of the program [21]. The educational material used should be defined by measurable objectives and indicators, frequently evaluated, modified, and updated as required. The practices of the patients should be individually monitored by a health care provider at each clinic visit, and patients should be encouraged to set realistic goals for subsequent visits [22]. Knowledge and self care practices should be frequently reassessed, as knowledge may not necessarily be translated into effective self care. An appropriate model of behavior change may be used, along with target indicators, for ongoing assessment of each patient's progress.

References

[1] Barcelo A, Rajpathak S. Incidence and prevalence of diabetes mellitus in the Americas. *Rev Panam Salud Publica* 2001; 10:300-308.

[2] Duff EMW, O'Connor A, McFarlane-Anderson N, Wint YB, Bailey EY, Wright-Pascoe R. Self-care, compliance and glycaemic control in Jamaican adults with diabetes mellitus. *West Indian Med J* 2006; 55(4):232-236

[3] Wint YB, Duff EMW, O'Connor A, McFarlane-Anderson N, Bailey EY, Wright-Pascoe R. Knowledge, motivation and barriers to diabetes control in adults in Jamaica. *West Indian Med J* 2006; 55(5):330-333

[4] O'Connor A, Duff EM, McFarlane-Anderson N, Wright-Pascoe R, Wint YB. High levels of F-2 Isoprostanes in Jamaican adults with diabetes mellitus. *Int J Diabetes & Metabolism* 2006; 14: 46-49

[5] Chutkan ME, Meeks-Gardner J, Wilks R. Concepts of obesity among outpatients of a Jamaican hospital. *Cajanus* 2001; 34: 127-134

[6] Pace AE, Ochoa-Vigo K, Caliri MHL, Fernandes APM. Knowledge on diabetes mellitus in the self care process. *Rev Latino-am Enfermagem* 2006; 14(5): 728-734

[7] Arauz AG, Sanchez G, Padilla G, Fernandez M, Rosello M, Guzman S. Intervencion educativa comunitaria sobre la diabetes en el ambito de la atencion primaria. *Rev Panam Salud Publica* 2001; 9(3): 145-153

[8] Lin EHB, Katon W, Von Korff M, et al. Relationship of depression and diabetes self-care, medication adherence, and preventive care. *Diabetes Care* 2004; 27:2154-2160

[9] Chlebowy DO, Garvin BJ. Social support, self-efficacy, and outcome expectations: impact on self-care behaviors and glycemic control in Caucasian and African American adults with type 2 diabetes. *Diabetes Edu* 2006; 32(5): 777-786

[10] Simmons D. Personal barriers to diabetes care: is it me, them or us? *Diabetes Spectrum* 2001; 14(1): 10-12

[11] UK Prospective Diabetes Study Group: Effect of intensive blood-glucose control with sulphonylureas or insulin compared with conventional treatment and risk of complications in patients with type 2 diabetes (UKPDS 33). *Lancet* 1998; 352: 837-853,

[12] Declaration of the Americas (DOTA); Standards for developing diabetes education programs in the Americas. *Pan Am J Public Health* 2001; 10: 349-353.

[13] Rachmani R, Slavacheski I, Beria M, Frommer-Shapira, Ravid Mordchai. Treatment of high-risk patients with diabetes: motivation and teaching intervention: a randomized, prospective 8-year follow-up study. *J Am Soc Nephrol* 2005;16:22-26

[14] Barcelo A, Robles S, White F, Jadue L, Vega J. An intervention to improve diabetes control in Chile. *Pan Am J Public Health* 2001;10: 328-333.

[15] Wolf AM, Conaway MR, Crowther JQ, et al. Translating lifestyle intervention to practice in obese patients with type 2 diabetes: Improving Control with Activity and Nutrition (ICAN) study. *Diabetes Care* 2004; 27(7): 1570-1576

[16] Gurka MJ, Wolf AM, Conaway MR, Crowther JQ, Nadler JL, Bovbjerg VE. Lifestyle intervention in obese patients with type 2 diabetes: impact of the patient's educational background. *Obesity* 2006;14:1085-1092

[17] American Diabetes Association: Standards of medical care in diabetes. *Diabetes Care* 2004; 27 (Suppl.1): S15-35

[18] Karter AJ, Ackerson LM, Darbinian J, D'Agostino R, Ferrara A. Self-monitoring of blood glucose levels and glycaemic control: the Northern California Permanente Registry. *Am J Med* 2001; 111:1-9.

[19] Karter AJ, Ferrara A, Darbinian JA, Ackerson LM, Selby JV. Self-monitoring of blood glucose: language and financial barriers in a managed care population with diabetes. *Diabetes Care* 2000; 23(4):477-483

[20] Holdip, J. Common Caribbean foods and your health. *Cajanus* 2006; 39(1): 1-58

[21] Badruddin N, Basit A, Hydrie MZI, Hakeem R. Knowledge attitude and practices of patients visiting a diabetes care unit. *Pakistan J Nutr.* 2002; 1(2): 99-102

[22] Duff EMW, Simpson SH, Whittle S, Bailey EY, Lopez SA, Wilks R. Impact on blood pressure control of a six-month intervention project. *West Indian Med J* 2000; 49: 307-311

In: Research Trends in Nutrition…
Editor: Johan P. Urster, pp. 7-51

ISBN: 978-1-60456-147-0
© 2008 Nova Science Publishers, Inc.

Chapter 1

Risk Modification of Inflammatory Bowel Diseases by Vitamin D, Calcium and Lactase/Lactose Interactions: Arguments Based on Relationships between IBD and Colorectal Cancer

Andrew Szilagyi[*]

Division of Gastroenterology, Sir Mortimer B Davis Jewish General Hospital,
McGill University School of Medicine, Montreal QC., Canada H3T 1E2.

Abstract

The inflammatory bowel diseases(IBD) and colorectal cancer(CRC) share common global geographic distributions. Similarly in both, pathogenesis depends on host and environmental influences. In particular, genetic background and intestinal microflora both contribute to disease formation. While diet is strongly implicated in CRC, such a pathogenic role is less clear in IBD. This focused review discusses the role of vitamin D obtained either through geographic exposure to sunlight or diet in both diseases as a modefier of risk, It reviews the evidence that risk of both disease is also linked epidemiologically to national dairy food consumption and the population prevalence of lactase status. The potential effector contribution of calcium is discussed. Based on these similarities in the two diseases, it is hypothesized that the observed paradoxical reduction in risk with dairy foods observed for CRC may also apply to IBD. If hypotheses put forth are supported, future studies on the effects of dairy foods on some diseases may need to consider lactase status and the use of lactose free products or digestive aids should be markedly reduced.

[*] E-mail address: aszilagy@gas.jgh.mcgill.ca ; Phone :514 340 8144 ; Fax: 514 340 8282.

Introduction

The Inflammatory Bowel (IBD) diseases (Crohn's ; CD, and Idiopathic ulcerative colitis; UC) affect patients of all ages. There are however 2 peaks of maximum incidence, more evident in UC. One is in young adulthood 20-30 and another smaller peak in patients over 60-70 years[1,2]. These diseases are usually lifelong and are marked by remissions and exacerbations in about half to two thirds of patients[1-5]. As such those patients acquiring their disease in childhood will likely continue to suffer some direct or indirect complication of the disease into middle age and beyond albeit at a reduced rate after the first decade of diagnosis[1,6].

Table 1. National yearly per capita intake of dairy foods(11) and national prevalence of Lactase nonpersistence (LNP)(12-14) of 26 countries are shown.

Country	Dairy KG/YR/CAP	LNP Status %
Finland	205.5	17
Ireland	198.6	6
Poland	195	37
Sweden	182	2
Norway	182	2
Denmark	149.7	4
New Zealand	146.1	9
United Kingdom	137.6	6
Switzerland	133.2	10
Czech	131.2	13
Canada	121.7	6
France	115.6	37
United States	115.4	15
Netherlands	114	4
Lithuania	112.3	32
Hungary	112.3	37
Austria	110.1	20
Spain	109	23
Australia	106.3	6
Germany	102.3	15
Italy	97.8	50
Israel	85.8	72
Mexico	43.2	70
Japan	42.9	93
Chile	23.5	70
China	7.7	93

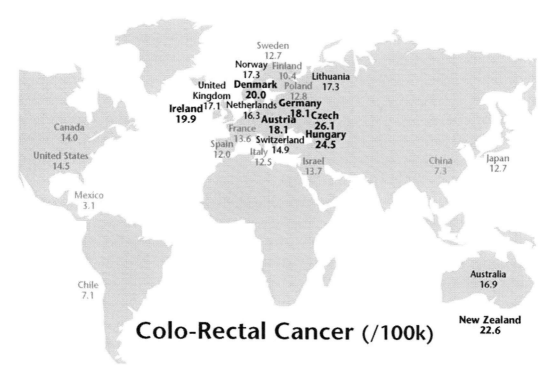

Figure 1a. National combined colorectal mortality rates (15) are shown distributed on the map.

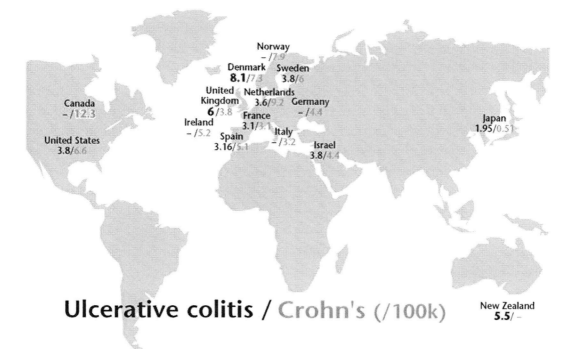

Figure 1b. National incidence rates(16-19) for Crohn's disease (N14) and Ulcerative colitis rates (N10) are shown on the map.

Crohn's disease and Idiopathic ulcerative colitis are distinguished on clinical and pathological criteria. Crohn's is a multisite disease with panmural inflammation and UC has variable colonic extension usually with epithelial restricted inflammation. Genetic and environmental factors are thought to play a role in disease causation. Both diseases share similar epidemiological features. As well colorectal cancer (CRC), closely linked with a Western type diet[7,8] and lifestyle[9,10] also shares epidemiological similarities with IBD (Table 1, Fig 1a and 1b). Colonic involvement with either CD or UC increases the risk of CRC after 2-3 decades of disease[20,21]. Although rates are less than previously reported[22,23].

A major feature shared by these diseases is their similar geographic distribution. There is increased incidence and prevalence in northwestern locations and diminishing incidence/prevalence in southeastern regions of the world (Fig 1b)[24]. The peculiar distribution has not been fully explained. However, a "Western" vs "Eastern" diet/ lifestyles are often quoted as in the case of CRC. Polarized distribution also raises the possible role of sunlight and ultraviolet radiation which affects synthesis of vitamin D. The distribution of sunlight and increased vitamin D is also accompanied by distribution of populations ability to digest lactose as discussed below. The interaction between the genetics of intestinal lactase and consumption of lactose containing foods (mainly dairy foods, DF) has not been extensively evaluated. Incremental risks with DF consumption and decremental risks with national prevalence of adult lactase non-persistence(LNP) status for a number of diseases however, have been described. Indeed such a relationship exists for both IBD and CRC (Shrier et al. Nutr Cancer in print). This review will discuss how the intervention of the epidemiological variables, vitamin D, and the lactase/lactose interactions could impact on risk modification of IBD and CRC. Calcium is a central player in this paradigm since its host effects are intimately related to vitamin D. However, dietary calcium is quantitatively highest in DFs. Because of the phenotypic division of the world's population into LNP and adult lactase persistent (LP) groups the 2 populations are exposed to different quantities of DFs and hence DF related calcium. Lactose is handled differently in the two populations.

Both IBD and CRC have complex etiologies. This review will address pathogenesis of IBD, discussed in the context of host/luminal abnormalities affecting intestinal mucosa. Similarly the pathogenesis of CRC will be elaborated. Non classical functions of vitamin D(not related to bone) as it pertains to immune modulation and antineoplastic effects will be discussed in relation to IBD and CRC. The potential function of lactose is discussed and review of current literature on the effects of DFs in IBD and CRC follow. Comparison of similarities in pathogenesis of both IBD and CRC will be emphasized. Arguments based on such similarities suggest that DFs should impact on IBD in a manner found for CRC.

Pathogenesis of IBD

The central target of IBD is destruction of intestinal mucosa. In UC the damage is superficial and uniform, beginning distally in the rectum[25]. In CD destruction is panmural and any area may be affected, but terminal ileum and cecum are most common. This is followed by the colon and small bowel or other unusual areas like the esophagus[26].

The beginning or relapse of clinical disease is often determined by an inciting event such as gastroenteritis(viral or bacterial), stress, nonsteroidal inflammatory agents, unknown dietary ingredients[27,28].Smoking is considered to be the strongest proven environmental risk factor for CD and cessation for UC[29,30]. Possible mechanisms include effects of nicotine on the inflammatory response[31,32]. Recently appendectomy has been noted to have a similar dual effect by reducing risk and severity of UC[33], but increasing risk and severity for CD[34]. The mechanism of risk modifying effect of appendectomy has not been clarified.

A second initiating event may be a breach in membrane permeability which can occur with inciting events as shown in models[35-37]. Permeability defects may also be present in families[38,39], may also have a genetic predisposition[40], and may precede relapse[41].

The increased permeability allows commensal bacteria to come in contact with the intestinal immune system. Genetic predisposition sets into motion an inappropriate immune response consisting of sequences of cytokines which lead to epithelial apoptosis. In addition there is a recruitment of a variety of white blood cells with subsequent contribution of cellular killing mechanisms. Ultimately these events result in destruction of the mucosal membrane. In CD the cytokine cascade leads to release of TNFα, INFγ IL-1, IL,2, IL6, IL-8 and IL-12 (T helper 1, Th1) response[42,43]. In UC it is IL-4, IL-5, IL-10 and IL-13(T helper 2, Th2) response[42-44]. Recently a new class of T cells(Th17) modulated by IL23 are investigatively emerging as a common mediator of inflammation in both CD and UC[45].

Initiation and continuation of the mucosal destruction may be approached mechanistically by describing a 2 compartment model in which disturbance in one, the other or both may result in disease. In this paradigm host abnormalities are intrinsic defects (autoimmune disorder). Alterations in luminal contents are extrinsic defects which may change host bacterial relationships(Fig 2).

Host Compartment

At least a dozen genetic polymorphisms for IBD have been described[45,46]. Interactions of these with other genes or gene products have not been completely worked out. Distribution of different genetic polymorphisms in populations suggests that a particular disposition is also not absolutely required for disease. Several genetic polymorphisms have been evaluated more extensively.

The best studied genetic polymorphism is the mutations in Nuclear Oligomerization Domain 2(NOD2/Caspase Activation Recruitment Domain15, CARD15) located on chromosome 16q12[47] with a variable population frequency about of 20%-50% in the patient population compared to 8-10% in non patients[45,48-50]. This intracellular signal receptor is distributed throughout the intestine, but has the highest concentration in Paneth cells of the terminal ileum. The receptor recognizes the universal bacterial antigen muramyl dipeptide[48]. In normal circumstances it may serve a function of modulating the central cytokine molecule NFκB. Activation or inhibition would depend on receptor signaling from the cell surface or feedback control via other cytokines like Tumor necrosis factor alpha (TNFα)[51]. Response serves to induce tolerance to the bacterial antigen or eradication of intracellular bacteria[51]. Interaction of NOD2/CARD15 with other Pattern Recognition Receptors(PRR), especially Toll-like receptors (TLRs) are thought to mediate protective mechanisms at the level of the intestinal mucosa[51,52].

There are at least 11 TLRs described, all with different functions[53-55]. The interaction with TLR2 (receptor for teichoic acid) serves to maintain barrier function[56] and abnormalities in this receptor could lead to alterations in permeability. Another receptor, TLR4 (endotoxin, LPS receptor) is also be intimately involved with recognition of bacterial invasion. Signaling between TLR4 and NOD2 appear to coordinate defense against invading bacteria. Patients with mutations on either NOD2 or TLR4 may increase NFκB activation through gain of function. A loss of function could also result in similar response through failure to inhibit NFκB activation by TLR2[53].

Generalized disturbances in immunity are also recognized in IBD. Currently there is a debate as to whether loss of oral tolerance leads to a variable effector response and hyper innate immunity[57]. Duchman et al showed that lamina propria cells in active disease from patients with IBD, proliferate in response to autologous microflora sonicates[58]. This response was inhibited by monoclonal antibody to MHC class 2 suggesting antigen driven response. In a mouse model of CD a similar autologous reaction was inhibited by either IL-10 or antibody to IL-12[59]. A more general defect in oral tolerance was demonstrated by Kraus et al. Response to oral feeding and subsequent immunization to keyhole limpet hemocyanin failed to dampen in vitro peripheral T-cell proliferation in both CD and UC patients compared with controls[60]. This defect could also be detected in primary relatives of patients with IBD suggesting a genetic component[61].

The other major finding in patients, especially with CD, is that decreased innate response is associated with secondary enhancement of adaptive immunity. This is less efficient in eradicating bacterial invasion[62]. Marks et al in an elegant set of experiments found a markedly attenuated polymorhonuclear leukocyte response in patients with CD both in the intestine and the skin. They showed that this poor response was associated with significantly lower levels of IL-8, a major cytokine involved with recruitment of leukocytes. This study clearly demonstrated a defect in innate immunity in patients with CD. They postulated that the chronic inflammation in CD is due to second line macrophage response (adaptive immunity), which fails to kill intra cellular bacteria. The reconciliation between these two defects, loss of oral tolerance with abnormal regulator T cell response or a diminished first line innate defense is not immediately obvious, and raises the notion that different pathways could lead to disease. In both cases however, cytokine sequences are activated.

Interspersed with these two possibilities are abnormalities described in antigen presenting dendritic cells which contribute to altered immune responses[63]. Whether these are primary or secondary to treatment is less clear[64].

Dietary factors like fatty acids have been also linked to a group of nuclear hormone receptors, Proteosome Proliferator-Activated Receptors (PPAR α,δ and γ). The PPAR γ in particular may interact with omega fatty acids and through signaling, could dampen the inflammatory response via NF-κB[65]. The anti-inflammatory effects of PPARγ may be therapeutically exploited. The ligand rosiglitazone(a PPARγ agonist) has been used in a pilot study and showed a 54% response rate with 12% remission rate after 12 weeks[66].

A link to immune defects with luminal events in IBD is the "old friends" a variation of the "hygiene" hypothesis[67]. According to these 2 related concepts, modern societies have dramatically reduced the possible exposure of infants and children to certain pathogens, such as parasites and simple infections which were common prior to modernization. As a result early in life, there is a failure to induce oral tolerance which leaves T reg cells unconditioned for future novel antigen encounters. Suggestion that parasites could dampen acute disease was shown by feeding of swine whipworms with either active UC or CD[68,69] through alteration of the respective immune response. However, not all studies have shown that early infections in children are protective, in fact these may increase risk of IBD[70].

Luminal Compartment

The human lower intestine contains some 400-500 species of bacteria, many of which have never been identified. Bacterial concentrations approach 10^{15}/ml[71]. After the neonatal period bacteria tend to remain stable[72] and usually do not adhere to mucosa[73]. The single layer of epithelial mucosa is responsible for sifting out pathogens from non-pathogens that breach the layer. As outlined above the first line innate immunity is instrumental in the type of defense. On the luminal side a layer of mucus synthesized by the epithelium participates in protection through physical and chemical means against invasion in the normal state[74]. There are 3 interrelated and ongoing debates about luminal events and IBD.

Table 2. Bacteria and viruses which have been evaluated as possible etiological agents for Inflammatory Bowel Disease. Symbol * suggests organisms role still debated, § more commonly either causes flare in immune compromised patients or is an innocent bystander, • more commonly causes flares.

Bacteria	(ref)	Viruses	(ref)
Mycobacterium * Avium Paratuberculosis	75-77	Paramyxovirus Measles	83,84
Listeria Monocytogenes	78	Mumps	84
Eschericia coli	78	Herpes simplex	84
Mycoplasma	79	Rubella	84
Clostridium difficile •	80-82	Cytomegalovirus §	85

The first question is whether IBD may be caused by a specific infectious agent(s). Table 2 outlines some infectious agents investigated to cause IBD, especially CD. Most have been rejected as primary candidates. However, among these, Mycobacterium Avium Paratuberculosis(MAP), which has been associated with Johne's disease of cattle and resembles CD[75,76] is still debated. Many reports seem to verify MAP's role in IBD[77,86,87], while others do not support its pathogenic potential in humans[88,89].We will discuss a possible role of MAP in the geographic distribution of CD below.

The central theme of the other 2 debates concerns the role of commensal bacteria that normally reside in the lumen. The 2 possibilities include: 1) Commensal flora penetrate protective mucus and tight junctions after a breach by a variety of inciting events mentioned above. Inflammation and a cycle of remission activation lead to marked alteration of luminal flora. 2) Commensal flora do the same as in 1, after the loss of other bacteria or organisms which previously prevented potential pathogenic commensals form activation of the inflammatory response. The markedly altered luminal flora is no longer able to function in limiting potential pathogen host interaction.

In the first of these arguments the loss of harmony between "protective" and "potentially pathogenic commensal" flora is a secondary event. In the second argument the loss of harmony is a primary event. The process has been termed as dysbiosis[90].

The notion that bacteria are important in causation of IBD derives from finding that most animal models do not work in germ free environment[91]. On a clinical level it has been observed that CD is much less likely to relapse after surgery if the fecal stream is not re-established[92]. The successful use of antibiotics[93,94] especially in CD colitis supports the role of bacteria in aggravating IBD.

Host bacteria interaction may be non specific and variable. A study of a germ free, IL-2 mouse model of CD, showed that Eschericia coli mpk but not Bacteroides vulgatus caused colitis[95]. In this model B. vulgatus given together with E. coli may have been protective. However, in a guinea pig model of carrageenan induced colitis addition of B.vulgatus to a germ free animal enhanced injury[96]. These studies demonstrate the possibility that bacteria may display probiotic properties under different environmental pressures.

In the last decade the concept of probiotics, (ingested live organisms that exert health benefits beyond their intrinsic nutritional value)[97], has been therapeutically applied to IBD with variable success[98]. However, since many probiotic bacteria (especially species of lactobacilli and bifidobacteria) reside in the human intestine, their potential role in disease risk modification under natural conditions is legitimately questioned.

Arguments for the first postulate; that dysbiosis is a secondary event to cyclical changes in IBD is supported by the following studies. Swidsinski et al reported that fecal type bacteria were found in apposition to inflamed mucosa in patients but not controls[99]. Surprisingly, greater numbers were found in apposition of uninflamed areas[99]. Similar high concentration was found in patients with infectious self limiting colitis and there was predominance of Bacteroides species[100]. The virtual absence of bacteria in mucus of healthy controls was reported by several groups[74,101]. However in active IBD biodiversity of species was markedly reduced[102]. Swidsinski et al showed that bacteria inversely correlate with presence of inflamed mucosa and the presence of polymorphonuclear leukocytes[74]. Together these studies imply that the loss of biodiversity may be directly related to the inflammatory response of the host.

The notion that dysbiosis is a primary event which reduces beneficial bacteria, leading to emergence of potentially harmful bacteria is not well studied. Madsen et al reported in the IL-10 knockout mouse model that development of colitis requires bacterial flora. This induces abnormal gut permeability prior to onset of the disease[103]. In humans it has been reported that both UC and CD are associated with reduced concentrations of Bifidobacteria[104,105] and loss of Lactobacilli may be important in UC[106]. Early dysbiosis was also found to predate pouchitis(a form of inflammatory bowel disease in the remaining neorectum after colectomy)[107]

What factors could alter distribution or ratio of different species of microbes? The more obvious are the use of antiobiotics which in addition to affecting pathogens could disturb normal flora[108]. Emergence of Clostridium difficile, spared by most antibiotics, could alter membrane permeability[109]. As well other medications like proton pump inhibitors, especially in older populations could favor emergence of C difficile[110]. These organisms have been linked with aggravating IBD[80-82] although, they have not been proven as a direct cause. The other potentially important influence on microbial flora is diet. In particular "prebiotics" (food elements, mostly carbohydrates, which are not digested by the host but instead reach the lower intestine and are then specifically metabolized by selective group(s) of bacteria with health benefits for the host beyond their intrinsic nutritional value[111]), can alter temporarily the composition of microflora and support protective organisms. Inulin in a number of vegetables can serve such a function[112] as can resistant starch[113]. Lactose in dairy foods may also serve such a purpose[114]. Therefore alteration in diets with reduced prebiotics may adversely influence lactic acid or as yet unknown bacterial populations. Prebiotics also have been shown to influence IBD[115].There may also be multiple effects of diet on bacterial metabolism which could result in abnormal effects [116,117]

In summary, the current concept of pathogenesis of IBD involves intrinsic genetic predisposition, to an abnormal immune response to commensal bacteria. The barrier breach may be due to either intrinsic genetic abnormalities or also to the effects of bacteria. Host signaling leads to an inappropriate inflammatory response resulting in destruction of mucosa in UC and as well, deeper layers in CD. A large part of the disease is due to abnormal host response, but it is recognized that altered events in the lumen must contribute in initiating or perpetuating abnormal inflammation. It seems logical also that luminal events should precede the abnormal host response. However, it is difficult to prove whether observations on intestinal flora are primary or secondary in nature.

Pathogenesis of Colorectal Cancer(CRC)

Like IBD, CRC shares similar geographic distribution with incidence highest in northwestern located countries and diminishing rates towards southeast locations (although not necessarily in individual countries). However, with "westernization", rates of cancer are increasing[118]. As well, just as with IBD, rates increase in immigrants from low prevalence to high prevalence regions[119].

Three major types of CRC are recognized, Familial, Sporadic and Inflammation related.

The pathogenesis of this cancer can also be viewed as a two compartment model. The internal compartment of CRC consists of genetic predisposition and growth promoting hormones(Fig 3).

Host Compartment

Genetic predisposition to CRC include Familial Adenomatous Polyposis syndromes (FAP)[120] and the Hereditary Non Polyposis Cancer(HNPC)[121,122] syndrome as well as a few others[123,124]. These make up 5-6 % of cancers. Familial occurrence is more common in apparent sporadic cancer, but without clear genetic predisposition. Somatic genetic mutations are induced by several mechanisms in all cases of non familial CRC.

The initial breakthrough in understanding of the sequential genetic mutations was reported by Fearon and Vogelsteins group[125,126]. In this sequence somatic mutations at the chromosomal level lead to mutations in the "gate keeper APC" gene, subsequently k-RAS mutations follow. Inhibition of tumor suppressor gene p53 and subsequently mutations of the

DCC gene lead to metastatic disease. These alterations are thought to result in a sequence of hyperproliferative foci in the colon crypts(Aberant Crypt Foci), leading to small polyp formation, growth and cancer development with subsequent metastases over a period of several years. The APC suppressor gene, is also involved in sporadic cancer, where one function is to regulate β-catenin, which together with E-cahedrin affect cell-cell interactions. Cytoplasmic β-catenin, normally controlled, under- goes phosphorylation, ubiquination and subsequent degradation. When it is stabilized by loss of function of the APC gene, it is translocated to the cell nucleus where it activates the canonical Wingless-Int (Wnt/Tcf) signaling pathway. The Wnt pathways of which there are at least 3, have a role in embryogenesis[127] but have been found to be involved in initiation of neoplastic transformation later in life[128-130]. A recent review of this model confirms most of the original findings, but also notes some differences. For example k-Ras mutations may preceed the APC mutation, initiating carcinogenic sequences. In addition the article outlines the role of TGFβ on cell cycling as it relates to the APC gene[131]

Further to the classical chromosomal induced instability (CIN; representing about 50% of cancers) epigenetic mechanisms have also been recognized[132]. One mechanism is the silencing of tumor suppressive genes. This involves the methylation of DNA promoter segments, CpG island methylator phenotype(CIMP; 35% of cancers) resulting in altered function of genes. The third mechanism involves hypermethylation of Miss Match Repair genes involved in DNA restitution. These involve microsatellite instability (MSI-High or Low or Stable) signatures. The majority of HNPC and 15% of sporadic cancers are attributed to this route of carcinogenesis. Because methylation of DNA seems important for carcinogenesis polymorphisms in the enzyme methylenetetrahydrofolate reductase has been sought to determine whether there is any increased risk. To date only the 677TT genotype in association with low folate levels[133] or in actively alcohol consuming subjects showed an increased risk[134].

An integrative classification based on the presence of CIMP high or low, MSI high low or stable and several other genetic alterations such as the BRAF,KRAS, and MLH1 mutations is proposed to account for novel mechanisms leading to CRC[135].

Cancer associated with inflammation is recognized in colitis and represents about 5% of all CRC. Genetic alterations in IBD related CRC are similar to those in sporadic cancer but sequences are different. For example, the p53 suppressor gene silencing occurs early, while the APC mutation is late. Additional differences as well are reviewed by Rhodes and Campbell in [136].

A link between sporadic and IBD related colon cancer which may be common to both is an abnormality of surface glycosylation which could alter membrane adherence characteristics [137,138]. Further links with sporadic cancers are supported.

Prostaglandins (especially PGE$_2$) exert effects on cellular proliferation, immune surveillance and inhibit apoptosis[139]. Research in this area has been fuelled by clinical studies which show that aspirin[140,141], nonsteroidal antiinflammatory agents[142] and selective COX2 inhibitors[143] decrease colonic neoplasms. Induction of PG synthesis is under Cyclooxygenase (COX) 1 and 2. The latter has been shown to be upregulated in both inflammation and neoplasms. The inducible COX2 enzyme is under control of the APC suppresor gene. As such mutations of this gene also lead to increased COX2 expression and consequent potentiation of carcinogenesis[139].

Toll-like receptors play a role in pathogenesis of neoplastic transformation as well. However, their role is unclear because in some experimental models TLRs promote while in others TLRs may protect against epithelial injury[139,144]. A link between TLR4 and up regulation of the COX2 inducible enzyme has been established. In a mouse model of colitis where an adaptor protein for normal TLR4 function, MyD88 gene product, was deleted, COX2 enzyme failed to be upregulated[145]. The authors hypothesized that an intact TLR4 signaling leads to inhibition of apoptosis via the COX2 system. This effect could be helpful in preserving epithelial integrity and limit injury in IBD but in the long run, might participate in carcinogenesis. The TLRs(TLR2 and 4) can induce an inflammatory response through activation of NF-κB. Activation involves dissociation and degredation of the migratory inhibitor IKKβ. In an interesting mouse model of colitis induced cancer, IKKβ knockout mice had a 75% reduction in tumor development. The authors also showed that IKKβ promoted cancer development independent of inflammation possibly through induction of the apoptosis inhibitor protein family of Bcl-xl[146]. Another intriguing study showed that TLR4 which recognizes endotoxin(LPS), also activates NF-κB in response to saturated fatty acids, an important component of LPS. The response did not occur with unsaturated fatty acids[147]. This observation could be exploited to evaluate whether dietary saturated fatty acids could act through this receptor. TLR2 appears to function in maintenance of the mucosal barrier and also activates NF-κB[56]. Recently genetic polymorphisms in TLR2 and TLR4 have been found to increase risk for colorectal cancer in Croatian patients, suggesting clinical relevance[148].

Pattern recognition receptors are aso involved in inhibiting carcinogenesis[149]. The receptor TLR4 is downregulated in metastatic colon cancer cell lines. LPS stimulation results in increased expression. In normal tissue and non metastatic cells TLR4 is normally expressed suggesting that the receptor may prevent advancement of tumor progression via normal bacterial signaling[150].

The second important contributors to CRC are the role of growth factors. Giovannucci suggested in 1995 that insulin, obesity and insulin resistance leading to high serum levels could promote neoplastic growth[151]. Since then, many studies have supported this hypothesis and as well the mechanisms of promotion have been better defined[152]. More precise role in carcinogenesis of insulin-like growth factors have been also described, but mainly in models or in vitro. Promoting effect of both IGF-1 and IGF-2 are mediated through receptors. The bioavailability of IGFs are regulated by binding proteins in the serum and CRC cells are able to degrade IGFBP by producing proteases[153]. Some clinical studies do support the importance of elevated IGF-1 as a risk for CRC[154,155].

Other growth promoting factors include gastrin, usually produced by antral G cells of the stomach. Elevated gastrin levels have been found in association with Helicobacter pylori, but the levels of hormone rather than bacteria correlate with the presence of mostly distal polyps[156] or cancer[157]. Gastrin 17 in vitro colon cancer cell line upregulates β-catenin/Tcf signaling, thus linking the hormone to possible tumor promoting status[158].

Human growth hormone may also promote polyps and CRC. Patients with acromegaly may have an increased risk for hyperplastic, adenomatous polyps and cancer[159,160]. However, the failure to note increased prevalence of these neoplasms in an Indian study[161], suggests that such a predisposition may be environmentally altered.

Hormonal promoters may act through the nuclear hormonal superfamily including the peroxisome proliferator-activated receptors. These ligand activated transcription factors consist of 3 types PPAR-α, δ and γ, each with different functions. All are involved with lipid metabolism. PPAR-γ is involved with glucose insulin response and adipocyte differentiation[162-164]. PPAR-δ enhances fat metabolism[165,166], but the receptors are also involved with immunity and cellular differentiation[162-164]. PPAR-γ is shown to inhibit colon cancer cell lines in vitro[167,168] and in clinical studies polymorphisms of PPAR-γ, together with Insulin and vitamin D receptor genes affect CRC[169]. The role of PPAR-δ in carcinogenesis is controversial. However recent reports show that in cancer cell lines communications occur with vascular endothelial growth factor(VEGF)[170] and PPAR-δ[171]. Prostacyclin activates this receptor in CRC models suggesting an important function. The latter finding connects PPAR-δ to the COX2 system which is 80% upregulated in CRC. As well, recently β-catenin transactivation has been shown to target PPAR-δ[172]. These connect diet with cell signaling events in carcinogenesis.

Luminal Compartment

The potential role of pattern receptors in carcinogenesis highlights possible importance of infectious agents in CRC pathogenesis. There are indeed several contenders within the intestinal lumen which could participate (Table 3). Although, a few viruses like human papiloma[173] herpes simplex virus[174] and JC[175] virus have been suspected of carcinogenesis in CRC, proof of effect has not been forthcoming in some[176]. Instead the role of the commensal flora and several particular or groups of bacteria or their metabolic products of luminal ingesta are suspected of contributing to CRC pathogenesis[177,178].

The notion that bacteria may promote cancer was proposed by Hill's group[179,180]. It was hypothesized that bacteria could convert bile salts into carcinogenic steroids in conjunction with a high fat diet[181,182]. High risk populations do contain more fecal bile salts than low risk groups[178]. In addition the secondary bile salt Deoxycholic acid (produced by 7-alpha dehydroxylation of cholic acid by bacteria) was shown to promote carcinogenesis through cell signaling[178]. Other groups, such as sulfate reducing bacteria, hypothesized to play a possible role in pathogenesis of ulcerative colitis also, are thought to metabolize hydrogen sulfate and produce sulfide which may be genotoxic through free radical formation[183]. The notion of free radicals inducing CIN is also supported by a study showing that $.0_2^-$ radical produced by Enterococcus faecalis will induce CIN in vitro. Development of chromosomal abnormalities was prevented by using either superoxide dismutase or a COX-2 inhibitor[184]. The presence of adherent E. coli in mucosal samples of patients with CD or CRC which induce IL-8 secretion in in vitro cell lines suggest a possible common infectious cause to these diseases[185]. Several small animal models of CRC also have been described where disease modification occurred in the germ free state[186-188].

In summary, pathogenesis of CRC involves host genetic predisposition and growth factors, the most important responding to dietary intake. At the epithelial level sequential genetic alterations in several different pathways are essential for initiation and promotion of carcinogenesis. The luminal contribution to carcinogenesis is putatively through multiple factors either dietary fats and antigens, bacterially altered antigens, bile salts, or biologic agent like bacteria or possibly viruses. A common theme however, is abnormal cell signaling between host and luminal contents, which at least are accomplices to carcinogenesis.

Table 3. Potential Bacterial and viral causes and associations with colorectal cancer. The asterisk denotes potential pathogen in small animal models only. Based on references as shown. (refs).

Bacteria	(refs)	Viruses	(refs)
Streptoccus infantarius(bovis)	(177)	Papiloma virus	(173)
Clostridium septicum	(177)	Herpes simplex	(174)
Helicobacter hepaticus*	(177)	JC virus	(175)
Citrobacter rodentium*	(177)		
Sulphate reducing group	(183)		
Entercoccus feacalis	(184)		
Adherent Escherichia coli	(185)		

Effect of Geographic Pattern of Disease on Modification of Risk

The geographic distribution of both IBD and CRC reflect high to low incidence and prevalence as described above. A mutual set of environmental factors which modify the risk of these diseases are postulated to account for the observations. These could represent common pathogenic variables, or common protective factors or a combination of both. As noted above sunlight and consequently vitamin D has been hypothesized to play this role in accounting for north to south reductions. However, sunlight may not be able to fully account for west to east reductions of disease risk. In addition to vitamin D the possible impact of genetic lactase/lactose interaction has not been adequately explored. Because both vitamin D and lactase/lactose are intimately related to calcium ingestion, it is difficult to separate possible interactive effects of these 3 variables. The following sections will describe the impact of vitamin D on the immune system and its antineoplastic effects as they apply to IBD and CRC. Subsequently the possible impact of lactase and lactose interactions will be described for these diseases. In the case of CRC, it is hypothesized that heat stable(ST) enterotoxin produced by Enterotoxigenic E.coli(ETEC) may also protect against this cancer and account for geographic distribution[189]. While this relationship is intriguing and deserves further exploration it is not clear at this time how it might account for the general geographic patterns observed for other diseases. The reported relationship does however suggest that there may be multiple reasons for pattern distribution of individual diseases(echoes of "hygiene hypothesis" for CRC?).

Impact of Vitamin D on Pathogenesis of IBD

The main function of vitamin D is regulation of calcium and phosphorus for maintenance of skeletal structure. It was found to be essential in preventing Rickets, but later it was found that exposure to sunlight (UV light) could compensate by synthesizing vitamin D_3 from 7-dehydrocholesterol in the skin[190]. Several foods contain vitamin D[190] and at least in North America vitamin D is added to certain food items, including milk. Detailed metabolism of vitamin D is reviewed by Dusso et al [191] and will be briefly outlined here. Activation of vitamin D requires hydroxylation of carbon 25 in the liver through the cellular cytochrome system. Further activation takes place predominantly in the kidneys via 1α-hydroxylase and parathyroid control. However, recently it has been discovered that this enzyme can be present at multiple extrarenal sites. Moreover, control of the enzyme at these sites relies on mechanisms different than that in the kidneys, and putatively depends on local autocrine/paracrine effects of 1,25, $(OH)_2D_3$. Vitamin D is carried in the circulation bound to a plasma protein (vitamin D binding protein). The actions of the 1,25$(OH)_2D_3$ require a specific vitamin D receptor(VDR) on cells which is under genetic control. A more rapid reacting membrane bound steroid receptor of 1,25 $(OH)_2D_3$ has also been reported accounting for some of the apparent non genetic mediated functions of calcitriol[192]. The primary actions of vitamin D involve regulation of calcium and phosphorus metabolism at the level of the gut, kidney, bone and parathyroid hormone[191]. However, many other sites contain VDR and 1α-hydroxylase (1,25$(OH)_2D_3$)[190,191].

Table 4. Non classical: non calcium homeostatic functions of vitamin D which may be protective against neoplastic and/or immunologic mediated diseases. Mechanistically these effects may occur via autocrine or paracrine routes, as well as by endocrine functions of 1,25-dihydroxy D3. This summary is based references(190,191,196,209).

Anti Neoplastic effect	Immune Modulatory effects
Induction of tumor suppressors	Facilitation of macrophage function
Inhibition of cell proliferation	Modulation of Th1 or Th2 cytokines with suppression of Th1 response
Regulation of apoptosis	Suppresion of lymphocyte function
Control of intracellular calcium which enhances apoptosis	Limits dendritic cell maturation thus facilitating oral tolerance
Genetic polymorphisms of the vitamin D receptor modulates neoplastic conversion	May enhance suppressor T cell concentrations
	Genetic polymorphisms of vitamin D receptor may affect risk of Crohn's

A number of diseases, particularly colon, prostate and breast cancer have been noted to be associated with vitamin D deficiency[191]. In addition immune mediated diseases have also been evaluated for this vitamin status[193,194]. Among them IBD has emerged as a potential group of diseases where the protective effects of the non classical actions of vitamin D may serve an important function[195]. Actions of vitamin D which could be involved in antineoplastic or anti-immune mediated disease effects are shown in Table 4. All immunomodulatory functions of vitamin D may impact on IBD.

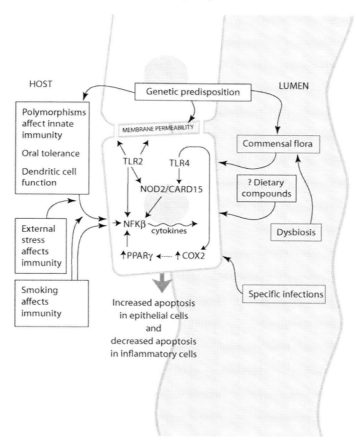

Figure 2. The central cell represents the colonic mucosa containing some receptors and effectors discussed in the text. The basic response leads to activation of NF-κB leading to cytokine cascades which participate in apoptosis of cells with resultant macro injury. Toll-like receptors are instrumental in both control of barrier function and cross communication with NOD2/CARD15 in eliminating invading bacteria. Dysfunction of the represented triangle could lead to increased bacterial translocations (or antigens), failure to eliminate intra cellular bacteria or inapropriate activation of NF-κB. Both COX2 and PPAR γ may participate in protection against epithelial apoptosis. On the host side a variety of genetic polymorphisms affecting either cell signaling, mucosal barrier function, innate immunity predispose to disease. It should be noted that the effect on innate immunity may decrease apoptosis of some inflammatory cells. Environmental factors o stress and smoking aggravate host malfunctions. On the luminal side commensal microflora the types of which are still avidly sought either initiate abnormal cell-cell communications or abet host deficiencies and participate in the sequences leading to mucosal cell apoptosis. The role of dysbiosis is of interest (see text). The search for specific infectious agents continues. Dietary factors are also considered but not clarified yet.

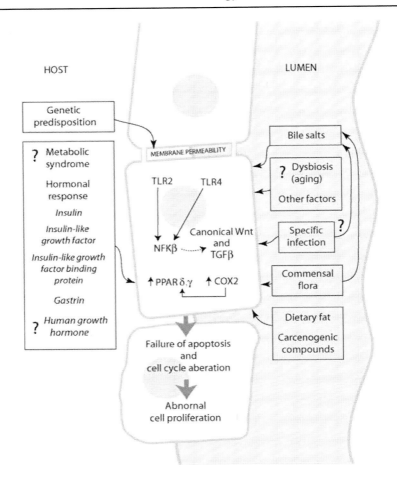

Figure 3. The central cell represents colonic mucosa containing some receptors discussed in the text. Toll-like receptors have among functions, of cell permeability control bacterial and perhaps dietary fat sensing (see text). Through different signaling pathways (see text) signal systems like the canonical Wnt/Tfc responsible for cell-cell contact and the TGFβ system responsible for cell-cycling are activated leading to failure of cellular apoptosis. The COX2 and Peroxiome Proliferator-Activating Receptor δ and PPARγ are upregulated and contribute to cell immortality. Enhanced production of PGI2 by COX2 is instrumental in upregulation of PPARδ. On the host side a small percentage of genetic polymorphisms lead to specific syndromes. The genetic predisposition in cases of other familial or sporadic cancers is an ongoing project. Hormonal growth factors contribute to promotion of carcinogenesis. The predominant response is through Insulin and Insulin-like growth factors which are in response to specific or mass calorie intake. On the luminal side conversion of primary bile salts to secondary bile salts, dietary fatty acids, specific carcinogens derived from cooked meats and dysbiosis due to variety of effects could initiate and promote carcinogenesis.

The best evidence to date of the role of vitamin D in modulation of IBD are based on in vitro data and animal models. In the IL-10 KO mouse model of spontaneous CD development deficiency of vitamin D accelerates the disease while the disease is delayed in vitamin D sufficient animals [196]. In a double IL-10/VDR KO model, fulminant colitis develops early and lymphoid producing organs are atrophied compared to the single IL-10 KO model with intact VDR[197]. This suggests an important T cell regulatory function for VDR. In vitro calcitriol inhibits production of IL-12 by macrophages and dendritic cells, interfering with the Th1 response [198]. A further variation of the IL-10 KO model is the observation that in addition to $1,25(OH)_2D_3$ supplement which delays and moderates severity the inclusion of calcium to diet has the greatest moderation effect on severity of colitis[199].

The IBDs are more common in the Northern than Southern parts of countries like the USA, suggesting a protective role for sunlight in this disease also[200]. However, data on vitamin D levels in patients with IBD have been largely evaluated for relationship to bone disease. Summer/winter differences have been reported, with the latter season showing lower values[201]. There has been a debate as to what constitutes low vitamin levels. However, Cantorna and Mahon argue that $25(OH)D_3$ levels which are associated with an increased risk for bone fractures (<50 nmol/L) are probably also associated with an increased risk for autoimmunity[194]. Low $25(OH)D_3$ levels in both CD and UC have been reported in 34.6% of young patients with a range of 24-70%[202]. These figures are modified by seasons, skin colour of the patient and whether they are taking supplements of vitamin D or not. Interestingly low vitamin D levels in patients with Crohn's disease have also been reported from Japan where large amount of fish (and relatively low quantities of DFs) are consumed in the diet[203].Vitamin D is not added to milk in Japan(personal communication 18th conference on dairy food science Tokyo 2003). In the report by Pappa et al duration and the activity of disease independently predicted low levels. An earlier study also suggested that poor nutrition (acquired by long duration of CD?) and disease activity accompanied low $25(OH)D_3$ plasma levels[204].Although not confirmed, a British study of European patients with CD, UC and controls found more homozygotes for Taq I, VDR polymorphisms in patients with CD than UC or controls. This suggests the possibility that such genetic alterations may confer susceptibility towards CD[205]. Recently a vitamin D analogue with reduced hypercalcemic effect was shown to inhibit NF-κB activation in peripheral blood mononuclear cells form patients with CD suggesting possible therapeutic use[206].

Based on the literature it seems reasonable to conclude that vitamin D may have a risk modulating effect on IBD. Following the 2 compartment paradigm of IBD pathogenesis vitamin D would be an environmental modulator of compartment 1, innate immune system exerting control over aggressive and inappropriate response directly and /or through control of intracellular calcium. There is insufficient evidence at this time to determine whether low vitamin D levels, genetic polymorphisms of VDR and/or low calcium levels in the predisease state augment the likelihood of clinical disease. It is very likely though that once disease has developed deficiencies would be aggravated.

Impact of Vitamin D on Pathogenesis of Colorectal Cancer

In 1980 Garland and Garland hypothesized that the geographic distribution of colon cancer in the USA suggested that sunlight and hence vitamin D could be protective against this disease[207]. Subsequently Garland et al reported that dietary intake of vitamin D and calcium were linked with a dose response reduction in colon cancer[208]. Basic research did confirm anti neoplastic effects of vitamin D. The multiple antineoplastic effects of vitamin D are listed in Table 4 and are reviewed in a number of articles in addition to those of

Zitterman[190] and Dusso[191,209]. In vitro and rodent models using the 1,2-dimethylhydrazine chemical induction of carcinogenesis have consistently shown reduced hyperproliferation of epithelium and reduction of tumor load in experiments using supplemental vitamin D alone or co-addition of calcium[210]. The inhibitory effects of a 1, 25 $(OH)_2D_3$ analogoue on an vitro mouse colon tumor cell line has also been demonstrated to be more active than the original[211]. Clinical mechanistic studies also support the antiproliferative effects of Vitamin D. For example in post polypectomy patients fasting 25(OH) D_3 levels were inversely correlated with crypt labeling indices and these were augmented in those on additional calcium supplement[212].

In keeping with the genetic abnormalities noted in colorectal cancer (discussed above) polymorphisms of VDR have been evaluated to determine any predisposition to colon cancer.

The presence of one polymorphism, the FokI FF genotype in conjunction with a "Western" type diet conferred increased susceptibility to cancer[213] and similarly the ff genotype increased risk in conjunction with low physical activity[214]. In a follow up study Murtaugh et al linked additional dietary constituents and VDR polymorphisms and insulin secretion especially in the FokI genotypes. The genotype Ff/ff together with a low consumption of sugar to high fiber ratio conferred a low risk while the consumption of red meat and FF genotype had the highest risks for colon cancer[215]. A recent report examined a possible protective effect of TaqI in conjunction with the FokI polymorphism. The study raised the possibility that The TT Ff or TtFf genotypes are associated with a protective effect because cancer patients exhibited a very low frequency of these genotypes[216].

Observational human studies of vitamin D and colorectal cancer to 2004 were reviewed by Grant and Garland [217]. They noted in an assembly of 24 studies on colorectal cancer and adenoma that combination intakes of studies on exposure to sunshine, dietary and supplemental vitamin D generally show reduced incidence of colorectal cancer. The effect is more pronounced in case-control studies as opposed to cohort studies. A more recent publication of the effect of calcium and vitamin D intake on distal colon adenomas in women suggested that vitamin A (retinol) attenuates the protective effect of vitamin D[218].

Relatively few interventional trials have been published using combination of vitamin D and calcium. Two recent such trials have been reported with different outcomes. The first, by Wactawski-Wende et al. carried out a prospective 7 yr trial on postmenopausal women. The active group took 1000 mg of calcium together with 400IU vitamin D against placebo. They did not find that this combination reduced risk of cancer[219]. However this report was criticized on several grounds[220]. It included participants who had higher than the national average intake of calcium and vitamin D, the subjects were particularly motivated toward a healthy life style, yet compliance was poor with medications. The follow up time was relatively short (7years) to allow for cancer development. Finally the vitamin D intervention of 400 IU is now considered too low for antineoplastic event.

An editorial by an eminent group of scientists argue that vitamin D intake should be increased for efficacy[221]. A recent publication which examined incident cancers of all types in postmenopausal women after a 4 yr intervention trial with about 1500mg calcium alone or with vitamin D 1100 IU/d or placebo did find a significant reduction in cancers in the calcium and vitamin D group. They also found a trend for reduction with calcium alone[222]. The results are difficult to generalize yet, as there were only a few cancers that developed in the groups under study.

Interaction of Lactose Consumption with Phenotypic Lactose Digestability on Fecal Microflora

The geographic distribution of IBD and CRC as discussed above, also has a relationship to distribution of populations, divided along phenotypic lactose digesters (LP) and maldigesters (LNP). A possible protective effect of the geographic distribution of LNP status against IBD was first reported by Nanji and Denardi. They noted an inverse relationship between national LNP prevalence and the incidence of both major forms of IBD[223]. Our group subsequently re-examined this finding and using a negative binomial model indeed confirmed statistically significant decremental risk of both CD and UC with increasing national LNP prevalence. We also noted a statistically significant incremental risk for UC with increasing national per capita DF consumption. In the case of CD the increased risk achieved a statistical trend (p<0.1)(Shrier et al., Nutr Cancer in print).

Ecological observations do not necessarily indicate a true relationship between the observed correlations. However, a mechanistic explanation how DFs and LNP/LP status interact can be based on the above outlined pathogenesis for IBD as well as CRC. The consumption of DFs is affected by the unique position of the milk sugar, lactose consisting of a galactose and a glucose molecule. In the second half of the twentieth century it was recognized that lactose digestion was under genetic influence[224,225]. Currently, 3 hypotheses are postulated to account for the phenotypic dichotomy. The most prominent by Simoons suggested that in ancient populations the continuing practice of dairy herding led to increased DF consumption and maintenance of intestinal lactase levels allowing a nutritional selective advantage[226]. Anderson and Vullo thought that based on geographic distribution of malaria LNP status together with a number of other genetic traits may protect against the disease[227]. The 3rd hypothesis postulated the LP and LNP status followed the distribution of sunlight and availability of vitamin D. In this case LP status allowed populations living in temperate climates to consume more DFs with high calcium content which then compensates for lack of sunlight[228]. This hypothesis links vitamin D to the genetics of lactase/lactose interactions and calcium.

The enzyme lactase phlorizin hydrolase(LPH) is distributed on the villi of the intestinal brushborder of the proximal part of the gut(duodenum and jejunum).The gene responsible for the enzyme is located on chromosome 2(2q21)[225]. In the majority of the worlds population the high lactase levels encountered in neonates eventually diminishes in a spotty fashion along the upper small bowel at various ages[229-231]. For example while Asians lose 90% of their LPH by the age of 2, Finnish children destined to be LNP do so when they are teenagers. The genetic polymorphism divides the world into those who can and those who cannot digest lactose. The former is a recessive[232] and the latter is a dominant trait[233] with the general geographic distribution described above.

In adults, it is generally agreed that LPH is non inducable by continued lactose consumption[234]. The control of the enzyme resides in the LPH promoter region and is mainly transcription regulated[235,236]. There may be a second mechanism possibly through translation[235]. To date several polymorphisms have been identified, but the predominant control mutations, except in some African populations, appears to be at bp C/T_{-13910}. In this locus T/T genotype is dominant and C/C is recessive[237,238].

A 90% loss of LPH allows less than 10g of lactose to be digested[239]. Consumption of lactose beyond this quantity in a single dose spills into the large intestine and is metabolized by bacteria into short chain fatty acids and gases hydrogen and carbon dioxide[240].In some subjects hydrogen is converted into methane(CH_4) or hydrogen sulfide (SH^-)[136,177,241]. Depending on quantity and the rate of entry of lactose into the colon many subjects suffer uncomfortable gas, bloating, cramps and occasionally diarrhea[242]. These symptoms together with cultural practices results in lower DF consumption in LNP compared with LP populations.

An unusual feature of lactose consumption is the observation that after continued regular ingestion, hydrogen gas production and the ellicitation of symptoms diminishes. This has been observed under epidemiological [243-245] and laboratory conditions as well[246].

While some consider improved symptoms to be largely a learned effect[247], others feel that some results cannot be explained in this manner. For example a dose effect of pretest dietary lactose on results of a single measurement of hydrogen and symptoms is difficult to attribute to learning[248], There should also be similar observations with other test sugars as well. However, this is not the case [249,250]. In addition, the adaptive process is accompanied by an increase in fecal measurement of β-galactosidase(bacterial lactase)[246].

Putatively the reduction of hydrogen with adaptation is due to expansion of lactic acid producing bacteria such as lactobacilli and bifidobacteria, but may include others. Evidence for this hypothesis has been provided in vitro[251,252] and in vivo with at least 1 study[253]. In LP populations lactose is digested and absorbed in the upper small bowel. Up to 8% of ingested lactose can still reach the lower intestine[254] and therefore contribute to alterations in the flora, provided high quantities of DFs are regularly consumed.

One other potential effect of lactose is the facilitation or enhanced bioavailabilty of Ca++ absorption mainly in the jejunum. Proof of this concept however is controversial, with some studies showing effect in models[255] or humans[256-258] and others failing to demonstrate this benefit[259,260]. It is not clear whether LNP status impacts on these findings. Lactose had no effect on zinc absorption in lactose intolerant post menopausal women[261]. There is no information on whether colonic adaptation impacts on calcium bioavailabilty.

Regular lactose consumption may promote a balanced intestinal flora as described. The effect in the host could result in modulation of disease such as IBD in a way that it is attenuated, delayed or modified. This process would be facilitated in LNP subjects who would require less lactose consumption to achieve luminal effects. In LP subjects greater amounts of DFs could exert similar effects through the small amount of lactose reaching the colon[254].

Dairy Foods and IBD

The current literature regarding the interaction of DFs and IBD with very few exceptions does not support any protective effects as suggested by the theoretical possibility outlined above. There are 5 separate topics which are relevant, and these are outlined in Table 5.

In the ecological report (above) we found that, yearly per capita DF consumption elevated risk for incidence of UC and approached a significant p value in CD (Shrier et al., MS submitted). While a direct pathogenic effect of DF is not evident in the literature, Cow's milk allergy can resemble IBD in children[262,263]. Could such allergy at a young age lead to adult IBD? Cow's milk sensitivity was evaluated in both forms of IBD[264-266]. In this study based on clinical history of Cow's milk sensitivity Glassman et al reported a 3 fold (8.5%) increase in CD compared with controls(2.8%). However, history of sensitivity rose to 20.9% in patients with UC. In other studies of older IBD patients, antibodies to lactoferrin in sera were detected[267,268]. A more recent general survey of gastrointestinal symptoms in adults evaluating the role of cow's milk sensitivity found the condition to be extremely rare[269]. As such, finding of milk protein antibodies in patients with IBD may reflect epiphenomena and unlikely to account for a significant number of cases.

Table 5.   Current published and hypothetical relationships between dairy food consumption and inflammatory bowel disease(IBD).

Early onset milk protein allergy	Relation to adult IBD
Passage of Mycobacterium in Pasteurized milk	A possible cause of Crohn's disease
Possible protective effect of carnitine on mutations of the Organic Cation Sodium Transporter OCTN	Dairy food contains carnitine; Can high intake protect against IBD
Lactose intolerance in IBD? Reduced intake in active disease	General avoidance of dairy foods could bias case-control studies.
Possible protective effect of dairy foods in IBD via prebiotic effects.	Regular consumption at lower doses in LNP and higher doses in LP may lead to bacterial adaptation.

Increased risk with DFs for CD may be more direct. The possible pathogenic role of Mycobacterium Avium Intracellulare spp Paratuberculosis(MAP) was discussed above.

The organism can be passed in milk and may enter the human food chain. There have been a number of queries whether MAP can be properly eliminated from milk by current pasteurization methods[270-273]. Hypothetically the organism has a potential to cause human disease.

An additional impetus to consider MAP as a CD pathogen is provided by recent finding that this organism and another potential pathogen Campylobacter jejuni share a 9 amino acid epitope in the human organic cation transporters(OCTN1)[274]. However, a recent case-control study from Britain, spanning 5 years failed to find any evidence of MAP present in milk or drinking water[275]. A recent therapeutic trial of anti MAP therapy for 2 years failed to maintain remission in CD[276]. These studies do not settle fully the controversy, but whether MAP is indeed pathogenic, it is questionable whether all affected sites in CD could be accounted for cause.

In fact, the British study showed that pasteurized milk was protective against CD[275]. A hypothetical explanation may relate to carnitine found in in DFs[277] and interaction with mutations in the OCTN transporters. Aggregates at chromosome locus 5q31 (genetic designation IBD5) have been linked with CD and UC[278,279]. The OCTN1 and OCTN2 transporters carry carnitine across mitochondrial membranes and facilitate both fatty acid oxidation and ATP generation[274]. In the presence of specific mutations the carriers function less well. The OCTN carriers are located throughout the small bowel and concentrated in the terminal ileum. The shared epitopes between MAP, Campylobacter jejuni and the OCTN1 carrier raises the hypothesis that an autoimmune response could be generated when susceptible patients get infected with these organisms[274]. As a result of either autoimmune damage or genetic polymorphism, abnormalities in carnitine transport could lead to IBD pathology. Indeed active CD is associated with low serum carnitine levels[280]. Lamonhwah et al suggest that the defect may be corrected with a high carnitine supplement[274]. Another British population study found a 49% prevalence of IBD5 haplotype in patients with CD[281], making the frequency sufficient to have a statistical impact if indeed carnitine can compensate for IBD5 defects. Possible impact of LNP/LP status was not specifically evaluated in the epidemiological study from Britain. A comparison with a Japanese (high prevalence LNP) population showed that the IBD5 haplotypes were rare [275].

The above discussion not withstanding, consumption of DFs in both patients with CD or UC are generally restricted[282-285]. The reason for restricting DFs is likely multifactorial, but it is less likely because of aggravation of the disease. In a prospective cohort study evaluating the effect of diet on relapse in UC, it was found that both UC patients in remission or relapse consumed about the same amount of DFs without a statistically significant difference[286].

There is some suggestion that in patients with small bowel involvement with CD, lactose intolerance is more severe and independent of ethnicity[287-289]. In cases of colon involvement in CD, severity of intolerance and ethnic influences are less dominant[288] than in UC [290,291]. In the case of UC with activity an increased sensitivity to lactose has been reported[291,292].

Nevertheless, much of the food interactions with IBD have not been clearly worked out and is thought to be based on personal and subjective experience[293]. Therefore, any protective effect of LNP status or high DF intake would be more difficult to detect.

Dairy Foods and CRC

In contrast to paucity of reports on the effect of dairy foods/calcium on IBD there are a dirth of studies on the topic for CRC. Early epidemiological publications often separated DF effect from that possibly attributed to calcium. However, it was suggested that DFs do reduce risk of CRC[294,295]. An important impetus to evaluate DFs was the observation that Ca^{++} is able to reduce neoplastic progression. Two major ways in which calcium is thought to be beneficial are the observations that Ca^{++} inhibits abnormal cellular proliferation in subjects with high risk familial colon cancer[296]. The other mechanism is intraluminal, in that binding of free fatty acids in high fat diets and bile salts could reduce mutagenesis of these compounds[297]. Initial assessment of observational studies of calcium effect have not been consistent [298]. However, the benefits of supplemental calcium have been reproduced in both animal models and clinical trials[299-301].

In addition there are other putative agents in dairy foods with antineoplastic potential, such as lactoferrin, conjugated linoleic acids and in fermented DFs, probiotics[302,303].

The effects of DFs on CRC have been reported to be variable. However, the main point of contention has been the consistent finding that while cohort studies report benefit these are not backed up by case-control studies[303,304]. The conventional argument for the discrepancy is that case-control methodology has a number of flaws related to dietary recall bias. However, as outlined above lactose may behave as a prebiotic[114], and models have demonstrated effects of prebiotics and probiotics against neoplasia[305-308]. With these concepts as background, we wondered whether DFs affect LNP/LP populations differently.

We noted that (as stated above) ecological studies suggest increased risk with DFs and diminished risk with increasing national prevalence of LNP status[309]. However, population studies tend to report DF benefit both in high DF consuming low LNP status countries as well as in low DF consuming, high LNP countries, but at consumed quantities of 3-6 fold difference[309]. The study by Zhuo and Watanabe is particularly interesting[310]. These authors evaluated food intake in a large number of provinces in China. They observed that the absence of DF intake was associated with an increased risk of CRC. This observation suggests that it is an ingredient in DFs which is required for effect and is not vitamin D. To our knowledge there is no addition of vitamin D to milk in China.

Based on the ecological/population reports, we evaluated 80 studies (cohort and case-control) related to DFs or Calcium(mainly but not exclusively derived from DFs) to determine what effect regional distribution might exert on outcome. While this is a crude analysis it was meant to evaluate lactose containing foods, since very few studies have actually examined this ingredient in DFs[311]. We assembled all studies regardless of CRC site into 3 world regions based on predominantly homogenous LNP, predominantly homogenous LP, and where the population consists of an average of 50% of each (range 21-79%). A previous analysis of biregional division of the world failed to add any clarification to then existing results of studies[298].

Taking into consideration LNP/ LP status we noted that in cohort studies in both homogenous regions confirmed DF benefit. Moreover, case-control studies in these regions approximated findings from cohort studies, albeit less well. In mixed populations (average 50%) there was an insignificant very modest protective effect with wide confidence intervals. In addition all studies were of the case-control type.

This analysis we feel removes some of the discrepancy between the 2 methodologies and suggests that perhaps other factors may play a role. We hypothesized that as lactose doses are increased and consumption continues colonic adaptation may exert antineoplastic effects as described in models[305-308]. Since large doses of calcium need to be ingested for potential effect, but these are not achieved by LNP, but are by LP populations. It is of interest that Ca++ at high doses in animal and human studies also exerts prebiotic effects[313-315]. At high DF intakes, as well, some lactose reaches the lower intestine in LP subjects[254]. It is therefore possible that at least part of DF effect even in LP populations may be through modification of fecal microflora.

Relationship between IBD, CRC and Expected Reduction of Disease Risk for IBD with DFs

The above outline attempts to point out similarities between pathogenesis of IBD and CRC.

These are summarized in Table 6. Similarities include geographic pattern, the requirement of pattern recognition sensors and hormonal nuclear receptors for aberrant siganling together with genetic predisposition, the attenuation of disease in germ free models, and the role of intra luminal commensal floral aberrant siganling. These suggest that the two diseases share some common pathogenic processes.

Table 6. Comparison of pathogenic similarities between Inflammatory bowel disease (IBD) and Colorectal cancer (CRC) is shown.

Similarities	Differences
Geographic distribution	Epidemiology; Age, CRC older
Variable details but partly genetic dependent	IBD; Immune CRC cell-cell adhesion, cell immortality
Dependence on microflora	? Dysbiosis of aging
Alteration of disease in germ free models	
Dependence on diet	Possibly more pathogenic with carcinogens in diet
Role of Vitamin D	
Calcium	Role not yet clearly defined beyond role in bones for IBD
Participation of Toll-like receptors	? different effectors activated
Participation of Peroxisome proliferator-activating Receptors	Emerging role of PPARγ in IBD
NF-κB dependent cytokine response	Relation to CRC needs more clarrification
Involvement of cyclooxygenase 2	upregulation protects IBD, promotes awry cell survival in CRC

A corollary question is also relevant. If IBD and CRC share so many similarities why are they not more commonly seen together. The answer is unclear but several points are evident.

The most obvious is that there may be subtle different causes. Different types of genetic predisposition or segregation with other genes regulate type of disease. Although there is an overlap in general, different age groups are affected. Aging affects both the host and luminal compartments. On the host side aging diminishes both immune response and through increased somatic genetic changes facilitates carcinogenesis[316]. On the luminal side aging promotes bacterial changes, perhaps leading to "natural" dysbiosis[317]. At the cell signaling level one wonders why APC/kRAS are not altered by stimuli that affect cell cytoplasm and nucleus, but p53 is affected early. COX2 which is upregulated in both diseases appear to share roles in IBD (prevention of destruction of mucosa) and CRC (immortalization of epithelial cells), through common mechanism of inhibition of apoptosis.

Common pathogenic processes may have geographic impact. The strongest example is the increased CRC rate in Japanese (low risk CRC) immigrants to Hawaii. This region is in the sun belt but has fully "Westernized" diet and lifestyle. However, the Hawaiian experience is noteworthy in that despite adequate sunshine, CRC frequency approach the "Western" prevalence rates, suggesting a relative homogenous distribution of any putative pathogen. The population is made up of multiethnic/racial background, but as recently reported, all three variables; calcium, vitamin D, and DFs were found to be protective in a multiethnic cohort study from Hawaii and southern California[318]. This study also suggests that the geographic dilution of pathogens(not bacteria exclusively) may be independent of the protective effects of these 3 agents.

In the case of IBD rates of disease in immigrants (from low risk) to western regions (high risk) also rise[319,320]. There is also evidence that vitamin D and Calcium likely exert anti-inflammatory effects on the host compartment. The apparent discrepancy is the effect of DFs on IBD. As outlined above ecological findings of the interaction of DFs and CRC are clearly false in both high LP and high LNP populations. In our previous analysis we argued that perhaps regional discrepancy in sufficiently mixed LNP/LP populations reflects an analytical bias related to non-separation of the 2 populations. If LNP subjects have a modified risk for CRC due to prebiotic effects of lactose compared with LP populations, discrepancies in outcome of studies could occur[309,311]. Based on the above argument, given the probable pathogenic importance of luminal microflora and the effects of beneficial commensal bacteria (probiotics and prebiotics) in both diseases, it may be expected that DFs exert benefit in IBD also. As well IBD should share a similar relationship to DF/LNP interactions as CRC. We would expect that studies would show reduced risk with DF consumption prior to disease development. Also, subjects with LNP status who consume DFs would be as protected as LP subjects with high intake of DF. It is the interaction between polymorphisms of lactase and lactose rather than the mere presence of the genetics that is likely to affect protective mechanisms[321,322]. As noted above patients with IBD generally reduce DF intake and are prone to develop vitamin D deficiency. Therefore case-control studies may not be the optimal way to evaluate any effect of LNP/LP/DF interactions. Rather, long term cohort studies are more likely to demonstrate hypothesized effects.

Summary and Conclusion

This review outlines pathogenic similarities between two complex diseases. The synthesis of the hypothesis is based both on laboratory results as well as clinical data, and these are identified as much as possible. An attempt is made to detail cellular, physiological and ecological relationships envisaged for comparison and it is realized that much detail has been omitted by necessity. Nevertheless, the primary emphasis is to argue that vitamin D (sunlight and diet dependent), Dairy food consumption including calcium and effects of the LNP/LP dichotomy may represent a general disease modifying system with an evolutionary background(fig 4).

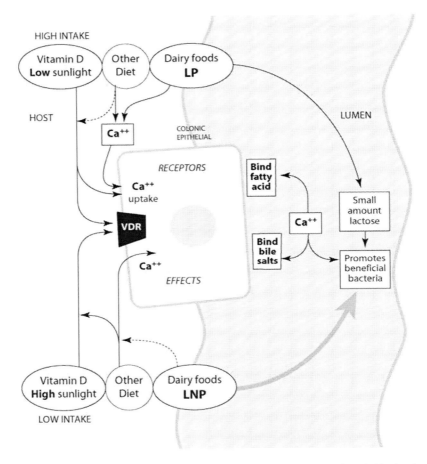

Figure 4. In northern areas, less vitamin D is obtained from sunlight and variable intake from diet. Adult lactase persistent (LP) populations are able to consume large amounts of dairy foods (DFs) which contain significant amount of calcium (Ca++). Both host compartment (see text) and luminal events could benefit from Ca++. In the lumen, binding of bile salts, dietary fatty acids and promotion of Lactic Acid Bacteria may contribute to both anti inflammatory and anti neoplastic effects (see text). In LP populations small amounts of lactose could also promote bacterial benefits (see text). Large intake of calcium could partly compensate for reduced vitamin D intake (limited dietary sources and reduced sunlight). In southern areas and high lactase persistent populations, high sunlight exposure and limited dietary sources may be sufficient for disease protection. As the Hawaiian/California experience shows however, calcium and DFs may be required as well. In these regions the excess lactose reaching the colon, through bacterial modification may compensate for some of the effects of calcium and vitamin D.

In this paradigm of three elements, Vitamin D is intimately involved with both calcium metabolism and several non-classical functions influencing innate immunological control and neoplastic transformation. Calcium is involved with the effector mechanism of vitamin D restricted to host events. However, calcium also has a function in modifying intraluminal events. These function as binding of fatty acids and bile salts, possibly modifying carcinogenesis, as well as, possibly, promoting at high doses, select populations of beneficial bacteria. The most abundant source of calcium are DFs but LNP populations do not usually achieve such high dietary intake of DFs. It is postulated that in LNP populations the consumption of regular, even modest to moderate amounts of DFs leads to colonic bacterial adaptation. This process could compensate for lack of higher calcium intake with consequent disease risk reduction. In LP populations with high individual DF intake, modest amounts of lactose reaching the colon could also provide stimulus for such beneficial bacteria. The combination and interactions of these 3 variables could potentially account for north/south and west/ /east disease risk distribution.

Confirmation of the impact of LNP/LP divide could lead to a number of practical modifications of analyzing data and dietary instructions. First, evaluation of the impact of DFs on diseases where microbial flora putatively contribute to pathogenesis may more accurately be identified if LNP/LP status is also taken into account. Secondly, the current practice of advising lactose free products and external lactase with DFs to treat lactose intolerance could be abandoned in favour of regular lower dose intake and adaptation, as initially suggested by Hertzler and Saviano[246]. Third, proof that CRC and IBD risk may be reduced through lactase/lactose interactions as outlined, would provide a clinical model for therapeutic impact of other currently studied prebiotics and probiotics. It is concluded that much more work should be carried out to evaluate potential impact of adaptation and possible prebiotic effects of lactose, and interactions with vitamin D and calcium.

References

[1]   Selby, W. The natural history of ulcerative colitis. *Baillieres Clin Gastroenterol.* 2007 11, 53-64.

[2]   Loftus, EV; Schoenfeld, P; Sandborn, WJ. The epidemiology and natural history of Crohn's disease in population-based patient cohorts from North America. *Aliment Pharmacol Ther.* 2002 16, 51-60.

[3]   Meyers, S; Janowitz, HD. The "natural history" of ulcerative colitis: an analysis of the lacebo response. *J Clin Gastroenterol.* 1989 11, 33-37.

[4]   Su, C; Lewis, JD; Goldberg, B; Brensinger, C; Lichtenstein, GS. A meta-analysis of the rates of remission and response in clinical trials of active ulcerative colitis. *Gastroenterology.* 2007 132. 516-526.

[5]   Su, C; Lichtenstein, GR; Krok, K; Brensinger, CM; Lewis, D. A meta-analysis of the placebo rates of remission and response in clinical trials of active Crohn's disease. *Gastroenterology.* 2004 126, 1257-1269.

[6]   Freeman, HJ. Natural history and clinical behavior of Crohn's disease extending beyond 2 decades. *J Clin Gastroenterol.* 2003 37, 216-219.

[7]   Slattery, ML; Boucher, KM; Caan, BJ; Potter, JD; Ma, KN. Eating patterns and risk of colon cancer. *Am J Epidemiol*. 1998 148, 4-16.

[8]   Willet, WC; Stampfer, MJ; Colditz, GA; Rosner, BA; Speizer, FE. Relation of meat, fat and fiber intake to the risk of colon cancer in a prospective study among women. *N Engl J Med*. 1990 323, 1664-1672.

[9]   Correa Lima, MP; Gomes-da-Silva, MH. Colorectal cancer: lifestyle and dietary factors. *Nutr Hosp*. 2005 20, 235-241.

[10] Larsson, SC; Rutegard, J; Bergkvist, L; Wolk, A. Physical activity, obesity, and risk of colon and rectal cancer in a cohort of Swedish men. *Eur J Cancer*. 2006 42, 2590-2597.

[11] Consumption statistics for milk and milk products. www.foodsci.uoguelph.ca/ dairyedu/intro.html.

[12] Kretchmer, N. Lactose and lactase. *Sci Am*. 1972, 71-78.

[13] Scrimshaw, NS; Murray, EB. The acceptability of milk and milk products in populations with high prevalence of lactose intolerance. *Am J Clin Nutr*. 1988 48S, 1079-1159.

[14] Cramer, DW; Xu, H. Lactase persistence, galactose metabolism and milk consumption as risk factors for ovarian cancer. In: Common food intolerances 2: Milk in human nutrition and adult-type hypolactasia. Auricchio, S; Semenza, G(eds). Basel, *Switzerland: Karger*. 1993, 52-60.

[15] Cancer around the world. CA Cancer *J Clin*. 1997 47, 26-27.

[16] Mayberry J, Mann R. Inflammatory bowel disease in rural sub-Saharan Africa: rarity of diagnosis in patients attending mission hospitals. *Digestion* 44, 172-176, 1989.

[17] Mayberry JF. Recent epidemiology of ulcerative colitis and Crohn's disease. *Int J Colorectal Dis* 4, 59-66, 1989.

[18] Russel MG, Stockbrugger RW. Epidemiology of inflammatory bowel disease: an update. *Scand J Gastroenterol* 31, 417-427, 1996.

[19] Director General of the European Health and Consumer Protection (http://europa.eu.int/comm/food/fs/sc/scah/out38_en.pdf).

[20] Tsianos, EV. Risk of cancer in inflammatory bowel disease(IBD). *Eur J Intern Med*. 2000 11, 75-78.

[21] Cosnes, SM; Beaugerie, L; Parc, R; Bennis, M; Tiret, E; Flejou, J-F. Colorectal neoplasia in Crohn's colitis: a retrospective comparative study with ulcerative colitis. *Histopathology*. 2007 50, 574-583.

[22] Winther, KV; Jess, Y. Langholz, E; Munkholm, P; Binder, V. Long-term risk of cancer in ulcerative colitis: A population-based cohort study from Copenhagen county. *Clin Gastroenterol Hepatol*. 2004 2, 1088-1095.

[23] Rutter, MD; Saunders, BP; Wilkinson, KH; Rumbles, S; Schofield, G; Kamm, MA; et al. Thirty-year analysis of a colonoscopic surveillance program for neoplasia in ulcerative colitis. *Gastroenterology*. 2006 130, 1030-1038.

[24] Karlinger, K; Gyorke, T; Mako, EO; Mester, A; Tarjan, Z. The epidemiology and pathogenesis of inflammatory bowel disease. *Euro J Radiol*. 2000 35, 154-167.

[25] Farmer, RG; Easley, KA; Rankin, GB. Clinical patterns, natural history, and progression of ulcerative colitis. A long-term follow-up of 1116 patients. *Dig Dis Sci*. 1993 38, 1137-1146.

[26] Farmer, RG; Hawk, WA; Turnbull, RB. Clinical patterns in Crohn's disease: a statistical study of 615 cases. *Gastroenterology*. 1975 68, 627-635.

[27] Halvarson, J; Jess, T; Magnuson, A; Montgomery, SM; Orholm, M; Binder, V; et al. Environmental factors in inflammatory bowel disease: a co twin study of a Swedish-Danish twin population. *Inflamm Bowel Dis.* 2006 12, 925-933.

[28] Miner, PB. Factors influencing the relapse of patients with inflammatory bowel disease. *Am J Gastroenterol.* 1997 92(12 Suppl). 1S-4S.

[29] Timmer, A. Environmental influences on inflammatory bowel disease manifestations. Lessons from epidemiology. *Dig Dis.* 2003 21, 91-104.

[30] Fraga, XF; Vergara, M; Medina, C; Casellas, F; Bermejo, B; Malagelada, JR. Effects of smoking on the presentation and clinical course of inflammatory bowel disease. *Eur J Gatroenterol Hepatol.* 1997 9, 683-687.

[31] Madretsma, S Wolters, LM; van Dijk, JP; Tak, CJ; Feyerabend, C; Wilson, JH; et al. In-vivo effect of nicotine on cytokine production by human non-adherent mononuclear cells. *Eur J Gastroenterol Hepatol.* 1996 8, 1017-1020.

[32] Guo, X; Wang, WP; Ko, JK; Cho, CH. Involvement of neutrophils and free radicals in the potentiating effects of passive cigarette smoking on inflammatory bowel disease in rats. *Gastroenterology.* 1999m 117, 884-892.

[33] Hallas, J; Gaist, D; Sorensen, HT. Does appendectomy reduce the risk of ulcerative colitis? *Epidemiology.* 2004 15, 173-178.

[34] Riegler, G; Caserta. L; Esposito, I; De Filippo, FR ; Bossa, F ; Esposito, P ; et al. Worse clinical course of disease in Crohn's patients with previous appendectomy. *Eur J Gastroenterol Hepatol.* 2005 17, 623-627.

[35] Madsen, KL; Malfair, D; Gray, D; Doyle, JS; Jewell, LD; Fedorak, RN. Interleukin-10 gene-deficient mice develop a primary intestinal permeability defect in response to enteric microflora. *Inflamm Bowel Dis.* 1999 5, 262-270.

[36] Fries, W; Mazzon, E; Squarzoni, S; Martin, A; Martines, D; Micali, A; et al. Experimental colitis increases small intestine permeability in rat. *Lab Invest.* 1999 79, 49-57.

[37] El Asmar, R; Panigrahi, P; Bamford, P; Berti, I; Not, T; Coppa, GV; et al. Host-dependent zonulin secretion causes the impairment of the small intestine barrier function after bacterial exposure. *Gastroenterology.* 2002 123, 1607-1615.

[38] Peeters, M; Geypens, B; Claus, D; Nevens, H; Ghoos, Y; Verbeke, G; et al. Clustering of increased small intestinal permeability in families with Crohn's disease. *Gastroenterology.* 1997 113, 802-807.

[39] Breslin, NP; Nash, C; Hilsden, RJ; Hershfield, NB. Price, LM; Meddings, JB; et al. Intestinal permeability is increased in a proportion spouses of patients with crohn's disease. *Am J Gastroenterol.* 2001 96, 2934-2938.

[40] Buhner, S; Buning, C; Genschel, J; Kling, K; Hermann, D; Dignass, A; et al. Genetic basis for increased intestinal permeability in families with Crohn's disease: role of Card15 3020ins C mutation? *Gut.* 2006 55, 342-347.

[41] D'Inca, R; Di Leo, V; Corrao, G; Martines, D; D'Odorico, A; Mestriner, C; et al. Intestinal permeability test as a predictor of clinical course in Crohn's disease. *Am J Gastroenterol.* 1999 94, 2956-2960.

[42] Neurath, MF; Finotto, S; Glimcher, LH. The role of Th1/Th2 polarization in mucosal immunity. *Nature Med.* 2002 8, 567-573.

[43] Dohi, T; Fujihashi, K. Type 1 an 2 T helper cell-mediated colitis. *Curr Opin Gastroenterol.* 2006 22, 651-657.

[44] Fuss, IJ; Heller, F Boirivant, M; Leon, F; Yoshida, M; Fichtner-Feigi, S; et al. Nonclassical CD1d-restricted NK T cells that produce IL-13 characterizes an atypical Th2 response in ulcerative colitis. *J Clin Invest.* 2004 113, 1490-1497.

[45] Fiocchi, C. Falling from grace: paradigm shifting in inflammatory bowel disease. *Curr Opin Gastroenterol.* 2007 23, 363-369.

[46] Gaya, DR; Russell, RK; Nimmo, ER; Satsangi, J. New genes in inflammatory bowel disease: lessons for complex diseases? *Lancet.* 2006 367, 1271-1284.

[47] Duerr, RH; Taylor, KD; Brant, SR; Rioux, JD; Silverberg, MS; Daly, MJ; et al. A genome-wide association study identifies IL23R as an inflammatory bowel disease gene. *Science.* 2006 314, 1461-1463.

[48] McGovern, DPB; Van Heel, DA; Jewell, DP. NOD2(CARD!%), the first susceptibility gene for Crohn's disease. *Gut.* 2001 49, 752-754.

[49] van Heel, DA; Ghosh, S; Butler, M; Hunt, KA; Lundberg, AMC; Ahmad, T; et al. Muramyl dipeptide and toll-like receptor sensitivity in NOD2-associated Crohn's disease. *Lancet.* 2005 365,17941796.

[50] Arnott, IDR; Nimmo, ER; Drummond, HE; Fennell, J; Smith, BRK; MacKinlay, E; et al. NOD2/CARD15, TLR4 and CD14 mutations in Scottish and Irish Crohn's disease patients: evidence for genetic heterogeneity within Europe. *Genes Immun.* 2004 5, 417-425.

[51] Rosensteil, P; Fantini, M; Brautigam, K; Kuhbacher, T; Waetzig, GH ; Seegert, D ; et al. TNF-α and INF-γ regulate the expression of the NOD2 (CARD15) gene in human intestinal epithelial cells. *Gastroenterology.* 2003 124, 1001-1009.

[52] Hisamatsu, T; Suzuki, M; Reinecker H-C; Nadeau, WJ; McCormick, BA; Podolsky, DA. CARD15/NOD2 functions as an antibacterial factor in human intestinal epithelial cells. *Gastroenterology.* 2003 124, 993-1000.

[53] Cario, E. Bacterial interactions with cells of the intestinal mucosa: Toll-like receptors and NOD2. *Gut.* 2005 54, 1182-1193.

[54] Harris, G; KuoLee, R; Chen, W. Role of toll-like receptors in health and diseases of gastrointestinal tract. *World J Gastroenterol.* 2006 12, 2149-2160.

[55] Cario, E; Podolsky, DK. Toll-like receptor signaling and its relevance to intestinal inflammation. *Ann N Y Acad Sci.* 2006 1072, 332-338.

[56] Cario, E; Gerken, G; Podolsky, DK. Toll-like receptor 2 controls mucosal inflammation by regulating epithelial barrier function. *Gastroenterology.* 2007 132, 1359-1374.

[57] Powrie, F. Immune regulation in the intestine; a balancing act between effector and regulatory T cell responses. *Ann N Y Acad Sci.* 2004 1029, 132-141.

[58] Duchman, R; Kaiser, I; Hermann, E; Mayet, W; Ewe, K; Meyer zum Buschenfelde, K-H. Tolerance exists towards resident intestinal flora but is broken in active inflammatory bowel disease. *Clin Exp Immunol.* 1995 102, 448-455.

[59] Duchman, R; Schmitt, E; Knolle, P; Meyer Zum Buschenfelde. K-H; Neurath, M. Tolerance towards resident intetsinal flora in mice is abrogated in experimental colitis and restored by treatment with interleukin-10 or antibodies to interleukin-12. *Eur J Immunol.* 1996 26, 934-938.

[60] Kraus, TA; Toy, L; Chan, L; Childs, J; Mayer, L. Failure to induce oral tolerance to a soluble protein in patients with inflammatory bowel disease. *Gastroenterology.* 2004 125, 1771-1778.

[61]   Kraus, TA; Cheifetz, A; Toy, L; Meddings, JB; Mayer, L. Evidence foe a genetic defect in oral tolerance induction in inflammatory bowel disease. *Inflamm Bowel Dis*. 2006 12, 82-88.

[62]   Marks, DJ; Harbord, MWN; MacAllister, R; Rahman, F; Young, J; Al-Lazikani, B; et al. Defective acute inflammation in Crohn's disease: a clinical investigation. *Lancet*. 2006 367, 668-678.

[63]   Kelsall, BL; Leon, F. Imvolvement of intestinal dendritic cells in oral tolerance, immunity to pathogens, and inflammatory bowel disease. *Immunol Rev*. 2005 206, 132-148.

[64]   Silva, MA; Lopez, CB; Riverin, F; Oligny, L; Menezes, J; Seidman, EG. Characterization and distribution of colonic dendritic cells in Crohn's disease. *Inflamm Bowel Dis*. 2004 10, 504-512.

[65]   Wild, GE; Drozdowski, L; Tartaglia, C; Clandin, T; Thomson, ABR. Nutritional modulation of the inflammatory response in inflammatory bowel disease- From the molecular to the integrative to the clinical. *World J Gastroenterol*. 2007 13, 1-7.

[66]   Lewis, JD; Lichtenstein, GR; Stein, RB; et al. An open-label trial of the PPAR-gamma ligand rosiglitazone for active ulcerative colitis. *Am J Gastroenterol*. 2001 96, 3323-3328.

[67]   Rook, GAW; Brunet, LR. Microbes, immunoregulation, and the gut. *Gut*. 2005 54, 317-320.

[68]   Summers, RW; Elliott, DE; Qadir, K; Urban, JF; Thompson, R; Weinstock, JV. Trichuris suis seems to be safe and possibly effective in the treatment of inflammatory bowel disease. *Am J Gastroenterol*. 2003 98, 2034-2041.

[69]   Summers, RW; Elliott, DE; Urban, JF; Thompsosn, R; Weinstock, JV. Trichuris therapy in Crohn's disease. *Gut*. 2005 54, 87-90.

[70]   Amre, DK; Lambrette, P; Law, L; Krupovers, A; Chotard, V; Costea, F; et al. Investigating the hygiene hypothesis as a risk factor in pediatric onset Crohn's disease: A case-control study. *Am J Gastroenterology*. 2006 101, 1005-1011.

[71]   Simon, GL; Gorbach, SL. The human intestinal microflora. *Dig Dis Sci*. 1986(suppl) 31,147S-162S.

[72]   Bornside, G. Stability of human fecal flora. *Am J Clin Nutr*. 1978 31, S141- S144.

[73]   van der Waaij, LA; Harmsen, HJM; Madjipour, M; Kroese, FGM; Zwiers, M; van Dulleman, HM; et al. Bacterial population analysis of human colon and terminal ileum biopsies with 16SrRNA-based fluorescent probes: Commensal bacteria live in suspension and have no direct contact with epithelial cells. *Inflamm Bowel Dis*. 2005 10, 865-871.

[74]   Swidsinski, A; Loening-Baucke, V; Theissig, F; Englehardt, H; Bengmark, S; Koch, S; et al. Comparative study of the intestinal mucous barrier in normal and inflamed colon. *Gut*. 2007 56, 343-350.

[75]   Burnham, WR; Lennard-Jones, JE; Stanford, JL; Bird, RG. Mycobacteria as a possible cause of inflammatory bowel disease. *Lancet*. 1978 2, 693-696.

[76]   Greenstein, RJ. Is Crohn's disease caused by a mycobacterium? Comparison with leprosy, tuberculosis, and Johne's disease. *Lancet Inf Dis*. 2003 3, 507-514.

[77]   Naser, S; Ghabrial, G; Valentine, JF. Culture of Mycobacterium avium subspecies paratuberculosis from the blood of patients with Crohn's disease. *Lancet*. 2004 364, 1039-1044.

[78] Liu, Y: Van Kruiningen, HJ; West, AB; Cartun, RW; Cortot, A; Colombel, J-F. Immunocytochemical evidence of Listeria, Escherichia coli, and Streptococcus Antigens in Crohn;s disease. *Gastroenterology.* 1995 108, 1396-1404.

[79] Kangro, HO; Chong, SKF; Hardiman, A; Heath, RB; Walker-Smith, JA. A prospective study of viral and mycoplasma infections in chronic inflammatory bowel disease. *Gastroenterology.* 1990 98, 549-553.

[80] Trnka, YM; LaMont, JT. Association of Clostridium difficile toxin with symptomatic relapse of chronic inflammatory bowel disease. *Gastroenterology.* 1981 80, 693-696.

[81] Rodeman, JF; Dubberke, ER; Reske, KA; Seo, DH; Stone, CD. Incidence of Clostridium difficile infection in inflammatoey bowel disease. *Clin Gastroenterol Hepatol.* 2007 5, 339-344.

[82] Issa, M; Vijayapal, A; Graham, MB; Beaulieu, DB; Otterson, MF; Lundeen, S; et al. Impact of Clostridium difficile on inflammatory bowel disease. *Clin Gastroenterol Hepatol.* 2007 5, 345-351.

[83] Wakefield, AJ; Ekbom, A; Dhillon, AP; Pittilo, M; Pounder, RE. Crohn's disease: pathogenesis and persistent and persistent measles virus infection. *Gastroenterology.* 1995 108, 911-916.

[84] Bernstein, CN; Blanchard, JF. Viruses and inflammatory bowel disease: Is there evidence for a causal association? *Inflamm Bowel Dis.* 2000 6, 34-39.

[85] Kandiel, A; Lashner, B. Cytomegalovirus colitis complicating inflammatory bowel disease. *Am J Gastroenterol.* 2006 101, 2857-2865.

[86] Polymeros, D; Bogdanos, DP; Day, R; Arioli, D; Vrgani, D; Forbes, A. Does cross-reactivity between mycobacterium avium paratuberculosis and human intestinal antigens characterize Crohn's disease. *Gastroenterology.* 2006 131, 85-96.

[87] Greenstein, RJ; Su, L; Harotunian, V; Shahidi, A; Brown, ST. On the action of methotrexate and 6-Mercaptopurine on M. avium subspecvies paratuberculosis. *Plos One.* 2007 2, e161.

[88] Ellingson, JLE. Absence of mycobacterium avium subspecies paratuberculosis components from Crohn;s disease intestinal biopsy tissues. *Clin Med Res.* 2003 1 217-226.

[89] Bernstein, CN; Blanchard, JF; Rawsthorne, P; Collinc, MT. Population-based case-control study of seroprevalence of Mycobacterium paratuberculosis in patients with Crohn's disease and ulcerative colitis. *J Clin Microbiol.* 2004 42, 1129-1135.

[90] Tamboli, CP; Neut, C; Desreumaux, P; Colombel, JF. Dysbiosis in inflammatory bowel disease. *Gut.* 2004 53, 1-4.

[91] Elson, CO; Sartor, RB; Tennyson, GS; Ridell, RH. Experimental models of inflammatory bowel disease. *Gastroenterology.* 1995 109, 1344-1367.

[92] Rutgeerts, P; Goboes, K; Peeters, M; Hiele, M; Penninckx, F; Aerts, R; et al. Effect of faecal stream diversion on recurrence of Crohn's disease in the neoterminal ileum. *Lancet.* 1991 338, 771-774.

[93] Isaacs, KL; Sartor, RB. Treatment of inflammatory bowel disease with antibiotics. *Gastroenterol Clin North Am.* 2004 33, 335-345.

[94] Rahimi, R; Nikfar, S; Rezaie, A; Abdollahi, M. A meta-analysis of broad-spectrum antibiotic therapy in patients with active Crohn's disease. *Clin Ther.* 2006 28, 1983-1988.

[95] Waldman, M; Bechtold, O; Frick, J-S; Lehr, H-A; Schubert, S; Dobrindt, U; et al. Bacteroides vulgatus protects against escherichia coli-induced colitis in gnotobiotic interleukin-2-deficient mice. *Gastroenterology*. 2003 125, 162-177.

[96] Onderdonk, AB; Franklin, ML; Cisneros, RL. Production of experimental ulcerative colitis in gnotobiotic guinea pigs simplified microflora. *Infect Immun*. 1981 32,225-231.

[97] Parker, RB. Probiotics the other half of the antibiotic story. *Anim Nutr Health*. 1974 29, 4-8.

[98] Fedorak, FN; Madsen, KL. Probiotics and the management of inflammatory bowel disease. *Inflamm Bowel Dis*. 2004 10, 286-299.

[99] Swidsinski, A; Ladhoff, A; Pernthaler, A; Swidsinski, S; Loening-Baucke, V; Ortner, M; et al. Mucosal flora in inflammatory bowel disease. *Gastroenterology*. 2002 122, 44-54.

[100] Swidsinski, A; Weber, J; Loening-Baucke, V; Hale, LP; Lochs, H. Spatial organization and composition of the mucosal flora in patients with inflammatory bowel disease. *J Clin Microbiol*. 2005 43, 3380-3389.

[101] Schultsz, C; Van Den Berg, FM; Ten Kate, FW; Tytgat, GNJ; Dankert, J. The intestinal mucus layer from patients with inflammatory bowel disease harbors high numbers of bacteria compared with controls. *Gastroenterology*. 1999 117, 1089-1097.

[102] Ott, SJ; Musfeldt, M; Wenderoth, DF; Hampe, J; Brant, O; Folsch, UR; et al. Reduction in diversity of colonic mucosa associated with active inflammatory bowel disease. *Gut*. 2004 53, 685-693.

[103] Madsen, KL; Malfair, D; Gray, D; Doyle, JS; Jewell, LD; Fedorak, RN. Interleukin-10 gene-deficient mice develop a primary intestinal permeability defect in response to enteric microflora. *Inflamm Bowel Dis*. 1999 5, 262-270.

[104] Favier, C; Neut, C; Mizon, C; Cortot, A; Colombel, JF; Mizon, J; et al. Fecal β-D-galactosidase production and bifidobacteria are decreased in Crohn's diseas. *Dig Dis Sci*. 997 42, 817-822.

[105] Macfarlane, S; Furrie, E; Kennedy, A; Cummings, JH; Macfarlane, GT. Mucosal bacteria in ulcerative colitis. *Br J Nutr*. 2005 93(suppl), S67-S72.

[106] Bullock, NRBooth, JC; Gibson, GR. Comparative composition of bacteria in the human intestinal microflora during remission and active ulcerative colitis. *Curr Issues Intest Micobiol*. 2004 5, 59-64.

[107] Komanduri, S; Gillevet, PM; Sikaroodi, M; Mutlu, E; Keshavarzian, A. Dysbiosis in pouchitis: Evidence of unique microbial patterns in pouch inflammation. *Clin Gastroenterol Hepatol*. 2007 5, 352-360.

[108] Hawrelak, JA; Myers, SPM. The causes of intestinal dysbiosis: A review. *Alternat Med Rev*. 2004 9,180-197.

[109] Berkes, J; Viswanathan, VK; Savkovic, SD; Hecht, G. Intestinal epithelial responses to enteric pathogens: effects on the tight junction barrier, ion transport, and inflammation. *Gut*. 2003 52, 439-451.

[110] Dial, S; Delaney, JA; Schneider, V; Suissa, S. Proton pump inhibitor use and the risk of community-acquired Clostridium difficile-associated disease defined by prescription for oral vancomycin therapy. *CMAJ*. 2006 175, 745-748.

[111] Gibson, GR; Roberfroid, MB. Dietary modulation of the human colonic microbiota: introducing the concept of prebiotics. *J Nutr*. 1995 125,1401-1412.

[112] Kleesen, B; Schw3arz, S; Boehm, A; Fuhrmann, H; Richter, A; Henle, T; et al. Jerusalem artichokes and chicory inulin in bakery products affect faecal microbiota of healthy volunteers. *Br J Nutr.* 2007, 1-10. doi: 1017/S0007114507730751.

[113] Silvi, S; Rumney, CJ; Cresci, A; Rowland, IR. Resistant starch modifies gut microflora and microbial metabolism in human flora-associated rats inoculated with faeces from Italian and UK donors. *J Appl Microbiol.* 1999 86, 521-530.

[114] Szilagyi, A. Redefining lactose as a conditional prebiotic. *Can J Gastroenterol.* 2004 18, 163-167.

[115] Szilagyi, A. Use of prebiotics for inflammatory bowel disease. *Can J Gastroenterol.* 2005 19, 505-510.

[116] Blaut, M; Clavel, T. Metabolic diversity of the intestinal: Implications for health and disease. *J Nutr.* 2007 137, 751S-755S.

[117] Bengmark, S. Bioecological control of inflammatory bowel disease. *Clin Nutr.* 2007 26, 169-181.

[118] Correa, P; Haenszel, W; The epidemiology of large bowel cancer. *Semin Oncol.* 1978 26, 1-141.

[119] Weisburger, JH. Causes relevant mechanisms and prevention of large bowel cancer. *Semin Oncol.* 1991 18, 316-336.

[120] Galiatsatos, P; Foulkes, WD. Familial adenomatous polyposis. *Am J Gastroenterol.* 2006 101, 385-398.

[121] Lynch, HT; Smyrk, TC; Watson, P; Lanspa SJ; Lynch JF; Lynch PM; et al. Genetics, natural history, tumor spectrum and pathology of hereditary non polyposis colorectal cancer: an updated review. *Gastroenterology.* 1993 104, 1535-1549.

[122] Boland, CR. Decoding hereditary colorectal cancer. *N Engl J Med.* 2006 354, 2815-2817.

[123] Gryfe, R; Swallow, C; Bapat, B; Redston, M; Gallinger, S; Couture, J. Molecular biology of colorectal cancer. *Curr Probl Cancer.* 1997 21, 233-300.

[124] Jeter, JM; Kohlmann, W; Gruber, SB. Genetics of colorectal cancer. *Oncology.* 2006 20, 369-376.

[125] Vogelstein, B; Fearon, ER; Hamilton, SR; Kern SE; Preisinger AC; Leppert M; et al. Genetic alterations during colorectal tumor development. *N Engl J Med.* 1988 319, 5250532.

[126] Fearon, ER; Vogelstein, B. A genetic model for colorectal tumorigenesis. *Cell.* 1990 61, 759-767.

[127] Requart, N; He, B; Taron, M; You, L; Jablons, DM; Rosell, R. The role of Wnt signaling and stem cells. *Fut Oncol.* 2005 6, 787-797.

[128] Taketo, MM. Wnt signalling and gastrointestinal tumorigenesis in mouse models. *Oncogene.* 2006 25, 7522-7530.

[129] Van der Flier, LG; Sabates-Bellver, J; Oving, I; Haegbarth, A; De Palo, M; Anti, M; et al. The intestinal Wnt/TCF signature. *Gastroenterology.* 2007 132, 628-632.

[130] Lugli, A; Zlobec, I; Minoo, P; Baker, K; Tornillo, L; Terracciano, L; et al. Prognostic significance of the wnt signalling pathway molecules APC, β-catenin and E-cadherin in colorectal cancer-a tissue microarray-based analysis. *Histopathology.* 2007 50,453-464.

[131] Arends, JW. Molecular interactions in the Vogelstein model of colorectal carcinoma. *J Pathol.* 2000 190, 412-416.

[132] Niv, Y. Microsatellite instability and MLH1 promoter hypermethylation in colorectal cancer. *World J Gastroenterol*. 2007 13, 1767-1769.

[133] Kono, S; Chen K. Genetic polymorphisms of methyltetrahydrofolate reductase and colorectal cancer and adenoma. *Cancer Sci*. 2005 96, 535-542.

[134] Giovannucci, E; Chen, J; Smith-Warner, SA; Rimm, EB; Fuchs, CS; Palomeque, C; et al. Methylenetetrahydrofolate reductase, alcohol dehydrogenase, diet, and risk of colorectal adenomas. *Cancer Epidemiol Biomark Prev*. 2003 12, 970-979.

[135] Jass, JR. Classification of colorectal cancer based on correlation of clinical, morphological and molecular features. *Histopathology*. 2007 50, 113-130.

[136] Rhodes, JM; Campbell, BJ. Inflammation and colorectal cancer: IBD-associated and sporadic cancer compared. *Trends Mol Med*. 2002 8,10-16.

[137] Rhodes, JM. Unifying hypothesis for inflammatory bowel disease and associated colon cancer: sticking the pieces together with sugar.

[138] Campbell, BJ; Yu, L-G; Rhodes, JM. Alterd glycosilation in inflammatory bowel disease: A possible role in cancer development. *Glycoconj J*. 2001 18, 851-858.

[139] Eisinger, AL; Prescoll, SM; Jones, DA; Stafforini, DM. The role of cyclooxygenase-2 and prostaglandins in colon cancer. *Prostagland Lipid Mediat*. 2007 82, 147-154.

[140] Chan, AT; Giovannucci, EL; Schemhammer, ES, Colditz, GA, Hunter, DJ; Willet, DJ; et al. A prospective study of aspirin use and the risk for colorectal adenoma. *Ann Intern Med*. 2004 140, 157-166.

[141] Cook, NR; Lee, I-M; Gaziano, JM; Gordon, D; Ridker, PM; Manson. JE: et al. Low-dose aspirin in the primary prevention of cancer: The women's health study: a randomized controlled trial. *JAMA* 2005 294, 47-55.

[142] Cruz-Correa, M; Hylind, LM; Romans, KE; Booker, SV; Giardiello, FM. Long-term treatment with sulindac in family adenomatous polyposis: a prospective cohort study. *Gastroenterology*. 2002 122, 641-645.

[143] Baron, JA; Sandler, RS; Bresalier, RS; Quan, H; Ridell, R; Lanas, A; et al. A randomized trial of rofecoxib for the chemoprevention of colorectal adenomas. *Gastroenterology*. 2006 131, 1674-1682.

[144] Rakoff-Nahoum, S; Paglino, J; Eslami-Varzaneh, F; Edberg, S; Medzhitov, R. Recognition of commensal microflora by toll-like receptors is required for intestinal homeostasis. *Cell*. 2004 118,229-241.

[145] Fukata, M; Chen, A; Klepper, A; Krishnareddy, S; Vamadeva, AS; Thomas, LS; et al. Cox-2 is regulated by toll-like receptor-4(TLR4) signaling: Role in proliferation and apoptosis in the intestine. *Gastroenterology*. 2006 131, 862-877.

[146] Greten, FR; Eckmann, L; Greten, TF; Park, JM; Li, Z-W; Egan, L; et al. IKKβ links inflammation and tumorigenesis in a mouse model of colitis-associated cancer. *Cell*. 2004 118, 285-296.

[147] Lee, JY; Sohn, KH; Rhee, SH; Hwang D. Saturated fatty acids but not unsaturated fatty acids, induce the expression of cyclooxygenase-2 mediated through toll-like receptor 4. *J Biol Chem*. 2001 276, 16683-16689.

[148] Boraska Jelavic, T; Barisic, M; Drmic Hofman, I; Boraska, V; Vrdoljak, E; Peruzovic, M; et al. Microsatelite GT polymorphism in the toll-like receptor 2 is associated with colorectal cancer. *Clin Genet*. 2006 70, 156-160.

[149] Clevers, H. At the crossroads of inflammation and cancer. *Cell*. 2004 118, 671-674.

[150] Simiantonaki, N; Kurzik-Dumke, U; Karyofylli, G; Jayasinghe, C; Michel-Schmidt, R; Kirkpatrick, CJ. Reduced expression of TLR4 is associated with the metastatic status of human colorectal cancer. *Int J Mol Med.* 2007 20, 21-29.

[151] Giovannucci, E. Insulin and colon cancer. *Cancer Causes Control.* 1995 6, 164-179.

[152] Giovannucci, E; Michaud, D. The role of obesity and related metabolic disturbances in cancers of the colon, prostate, and pancreas. *Gastroenterology.* 2007 132, 2208-2225.

[153] Durai, R; Yang, W; Gupta, S; Seifalian, AM; Winslet, MC. The role of the insulin-like growth factor system in colorectal cancer: review of current knowledge. *Int J Colorectal Dis.* 2005 20. 203-220.

[154] Slattery, ML; Murtaugh, M; Caan, B; Ma, KN; Neuhausen, S; Samowitz, W. Energy balance, insuli-related genes and risk of colon an rectal cancer. *Int J Cancer.* 2005 115, 148-154.

[155] Tripcovic, I; Tripkovic, A; Strnad, M; Capkun, V; Zekan, L. Role of insulin-like factor-1 in colon carcinogenesis: a case-control study. *Arch Med Res.* 2007 38, 519-525.

[156] Georgopoulos, SD; Polymeros, D; Triantafyllou, K; Spiliadi, C; Mentis, A; Karamanolis, DG; et al. Hypergastrinemia is associated with increased risk of distal colon adenomas. *Digestion.* 2006 74, 42-46.

[157] D'Onghia, V; Leoncini, R; Carli, R; Santoro, A; Giglioni, S; Sorbellini, F; et al. Circulating gastrin and ghrelin levels in patients with colorectal cancer: correlation with tumor stage, Helicobacter pylori infection and BMI. *Biomed Pharmacother.* 2007 61, 137-141.

[158] Cao, J; Yu, J-P; Liu, C-H, Zhou, L; Yu, H-G. Effects of gastrin 17 on β-catenin/Tcf-4 pathway in Colo320WT colon cancer cells. *World J Gastroenterol.* 2006 12, 7482-7487.

[159] Martino, A; Cammarota, G; Cianci, R; Bianchi, A; Sacco, E; Tilaro, L; et al. High prevalence of hyperplastic colonic polyps in acromegalic subjects. *Dig Dis Sci.* 2004 49, 662-666.

[160] Matano, Y; Okada, T; Suzuki, A; Yoneda, T; Takeda, Y; Mabuchi, H. Risk of colorectal neoplasm in patients with acromegaly and its relationship with serum growth hormone levels. *Am J Gastroenterol.* 2005 100, 1154-1160.

[161] Bhansali, A; Kochhar, R; Chawla, YK; Reddy, S; Dash, RJ. Prevalence of colonic polyps is not increased in patients with acromegaly: analysis of 60 patients from India. *J Gastroenterol Hepatol.* 2004 19, 266-269.

[162] Spiegelman, BM. Peroxisome proliferator-activated receptor gamma: A key regulator of adipogenesis and systemic insulin sensitivity. *Eur J Med Res.* 1997 2, 457-464.

[163] Spiegelman, BM. PPAR-gamma: adipogenic regulator and thiazolidinedione receptor. *Diabetes.* 1998 47, 507-514.

[164] Kliewer, SA; Lehman, JM; Milburn, MV; Willson, TM. The PPARs and PXRs: nuclear xenobiotic receptors that define novel hormone signaling pathways. *Recent Prog Horm Res.* 1999 54, 345-367.

[165] Oliver, WR; Shenk, JL; Snaith, MR; Russell, CS; Plunket, KD; Bodkin, NL; et al. A selective peroxisome proliferator-activated receptor delta agonist promotes reverse cholesterol transport. *Proc Natl Acad Sci.* 2001 98, 5306-5311.

[166] Evans, RM; Barish, GD; Wang, Y-X. PPARs and the complex journey to obesity. *Nat Med.* 2004 10, 1-7.

[167] Lin, MS; Chen, WC; Bai, X; Wang, YD. Activation of peroxisome proliferator-activated receptor gamma inhibits cell growth via apoptosis and arrest of the cell cycle in human colorectal cancer. *J Dig Dis* 2007 8, 82-88.

[168] Shen, D; Deng, C; Zhang, M. Peroxisome proliferator-activated receptor γ agonists inhibit the proliferation and invasion of human colon cancer cells. *Postgrad Med J.* 2007 83, 414-419.

[169] Slattery, ML; Curtin, K; Wolff, R; Ma, KN; Sweeney, C; Murtaugh, M; et al. PPARγ and colon and rectal cancer: association with specific tumor mutations, aspirin, ibuprofen and insuli-related genes. *Cancer Causes Control.* 2006 17, 239-249.

[170] Wang, D; Wang, H; Guo, Y; Ning, W; Katkuri, S; Wahli, W; et al. Crosstalk between peroxisome proliferator-activated receptor δ and VEGF stimulates cancer progression. *PNAS.* 2006 103, 19069-19074.

[171] Gupta, RA; Tan, J; Krause, WF; Geraci, MW; Wilson, TM; Dey, SK; et al. Prostacyclin-mediated activation of peroxisome proliferator-activated receptor δ in colorectal cancer. *PNAS.* 2000 97, 13275-13280.

[172] He, T-C; Chan, TA; Vogelstein, B; Kinzler, KW. PPARδ is an APC-regulated target of nonsteroidal anti-inflammatory drugs. *Cell.* 1999 99. 335-345.

[173] Bodaghi, S; Yamanegi, K; Xiao, SY; Da Costa, M; Palefsky, JM; Zheng, ZM. Colorectal papillomavirus infection in patients with colorectal cancer. *Clin Cancer Res.* 2005 11, 2862-2867.

[174] Konson, A; Ben-Kasus, T; Mahajna, JA; Danon, A Rimon, G ; Agbaria, R. Herpes simplex virus thymidine kinase gene transduction enhances tumor growth rate and cyclooxygenase-2 expression in murine colon cancer cells. *Cancer Gene Ther.* 2004 11, 830-840.

[175] Goel, A; Li, M-S; Nagasaka, T; Shin SK; Fuerst, F; Ricciardiello, L; et al. Association of JC virus with the methylator phenotype in sporadic colorectal cancers. *Gastroenterology.* 2006 130, 1950-1961.

[176] Lundstig, A; Stattin, P; Persson, K; Sasnauskas, K; Viscidi, RP; Gisle foss, RE; et al. No excess risk for colorectal cancer among subjects seropositive for the JC polyomavirus. *Int J Cancer.* 2007 on line PMID 17471560.

[177] Yang, L; Pei, Z; Bacteria, inflammation, and colon cancer. *World J Gastroenterol.* 2006 12, 6741-6746.

[178] McGarr, SE; Ridlon, JM; Hylemon, PB. Diet, Anaerobic bacterial metabolism, and colon cancer. *J Clin Gastroenterol.* 2005 39,98-109.

[179] Hill, MJ; Drasar, BS. Degradation of bile salts by human intestinal bacteria. *Gut.* 1968 9, 22-27.

[180] Aries, V; Crowther, JS; Drasar, BS; Hill, MJ; Williams, REO. Bacteria and the aetiology of cancer of the large bowel. *Gut.* 1969 10,334-335.

[181] Hill, MJ; Bacteria and the etiology of colonic cancer. *Cancer.* 1974 34, 815-818.

[182] Wynder, EL; Reddy, BS. Metabolic epidemiology of colorectal cancer. *Cancer.* 1974 34, 801-806.

[183] Attene-Ramos, MS; Wagner, ED; Gaskins, HR; Piewa, MJ. Hydrogen sulfide induces direct radical associated DNA damage. *Mol Cancer Res.* 2007 5, 455-459.

[184] Wang, X; Huycke, MM. Extarcellular superoxide production by Enterococcus faecalis promotes chromosomal instability in mammalian cells. *Gastroenterology.* 2007 132, 551-561.

[185] Martin, HM; Campbell, BJ; Hart, CA; Mpofu, C; Nayar, M; Singh, R; et al Enhanced Escherichia coli adherence and invasion in Crohn's disease and colon cancer. *Gastroenterology*. 2004 127, 80-93.

[186] Kuhn, R; Lohler, J; Rennick, D; Rajewsky, K; Muller, W. Interleukin-10-deficient mice develop chronic enterocolitis. *Cell*. 1993 22, 263-274.

[187] Kado, S; Uchida, K; Funabashi, H; Iwata, S; Nagata, Y; Ando, M; et al. Intestinal microflora are necessary for development of spontaneous addenocarcinoma of the large intestine in T-cell receptor β chain and p53 double-knockout mice. *Cancer Res*. 2001 61, 2395-2398.

[188] Engle, SJ; Ormsby, I; Pawlowski, S; Boivin, GP; Croft, J; Balish, E; et al. Elimination of colon cancer in germ-free transforming growth factor beta 1-deficient mice. *Cancer Res*. 2002 62, 6362-6366.

[189] Pitari, GM; Zingman, LV; Hodgson, DM; Alekseev, AE; Kazerounian, S; Bienengraeber, M; et al. Bacterial enterotoxins are associated with resistance to colon cancer. *PNAS*. 2003 100, 2695-2699.

[190] Zitterman, A. Vitamin D in preventive medicine: are we ignoring the evidence? *Br J Nutr*, 2003 89, 552-572.

[191] Dusso, AS; Brown, AJ; Slatopolsky E. Vitamin D. *Am J Renal Physiol* 2005 289, F8-F28.

[192] Khanal, R; Nemere, I. Membrane receptors for vitamin D metabolites. *Crit Rev Eukaryot Expr*. 2007 17, 31-47.

[193] Cantorna; MT. Vitamin D and autoimmunity: Is vitamin D status an environmental factor affecting autoimmune disease prevalence? *Proc Soc Exp Biol Med*. 2000 223, 230-233.

[194] Cantorna, MT; Mahon, BD. Mounting evidence for vitamin D as an environmental factor affecting autoimmune disease prevalence. *Exp Biol Med* 2004 229, 1136-1142.

[195] Froicu, M; Cantorna, MT. Vitamin D and the vitamin D receptor are critical for control of the innate immune response to colonic injury. *BMC Immunology*. 2007 8, doi: 10.1186/1471-2172-8-5.

[196] Cantorna; MT. Vitamin D and its role in immunology: Multiple sclerosis, and inflammatory bowel disease. *Prog Biophys Mol Biol*. 2006 92, 60-64.

[197] Froicu, M; Zhu, Y; Cantorna, MT. Vitamin D receptor is required to control gastrointestinal immunity in IL-10 knockout mice. *Immunology*. 2006 117, 310-318.

[198] D'Ambrosio, D; Cipitelli, M; Cocciolo, MG; Mazzeo, D; Di Lucia, P; Lang, R; et al. Inhibition of IL-12 production by 1, 25-Dihydroxyvitamin D_3 involvement of NF-κB downregulation in transcriptional repression of the p40 gene. *J Clin Invest*. 1998 10, 252-262.

[199] Zhu,Y; Mahon, BD; Froicu, M; Cantorna, MT. Calcium and 1 alpha, 25-dihydroxyvitamin D_3 target the TNF-alpha pathway to suppress experimental inflammatory bowel disease. *Eur J Immunol*. 2005 35, 217-224.

[200] Sonnenberg, A; McCarty, DJ; Jacobsen, SJ. Geographic variation of inflammatory bowel disease within the United States. *Gastroenterology*. 1991 100, 143-149.

[201] McCarty, D; Duggan, P; O'Brien, M; Kiely, M; McCarthy, J; Shanahan, F; et al. Seasonality of vitamin D status and bone turnover in patients with Crohn's disease. *Aliment Pharm Ther*. 2005 21, 1073-1083.

[202] Pappa, HM; Gordon, CM; Saslowsky, TM; Zholudev, A; Horr, B; Shih, M-C; et al. Vitamin D status in Children and young adults with inflammatory bowel disease. *Pediatrics*. 2006 118,1950-1961.

[203] Tajika, M; Matsuura, A; Nakamura, T; Suzuki, T; Sawaki, A; Kato, T; et al. Risk factors for vitamin D deficiency in patients with Crohn's diseases. *J Gastroeneterol*. 2004 39, 527-533.

[204] Harries, AD; Brown, R; Heatley, RV; Williams, LA; Woodhead, S; Rhodes, J. Vitamin D status in Crohn's disease: association with nutrition and disease activity. *Gut*. 1985 26, 1197-1203.

[205] Simmons, JD; Mullighan, C; Welsh, KI; Jewell, DP. Vitamin D receptor gene polymorphism: association with Crohn's disease susceptibility. *Gut*. 2000 47, 211-214.

[206] Stio, M; Martinesi, M; Bruni, S; Treves, C; Mathieu, C; Verstuyf, A; et al. The vitamin D analogue TX 527 blocks NF-κB activation in peripheral blood mononuclear cells of patients with Crohn's disease. *J Steroid Biochem Mol Biol*. 2007 103, 51-60.

[207] Garland, CF: Garland , FC. Do sunlight and vitamin D reduce the likelihood of colon cancer? *Int J Epidemiol*. 1980m 9, 227-231.

[208] Garland, C: Sekelle, RB; Barrett-Conor, E; Criqui, MH; Rossof, AH; Paul, O. Dietary vitamin D and calcium and risk of colorectal cancer: a 19 –year prospective study in men. *Lancet*. 1985 1,307-309.

[209] Lamprecht, SA: Lipkin, M. Cellular Mechanisms of calcium and vitamin D in the inhibition of colorectal carcinogenesis. *Ann N Y Acad Sci* 2001 952, 73-87.

[210] Harris, DM: Go, VLW. Vitamin D and colon carcinogenesis. *J Nutr*. 2004 134,3463S-3471S.

[211] Spina, CS; Ton, L; Yao, M; Maehr, H; Wolfe, MM; Uskovic, M; et al. Selective vitamin D receptor modulators and their effects on colorectal tumor growth. *J steroid Biochem Mol Biol*. 2007 103, 757-762.

[212] Holt, PR; Arber, N; Halmos, B; Forde, K; Kissileff, H; McGlynn, KA; et al. Colonic epithelial cell proliferation decreases with increasing levels of serum 25-hydroxy vitamin D. *Cancer Epidemiol Biomark Prev* 2002 11,113-119.

[213] Slattery, M; Murtaugh, M; Caan, B; Ma, K; Samowitz, W. Association between dietary fats and VDR genotype and colorectal cancer. *Int J Cancer Prev*. 2005 1, 193-205.

[214] Slattery, ML; Murtaugh, M; Caan, B; Ma, K-N; Wolff, R; Samowitz, W. Association between BMI, energy intake, energy expenditure, VDR genotype and colon and rectal cancers. *Cancer Cause Control*. 2004 15, 863-872.

[215] Murtaugh, M; Sweeney, C; Ma, K-N; Potter, JD; Caan, BJ; Wolff, RK; et al. Vitamin D receptor gene polymorphisms, dietary promotion of insulin resistance, and colon and rectal cancer. *Nutr Cancer*. 2006 55, 35-43.

[216] Yaylim-Eraltan, I; Arzu Ergen, H; Arikan, S; Okay, E; Ozturk, O; Bayrak, S; et al. Investigation of the VDR gene polymorphisms association with susceptibility to colorectal cancer. *Cell Biochem Funct*. 2007 25, 731-737.

[217] Grant, WB; Garland, CF. A critical review of studies on vitamin D in relation to colorectal cancer. *Nutr Cancer*. 2004 48 115-123.

[218] Oh, K; Willett, WC; Wu, K; Fuchs, CS; Giovannucci, EL. Calcium and vitamin D intakes in relation to risk of distal colorectal adenoma. *Am J Epidemiol*. 2007 165, 1178-186.

[219] Wactawski-Wende, J; Morley Kotchen, J; Anderson, GL; Assaf, AR. Brunner, RL; O'Sullivan, MJ; et al. Calcium plus vitamin D supplementation and the risk of colorectal cancer. *N Engl J Med*. 2006 354, 684-696.

[220] Newmark, HL; Heaney, RP; Calcium, vitamin D, and risk reduction of colorectal cancer. *Nutr Cancer*. 2006 56, 1-2.

[221] Vieth, R; Bischoff-Ferrari, H; Boucher, B; Dawson-Hughes, B; Garland, CF; Heaney, RP; et al. The urgent need to recommend an intake of vitamin D that is effective. *Am J Clin Nutr*. 2007 85, 649-650.

[222] Lappe, JM; Travers-Gustafson, D; Davies, KM; Recker, RR; Heaney, RP. Vitamin D and calcium supplementation reduces cancer risk: results of a randomized trial. *Am J Clin Nutr*. 2007 85, 1586-1591.

[223] Nanji, AA; Denardi, FG. Primary adult lactose intolerance protects against development of inflammatory bowel disease. *Med Hypotheses*. 1986 19, 1-6.

[224] Auricchio, S; Rubino, A; Landolt, M; Semenza, G; Prader, A. Isolated intestinal lactase deficiency in the adult. *Lancet*. 1963 2, 324-326.

[225] Kruse, TA; Bolund, C; Grzeschik, KH; Ropers, HH; Sjostrom, H; Noren, O; et al. The human lacrase-phlorizin gene is located on chromosome 2. *FEBS Lett*. 1988 240, 123-126.

[226] Simoons, FJ. The geographic hypothesis and lactose malabsorption. A weighing of the evidence. *Dig Dis Sci*. 1978 23, 963-980.

[227] Anderson, B; Vullo, C. Did malaria select for primary adult lactase deficiency? *Gut*. 1994 35, 1487-1489.

[228] Flatz, G; Rotthauwe, HW. Lactose nutrition and natural selection. *Lancet*. 1973 2, 76-77.

[229] Maiuri, L; Raia, V; Potter J; Swallow D; Ho MW; Fiocca R; et al. Mosaic pattern of lactase expression by villous enterocytes in human adult-type hypolactasia. *Gastroenterology*. 1991 100, 123-126.

[230] Rossi, M; Maiuri, L; Fusco, MI; Salvati VM; Fuccio A; Auricchio S; et al. Lactase persistence versus decline in human adults: multifactorial events are involved in down-regulation after weaning. *Gastroenterology*. 1997 112, 1506-1514.

[231] Wang, Y; Harvey, CB; Hollox, E; Phillips AD; Poulter M; Clay P; et al. The genetically programmed down-regulation of lactase in children. *Gastroenterology*. 1998 114, 1230-1236.

[232] Sahi, T; Isokoski, M; Jussila, J; Launiala K; Pyörälä K. Recessive inheritance of adult-type lactose malabsorption. *Lancet*. 1973 2, 823-826.

[233] Gilat, T. Lactase deficiency: the world pattern today. *Isr J Med Sci*. 1979 15, 369-373.

[234] Gilat, T; Russo, S; Gelman-Malachi, E; Aldor, TA. Lactase in man: a non adaptable enzyme. *Gastroenterology*. 1972 62, 1125-1127.

[235] Lloyd, ML. The regulation of lactase expression in adult life. In: Auricchio, S; Semenza, G. eds. Common Food Intolerances 2: Milk in Human Nutrition and Adult-Type Hypolactasia. *Basel: Karger*. 1993. 124-131.

[236] Kuokkanen, M; Enattah, NS; Oksanen, A; Savilahti E; Orpana A; Järvelä I. Transcriptional regulation of the lactase-phlorizin hydrolase gene by polymorphisms associated with adult-type hypolactasia. *Gut*. 2003 52, 647-652.

[237] Enattah, NS; Sahi, T; Savilahti, E; Terwilliger JD; Peltonen L; Jarvela I. Identification of a variant associated with adult-type hypolactasia. *Nat Genet*. 2002 30, 233-237.

[238] Rasinspera, H; Savilahti, E; Ennatah, NS; Kuokkanen M; Tötterman N; Lindahl H. et al. A genetic test which can be used to diagnose adult-type hypolactasia in children. *Gut.* 2004 53, 1571-1576.

[239] Oku, T; Nakamura, S; Ichinose, M. Maximum permissive dosage of lactose and lactitol for transitory diarrhea and utilizable capacity for lactose in Japanese female adults. *J Nutr Sci Vitaminol.*2005 51, 51-57.

[240] Siigur, U; Tamm, A; Tammur, R. The faecal SCFAs and lactose intolerance in lactose malabsorbers. *Eur J Gastroenterol Hepatol.* 1991 3, 321-324.

[241] Kajs, TM; Fitzgerald, JA; Buckner, RY; Coyle GA; Stinson BS; Morel JG. et al. Influence of a methanogenic flora on the breath H_2 and symptom response to ingestion of sorbitol or oat fiber. *Am J Gastroenterol.* 1997 92, 89-94.

[242] Kitts, D; Yuan, Y; Joneja, J; Scott, F; Szilagyi, A; Amiot, J; et al. Adverse reactions to food constituents: allergy, intolerance, and autoimmunity. *Can J Physiol Pharmacol.* 1997 75:241-254.

[243] Habte, D; Sterby, G; Hijalmarsson, B. Lactose malabsorption in Ethiopian children. *Acta Pediatr Scand.* 1973 62, 649-654.

[244] Sadre, M; Karbasi, K. Lactose intolerance in Iran. *Am J Clin Nutr.* 1979 32, 1948-1954.

[245] Villar, J; Kestler, E; Castillo, P; Juarez, A; Menendez, R; Solomons, NW. Improved lactose digestion during pregnancy: a case of physiologic adaptation? *Obstet Gynecol.* 1988 71, 697-700.

[246] Hertzler, SR; Savaiano, DA. Colonic adaptation to daily lactose feeding in lactose maldigesters reduces lactose intolerance. *Am J Clin Nutr.* 1996 64, 232-236.

[247] Briet, F; Pochart, P; Marteau, P; Flourie, B; Arrigoni, E; Rambaud, JC. Improved clinical tolerance to chronic lactose ingestion in subjects with lactose intolerance: A placebo effect? *Gut.* 1997 41, 632-635.

[248] Szilagyi, A; Malolepszy, P; Yesovitch, S; Nathwani, U; Vinokuroff, C; Cohen, A; et al. Inverse dose effect of pretest dietary hydrogen results and symptoms in lactase nonpersistent subjects. *Dig Dis Sci.* 2005 50, 2178-2182.

[249] Briet, F; Achour, L; Flourie, B; et al. Symptomatic response to varying levels of fructo-oligosaccharides consumed occasionally or regularly. *Eur J Clin Nutr.* 1995 49, 501-507.

[250] Szilagyi, A; Malolepszy, P; Yesovitch, S; Vinokuroff, C; Nathwani, U; Cohen, A; et al. Fructose malabsorption may be gender dependent and fails to show compensation by colonic adaptation. *Dig Dis Sci.* 2007 52, 2999-3004.

[251] Jiang, T; Savaiano, DA. In vitro lactose fermentation by human colonic bacteria is modified by Lactobacillus acidophilus supplementation. *J Nutr.* 1997 1237, 1489-1495.

[252] Jiang, T; Savaiano, DA. Modification of colonic fermentation by bifidobacteria and pH in vitro. Impact on lactose metabolism, short-chain fatty acid, and lactate production. *Dig Dis Sci.* 1997 42, 2370-2377.

[253] Ito, M; Kimura, M. Influence of lactose on faecal microflora in lactose maldigesters. *Microb Ecol Health Dis.* 1993 6, 73-76.

[254] Bond, JH; Levitt, MD. Quantitative measurement of lactose absorption. *Gastroenterology.* 1976 70, 1058-1062.

[255] Buchowski, MS; Miller, DD. Lactose, calcium source and age affect calcium bioavailability in rats. *J Nutr.* 1991 121, 1746-1754.

[256] Schuette, SA; Knowles, JB; Ford, HE. Effect of lactose or its component sugars on jejunal calcium absorption in adult man. *Am J Clin Nutr.* 1989 50, 1084-187.

[257] Schuette, SA; Yasillo, NJ; Thompson, CM. The effect of carbohydrates in milk on the absorption of calcium by postmenopausal women. *J Am Coll Nutr.* 1991 10,132-139.

[258] Abrams, SA; Griffin, IJ; Davila, PM. Calcium and zinc absorption from lactose-containing and lactose-free infant formulas. *Am J Clin Nutr.* 2002 76, 442-446.

[259] Brink, EJ; van Beresteijn, EC; Dekker, PR; Beynen, AC. Urinary excretion of magnesium and calcium as an index of absorption is not affected by lactose intake in healthy adults. *Br J Nutr.* 1993 69, 863-870.

[260] Zitterman, A; Bock, P; Drummer; C; Scheld, K; Heer, M; Stehle, P. Lactose does not enhance calcium bioavailability in lactose-tolerant healthy adults. *Am J Clin Nutr.* 2000 71, 931-936.

[261] Wood, RJ; Hanssen, DA. Effect of milk and lactose in zinc absorption in lactose intolerant postmenopausal women. *J Nutr.* 1988 118, 982-986.

[262] Wilson, NW; Self, TW; Hamburger, RN. Severe cow's milk induced colitis in an exclusively breast-fed neonate. Case report and clinical review of cow's milk allergy. *Clin Pediatr.* 1990 29, 77-80.

[263] Kumar, D; Repucci, A; Wyatt-Ashmead, Chelmisky, G. Allergic colitis presenting in the first day of life: Report of three cases. *J Pediatr Gastroenterol Nutr.* 2000 31, 195-197.

[264] Glassman, MS; Newman, LJ; Berezin, S; Gryboski, JD. Cow's milk protein sensitivity during infancy in patients with inflammatory bowel disease. *Am J Gastroenterol.* 1990 85, 838-840.

[265] Biancone, L; Paganelli, R; Fais, S; Squarcia, O; D'Offizi, G; Pallone, F. Peripheral and intestinal lymphocyte activation after in vitro exposure to cow's milk antigens in normal subjects with Crohn's disease. *Clin Immunol Immunopathol.* 1987 45, 491-498.

[266] Paganelli, R; Pallone, F; Montano, S; Moli, S; Matricardi, PM; Fais, S; et al. Isotypic analysis of antibody response to a food antigen in inflammatory bowel disease. *Int Arch Allergy Appl Immunol.* 1985 78, 81-85.

[267] Skogh, T; Peen, E. Lactoferrin antibodies and inflammatory disease. *Adv Exp Med Biol.* 1993 336, 533-538.

[268] Peen, E; Almer, S; Bodemar, G; Ryden, BO; Sjolin, C; Tejle, K; et al. Anti-lactoferrin antibodies and other types of ANCA in ulcerative colitis, primary sclerosing Cholangitis, and Crohn's disease. *Gut.* 1993 34, 56-62.

[269] Paajanen, L; Korpela, R: Tuure, T; Honkanen, J; vela, I; Ilonen, J; et al. Cow milk is not responsible for most gastrointestinal immune-like syndromes-evidence from a population-based study. *Am J Clin Nutr,* 2005 82, 1327-1335.

[270] Collins, MT. Mycobacterium paratuberculosis: A potential Food-borne pathogen? *J Dairy Sci.* 1997 80, 3445-3448.

[271] Herman-Taylor, J; Bull, T. Crohn's disease caused by Mycobacterium avium subspecies paratuberculosis: apublic health tragedy whose resolution is long overdue. *J Med Microbiopl.* 2002 51, 3-6.

[272] Corti, S; Stephan, R. Detection of Mycobacterium avium subspecies paratuberculosis specific IS900 insertion sequences in bulk-tank milk samples obtained from different regions throughout Switzerland. *BMC Microbiol.* 2002 2, 15-22.

[273] Stabel, JR; Lambertz, A. Efficacy of pasteurization conditions for the inactivation of Mycobacterium avium subsp. Paratuberculosis in milk. *J Food Prot.* 2004 67, 2719-2726.

[274] Lamhonvah, A-M; Ackerley, C; Onizuka, R; Tilups, A; Lamhonvah, D; Chung, C; et al. Epitope shared by functional variant of organic cation/carnitine transporter, OCTN1, Campylobacter jejuni and Mycobacterium paratuberculosis may underlie susceptibility to Crohn's disease at 5q31. *Biochem Biophys Res Commun.* 2005 337, 1165-1175.

[275] Abubakar, I; Myhill, DJ, Hart, AR; Lake, IR, Harvey, I; Rhodes, JM; et al. A case-control study of drinking water and dairy products in Crohn's disease—further investigation of the possible role of Mycobacterium avium paratuberculosis. *Am J Epidemiol.* 2007 165, 776-783.

[276] Selby, W; Pavli, P; Crotty, B; Florin, T; Radford-Smith, G; Gibson, P; et al. Two-year combination antibiotic therapy with clarithromycin, rifabutin and clofazimine for Crohn's disease. *Gastroenterology.* 2007 132, 2313-2319.

[277] Penn, D; Dolderer, M; Schmidt-Sommerfeld, E. Carnitine concentrations in the milk of different species and infant formulas. *Biol Neonate.* 1987m 52, 70-79.

[278] Giallourakis, C; Stoll, M; Miller, K; Hampe, J; Lander, ES; Daly, MJ; et al. IBD5 is a general risk factor for inflammatory bowel disease: Replication of association with Crohn's disease and identification of a novel association with ulcerative colitis. *Am J Hum Genet.* 2003 73, 205-211.

[279] Latiano, A Palmieri, O; Valvano, RM; Dinca, R; Vecchi, M; Ferraris, A; et al. Contribution of IBD5 locus to clinical features of IBD patients. *Am J Gastroenterol.* 2006 101, 318-325.

[280] Bohmer, T; Rydning, A; Solberg, HE. Carnitine levels in human serum in health and disease. *Clin Chim Acta.* 1974 57, 55-61.

[281] Negoro, K; McGovern, DPB; Kinouchi, Y; Takahashi, S; Lench, NJ; Shimosegawa, T; et al. Analysis of the IBD5 locus and potential gene-gene interactions in Crohn's disease. *Gut.* 2003 52, 541-546.

[282] Hunter, JO. Nutritional factors in inflammatory bowel disease. *Eur J Gastroenterol Hepatol.* 1998 10, 235-237.

[283] Green, TJ: Issenman, RM; Jacobson, K. Patients' diets and preferences in a pediatric population with inflammatory bowel disease. *Can J Gastroenterol.* 1998 12. 544-549.

[284] Joachim, G. The relationship between habits of food consumption and reported reactions to food in people with inflammatory bowel disease. *Nutr Health.* 1999 13, 69-83.

[285] Jowett, SL; Seal, CJ; Phillips, E; Gregory, W; Barton, JR; Welfare, MR. Dietary beliefs of people with ulcerative colitis and their effect on relapse and nutrient intake. *Clin Nutr.* 2004 23, 161-170.

[286] Jowett, SL; Seal, CJ; Pearce, MS; Phillips, E; Gregory, W; Barton, JR; et al. Influence of dietary factors on the clinical course of ulcerative colitis: a prospective cohort study. *Gut.* 2004 53, 1479-1484.

[287] Pironi, L; Callegari, C; Cornia, GL; Lami, F; Miglioli, M; Barbara, L. Lactose malabsorption in adult patients with Crohn's disease. *Am J Gastroenterol.* 1988 93, 1267-1271.

[288] Mishkin, B; Yalovsky, M; Mishkin, S. Increased prevalence of lactose malabsorption in Crohn's disease patients at low risk for lactose malabsorption based on ethnic origin. *Am J Gastroenterol.* 1997 92, 1148-1153.

[289] von Tirpitz, C; Kohn, C; Steinkamp, M; Geerling, I; Maer, V; Moller, S; et al. Lactose intolerance in active Crohn's disease, clinical value of duodenal lactase analysis. *J Clin Gastroenterol.* 2002 34, 49-53.

[290] Bernstein, CN; Ament, M; Artinian, L; Ridgeway, J; Shanahan, F. Milk tolerance in adults with ulcerative colitis. *Am J Gastroenterol.* 1994 89, 872-877.

[291] Kochhar, R; Mehta, SK; Goenka, MK; Mukherjee, JJ; Rana, SV; Gupta, D. Lactose intolerance in idiopathic ulcerative colitis in north Indians. *Indian J Med Res.* 1993 98, 79-82.

[292] Samuelsson, M; Ekbom, A; Zack, M; Helmick, CG; Adami, HO. Risk factors for extensive ulcerative colitis and ulcerative proctitis: a population based case-control study. *Gut.* 1991 32, 1526-1530.

[293] Mishkin, S. Dairy sensitivity, lactose malabsorption, and elimination diets in inflammatory bowel disease. *Am J Clin Nutr.* 1997 65, 564-567.

[294] Jensen, OM; MacLennan, R; Wahrendorf, J. Diet, bowel function, fecal characteristics and large bowel cancer in Denmark and Finland. *Nutrition Cancer.* 1982 4, 5-19.

[295] International Agency for Research Group. Dietary fibre, transit-time, faecal bacteria, steroids, and colon cancer in two scandinavian populations. *Lancet.* 1977 2, 207-211.

[296] Lipkin, M; Newmark, H. Effect of added dietary calcium on colonic epithelial-cell proliferation in subjects at high risk for familial colonic cancer. *N Engl J Med.* 1985 313, 1381-1384.

[297] Nemark, HL; Wargovich, MJ; Bruce, WR. Colon cancer and dietary fat, phosphate, and calcium: a hypothesis. *J Natl Cancer Inst.* 1984 72, 1323-1325.

[298] Martinez, ME; Willet, WC. Calcium, vitamin D, and colorectal cancer: a review of the epidemiological evidence. *Cancer Epidemiol Biomarkers Prev.* 1998 7, 163-168.

[299] Pence, BC. Role of calcium in colon cancer prevention: Experimental and clinical studies. *Mut Res/Fund Mol Mech Muts.* 1993 290, 87-95.

[300] Grau, MV; Rees, JR; Baron, JA. Chemoprevention in gastrointestinal cancers: Current status. *Basic Clin Pharm Toxicol.* 2006 98, 281-287.

[301] Shaukat, A; Scouras, N; Schunemann, J. Role of supplemental calcium in the recurrence of colorectal adenomas: A meta analysis of randomized controlled trials. *Am J Gastroenterol.* 2005 100, 390-394.

[302] Holt, PR. Dairy foods and prevention of colon cancer: Human studies. *J Am Coll Nutr.* 1999 5, 379S-391S.

[303] Norat, R; Riboli, E. Dairy products and colorectal cancer. A review of possible mechanisms and epidemiological evidence. *Euro J Clin Nutr.* 2003 57, 1-17.

[304] Cho, E; Smith,-Warner, SA; Spiegelman, D; Beson, WL; van den Brandt, PA: Colditz GA: et al. Dairy foods, calcium and colorectal cancer: a pooled analysis of 10 cohort studies. *J Natl Cancer Inst.* 2004 96, 1015-1022.

[305] Burns, AJ; Rowland, IR. Anti-carcinogenicity of probiotics and prebiotics. *Curr Issues Intest Microbiol.* 2000 1, 13-24.

[306] Wollowski, I; Rechkemmer, G; Pool-Zobel, BL. Protective role of probiotics and prebiotics in colon cancer. *Am J Clin Nutr.* 2001 73(suppl 2), 451S-455S.

[307] Rafter, J; Lactic acid bacteria and cancer: mechanistic perspective. *Br J Nutr.* 2002 88(Suppl 1), S89-S94.

[308] Burns, AJ; Rowland, IR. Antigenotoxicity on faecal water-induced DNA damage in human colon adenocarcinoma cells. *Mutat Res,* 2004 551, 233-243.

[309] Szilagyi, A; Nathwani, U; Vinokuroff, C; Correa, JA; Shrier, I. Evaluation of relationships among national colorectal cancer mortality rates, genetic lactase non-persistence status, per capita yearly milk and milk product consumption. *Nutr Cancer.* 2006 55, 151-156.

[310] Zhuo, X-G: Watanabe, S. Factor analysis of digestive cancer mortality and food consumption in 65 Chinese counties. *J Epidemiol.* 1999 9, 275-284.

[311] Jarvinen, R; Knekt, P; Hakulinen, T; Aromaa, A. Prospective study on milk products, calcium and cancers of the colon and rectum. *Eur J Clin Nutr.* 2001 55, 1000-1007.

[312] Szilagyi, A; Nathwani, U; Vinokuroff, C; Correa JA; Shrier, I. The effect of lactose maldigestion on the relationship between dairy food intake and colorectal cancer: A systematic review. *Nutr Cancer.* 2006 55, 141-150.

[313] Bovee-Oudenhoven, IM; Wissink, ML; Wouters, JT; Van der Meer, R. Dietary calcium phosphate stimulates intestinal lactobacilli and decreases the severity of a salmonella infection in rats. *J Nutr.* 1999 129, 607-612.

[314] Bovee-Oudenhoven, IM; Termont, DS; Weerkamp, AH; Faassen-Peters, MA; Van der Meer, R. Dietary calcium inhibits the intestinal colonization and translocation of Salmonella in rats. *Gastroenterology.* 1997 113, 550-557.

[315] Bovee-Oudenhoven, IM; Lettink-Wissink, ML; Van Doesburg, W; Witteman, BJ; Van Der Meer, R. Diarrhea caused by enterotoxigenic Escherichia coli infection of humans is inhibited by dietary calcium. *Gastroenterology.* 2003 125, 469-476.

[316] Schmucker, DL; Heyworth, MF; Owen, RL; Daniels CK. Impact of aging on gastrointestinal mucosal immunity. *Dig Dis Sci.* 1996 41, 1183-1193.

[317] Hopkins, MJ; Sharp, R; Macfarlane, GT. Age and disease related changes in intestinal bacterial populations assessed by cell culture, 16S rRNA abundance, and community cellular fatty acid profiles. *Gut.* 2001 48, 198-205.

[318] Park, S-Y; Murphy. SP; Wilkens, LR; Nomura, AMY; Henderson, BE; Kolonel, LN. Calcium and vitamin D intake and risk of colorectal cancer: the multiethnic cohort study. *Am J Epidemiol.* 2007 165, 784-793.

[319] Benfield, GF; Montgomery, RD; Asquith, P. Ulcerative colitis in Asian immigrants. *Postgrad Med J.* 1987 63, 629-635.

[320] Carr, I; Mayberry, JF. The effects of migration on ulcerative colitis: a three-year prospective study among Europeans and first-and second- generation South Asians in Leiseter (1991-1994). *Am J Gastroenterol.* 1999 10, 2918-2922.

[321] Rasinspera, H; Forsblom, C; Enattah, NS; Halonen, P; Salo, K; et al. The C/C-13910 genotype of adult-type hypolactasia is associated with an increased risk of colorectal cancer in the Finnish population. *Gut,* 2005 54. 643-647.

[322] Buning, C; Ockenga, J; Kruger, S; Jurga, J; Baier, P; Dignass, A; et al. The C/C(-13910) and G/G(-22018) genotypes for adult-type hypolactasia are not associated with inflammatory bowel disease. *Scand J Gastroenterol.* 2003 38, 538-542.

In: Research Trends in Nutrition…
Editor: Johan P. Urster, pp. 53-128

ISBN: 978-1-60456-147-0
2008 Nova Science Publishers, Inc.

Chapter 2

Nutrition-Related Cardiovascular Risk Factors and Dietary Intervention in Middle-Aged and Older People: Is There a Gender Connection?

Hana Castel[1,*], Ilana Harman-Boehm[1,†] and Niva Shapira[2,§]

[1]Soroka University Medical Center and the Faculty of Health Sciences,
Ben Gurion University of the Negev, Beer Sheva, Israel
[2]Stanley Steyer School of Health Professions, Tel Aviv University, Ramat Aviv, Israel

Abstract

Cardiovascular disease, a leading cause of mortality in most industrialized countries, is associated with non-modifiable and modifiable risk factors. For some of the modifiable risk factors (hypertension, dyslipidemia, obesity and type 2 diabetes mellitus) nutritional therapy is recommended. The prevalence of these diet-modifiable risk factors, as well as of CVD, increases in middle-aged and older people. A body of evidence is accumulating that gender has an impact on the presentation, management and outcomes of CVD. It also has an impact on the modifiable risk factors and on the way they affect CVD risk and outcomes in this population. Gender differences exist also in relation to nutrition and may affect the nutrition-CVD risk factors interrelation in several ways: The sexes differ in the effect of nutrients and diet patterns on CVD risk, in the establishment of dietary habits, in the outcome of nutritional interventions and in compliance with dietary modification. Understanding of the impact of gender on the influence of nutrition on CVD and on the contributing risk factors may improve nutritional interventions in the primary and secondary prevention of CVD.

---

[*] E-mail address: castel@bgu.ac.il; Current address: Soroka University Medical Center, PO Box 105, Beer Sheva 84105, Israel (Corresponding author)
[†] E-mail address: ilanahb@bgu.ac.il; Current address: Soroka University Medical Center, PO Box 105, Beer Sheva 84105, Israel
[§] E-mail address: nivnet@inter.net.il; Current address: Stanley Steyer School of Health Professions, Tel Aviv University, Ramat Aviv 69978, Israel

This chapter will include a short overview of the CVD risk factors, modifiable by diet and their gender-related aspects. We will emphasize the rationale for the dietary recommendations for primary and secondary prevention of CVD.

Introduction

Coronary heart disease is a leading cause of morbidity and mortality. One in 3 American adults has one or more types of cardiovascular [CVD]; 48% of these are estimated to be age 65 or older. Coronary heart disease [CHD] is the single largest killer in the US where it caused 1 in every 2.8 deaths in 2004 [1]. Accumulating comprehension of CVD and related factors has led to a progressive decline in the death rate from CVD. Overall death rates, non-sudden CHD rates, and sudden cardiac death rates in the US have decreased during the years 1950-1999 by 59%, 64% and 49% respectively [2]. The death rate from CVD and stroke decreased during the years 1993-2003 by 22.2%. 29.3% and 19.5%, respectively [1]. This decline in CVD-related mortality reflects the progress in the management and prevention of CVD and CVD risk factors. Some of the CVD risk factors are modifiable by diet. CVD, CVD risks, nutritional state and intervention outcome – are all affected by gender. The overgrowing understanding of these aspects of CVD and CVD risk factors raises the question whether the CVD risk/nutrition relationship is gender-dependent, and should CVD risk-management be gender-oriented.

Coronary Heart Disease and the Impact of Gender

Information about CVD and the factors contributing to it has been derived from many studies, some of them large, population-based studies including the Framingham Heart Study (FHS) - a prospective investigation of cardiovascular disease [3], the Framingham Offspring Study (FOS) – which focused on cardiovascular disease and its risk factors [4], the National Health Examination Survey (NHES) and the National Health and Nutrition Examination Surveys (NHANES) I – III, a series of cross-sectional health examination surveys [5], The Atherosclerosis Risk in Communities (ARIC) study - a prospective study to investigate atherosclerosis [6, 7], the Cardiovascular Health Study (CHS), which focused on the older population [8], the Behavioral Risk Factor Surveillance System (BRFSS), designed to provide life style risk behavior information [9], and many others. The incidence of first major vascular events increases with age. About 83% of people who die of CHD, are at age 65 or older (NCHS) [1]. The aging of the population is associated with an increased incidence of chronic diseases, including CHD, heart failure and stroke [10]. Despite a decrease in age-adjusted cardiovascular death rates in several developed countries, rates of CVD have risen significantly in low income and middle income countries [11].

Compelling data from epidemiological studies and randomized clinical trials show that CHD is largely preventable. Assessment and management of risk factors should be cost-effective, stressing the importance of gender as an interrelating factor.

Gender-Related Aspects of CVD

Since the first description of sex bias in treating women with suspected or diagnosed coronary artery disease (CAD) in 1987 [12], the influence of gender on the prevalence, prognosis and manifestation of CVD has been described in multiple studies. Differences in the use of diagnostic and therapeutic measures have also been described. Although many of the risk factors for CVD and strategies for preventing disease are similar for men and women, the magnitude of their effects may differ depending on sex.

Gender differences in CVD morbidity and mortality: the incidence of CAD follows a different pattern in men and women: among subjects aged 35 to 84 years, men have about twice the total incidence of morbidity and mortality of women. The sex gap in morbidity tends to diminish during the later years, mainly because of a surge in growth of female morbidity after age 45 [13]. The sexes differ in the remaining lifetime risks for CHD among subjects free of disease, which favors women but changes with age [3]. The death rate from CVD has been declining progressively; the slower decline in women is explained in part by greater delay to diagnosis and less aggressive management. Serious cardiovascular events, such as myocardial infarction and sudden cardiac death, occur in women later than in men, but once women develop CVD, their prognosis is worse. Data from the FHS indicate that an approximate 10-year lag between the sexes persists in mortality rates throughout the life span, women dying later than men. The relative health advantage held by women, however, is countered by a case fatality rate from coronary attacks that exceeds the male rate (32% versus 27%) [13].

Women with acute myocardial infarction have a higher hospital mortality rate than men. This difference has been ascribed to their older age, more frequent comorbidities, and less frequent use of revascularization [1]. Most of cases of sudden cardiac deaths occur in men, and the annual incidence is 3 to 4 times higher in men than in women. This disparity decreases with advancing age [1].

Sex-based differences in early mortality after myocardial infarction, varying according to age, have been reported. The overall mortality rate during hospitalization was 16.7% among women and 11.5% among men; the younger the age of the patients, the higher the risk of death among women relative to men [14]. In another study, the higher rate of hospital mortality in women (14.8% versus 6.1%) following acute myocardial infarction was ascribed largely to the different age structure of these populations: The higher age-adjusted hospital mortality for women was associated with a lower rate of percutaneous coronary intervention [15].

Gender differences in CVD presentation: The Framingham study, starting with the early publications, emphasized the gender differences in the presentation of coronary heart disease: Myocardial infarction is more likely to be unrecognized in women than in men (34% versus 27%). Sudden death comprises a greater proportion of male deaths than female deaths (50% versus 39%); when sudden death occurs, it is not preceded by previous symptoms of CHD in 50% of men and in 64% of women [1].

According to NHANES data the age-adjusted prevalence of MI among Americans age 40-75, is higher among men than women, but prevalence of angina pectoris is higher in women than men [16]. Before age 75, a higher proportion of CVD events due to CHD occur in men than in women, and a higher proportion of events due to CHF occur in women than in men [1].

Gender differences in management of CVD: Women with acute an coronary event are less likely than men to be referred for invasive evaluation and procedures, and are more likely to have normal coronary arteries on coronary angiography. They have more bleeding complications following these procedures than men [17]. Female sex behaves as an independent adverse short-term prognostic factor on a combined outcome, including death, reinfarction, post-infarction angina, and stroke during hospitalization [18]. Sex differences in medical and invasive coronary procedures have been repeatedly investigated and discussed [17, 19, 20]. Despite improvements in angioplasty outcomes with time, women remain at significantly higher risk of in-hospital death than men after elective PCI. This increased mortality is observed in every age group, even after adjusting for other significant comorbidities [21]. On the other hand, other investigators have found that although revascularization was more often performed in men, there was no gender difference in the in-hospital or 30-days mortality, and at 1 year male gender was associated with higher mortality [22].

Gender-related differences in pathophysiologic findings: Recognition of gender as a contributing factor to the incidence and progression of CVD and CVD-related risk factors over the last 2 decades has led to a growing interest in the gender sensitive character of the disease. As a consequence of accelerated research in the area of cardiovascular disease, extensive sex-specific data has accumulated. Men and women differ in normal [23, 24] and abnormal [25, 26] cardiac physiology and electrophysiology [27, 28] and in processes related to aging [29, 30]. Gender-based pathophysiologic findings have been related to the demonstrated differences in the presentation and outcome of acute coronary events between the sexes secondary to gender-based difference in the vascular wall, metabolic alterations and atherosclerotic plaque deposition [31]. Microvascular dysfunction may account for the relatively low prevalence of obstructive findings on coronary angiography in women presenting with angina [32].

Gender differences in the occurrence, presentation and outcome of CVD underscore the importance of sensitivity to gender issues in the domain of CVD prevention. Major risk factors for coronary heart disease, such as hypercholesterolemia, hypertension, and smoking [33] are modifiable, in part via nutritional interventions, the effectiveness of which is also gender dependent.

Conventional Risk Factors for CVD/CHD

The Framingham study has established the risk factors for CHD: hypercholesterolemia, hypertension, diabetes mellitus, obesity greater than 30% over ideal body weight, family history and cigarette smoking [34]. According to a case-control study of 52 countries (INTERHEART), 9 easily measured and potentially modifiable risk factors account for over 90% of the risk of an initial acute MI. The effect of these risk factors is consistent in men and women, across different geographic regions, and by ethnic group, making the study applicable worldwide. These 9 risk factors include cigarette smoking, abnormal blood lipid levels, hypertension, diabetes, abdominal obesity, a lack of physical activity, low daily fruit and vegetable consumption, overconsumption of alcohol, and psychosocial index [35]. According to data from 3 prospective cohort studies, 87%-100% of patients with fatal CHD had at least one major antecedent CHD risk factor [33]. Taking into account CHD risk factors in combination provides a very potent predictor of 10-year risk of CHD compared with individual risk factors (NHANES III) [36]. The Framingham risk score has been used for CHD risk assessment. Recently, additional risk factors, not included in the Framingham algorithm, have received much attention and may help improve risk assessment. These include lifestyle risk factors (body mass index and waist circumference) and emerging risk factors: C-reactive protein (CRP), white blood cell count, fibrinogen, homocysteine, glycosylated hemoglobin, and albuminuria. The odds of being in the highest CHD risk group are greater at the upper levels of the examined risk factors. Means for most risk factors were slightly higher for women than men. All examined CHD risk factors were significantly associated with increasing 10-year CHD risk among men and women; therefore, all of them may be important in CHD risk assessment [37]. The prevalence of persons reporting 2 or more risk factors for heart disease and stroke increased among successive age groups (BRFSS) [38]. The aging of the population results in an increased incidence of chronic diseases, including coronary artery disease, heart failure and stroke [10].

The relative and absolute contribution of the major risk factors (blood pressure, levels of LDL-C and HDL-C, glucose intolerance, and smoking) by intensity, to the first coronary event, was estimated in the NHANES III data. More than 90% of events occur in persons having 1 or more elevated risk factors and 8% with a borderline level of multiple factors. Borderline risk factors contributed incrementally to CHD risk in the presence of other elevated risk factors, and this was more consistent in women than in men [39].

The lifetime risk for atherosclerotic cardiovascular disease and the effect of risk factor burden on lifetime risk has been evaluated using the FHS data [40]. The absence of established risk factors at 50 years of age was associated with very low lifetime risk for CVD and markedly longer survival. With more adverse levels of single risk factors, lifetime risks increased and median survivals decreased. Compared with participants with > or =2 major risk factors, those with optimal levels had substantially lower lifetime risks (5.2% versus 68.9% in men, 8.2% versus 50.2% in women) and markedly longer median survivals (>39 versus 28 years in men, >39 versus 31 years in women). The predictive power of risk factors may change during life: it has been reported that it decreases sharply with age for the three major risk factors hypertension, hypercholesterolemia, and cigarette smoking, however cholesterol continues to be a significant independent predictor of ischemic heart disease mortality at older ages for both men and women [41].

The Influence of Gender

The prevalence of individual risk factors differs between the sexes both in the strength of association between the risk factor and CVD, and in the existence of other, novel "non-classical" gender-related factors.

Gender difference in the prevalence of CVD risk factors: The differences in the levels of common CHD risk factors reported in several studies [36, 37] do not explain the gender gap, since adjustment for those differences does not alter the the sex -dependence in incidence rates of CVD [42]. Usually, men have less favorable heart disease risk profiles than women. According the NHANES III study, among participants age 60 and over, 40.3% of men and 8.2% of women were at "intermediate risk" (10% to 20%) of CHD. The proportion of participants with a 10-year risk of CHD of >20% increased with advancing age and was higher among men than women but varied little with race or ethnicity [36]. According to reports from the US, the trends in some of CVD risk changes are unfavorable for women: Smoking rates are declining less for women than for men. Along with increasing prevalence of obesity, more women report no regular sustained physical activity and ≈40% of women >55 years old have elevated serum cholesterol [43]. The prevalence of hypertension is higher in men than in women below the age of 35 years but by the age of 65 years the prevalence is higher in women [44].

Absolute 10-year CHD risk exceeded 10% in men older than 45 with 1 elevated risk factor and 4 more borderline risk factors and in those who had at least 2 elevated risk factors. In women, absolute CHD risk exceeded 10% only in those over age 55 who had at least 3 elevated risk factors [39]. In another large study most of the risk factors were more favorable in women, but the sex difference in risk factor levels diminished with increasing age. Differences in risk factors between sexes, particularly in HDL cholesterol and smoking, explained nearly half of the difference in CHD risk between men and women. Differences in serum total cholesterol level, blood pressure, body mass index, and diabetes prevalence explained about one-third of the age-related increase in CHD risk among men and 50% to 60% among women. The investigators concluded that differences in major cardiovascular risk factors explained a substantial part of the sex difference in CHD risk [45]. Less favorable levels of cigarette smoking, dietary fiber, vitamin C, blood viscosity, uric acid, HDL cholesterol, and triglycerides in men compared to women were reported in the Edinburgh Artery Study: Only three presumably cardioprotective factors were significantly more prevalent in men than women - men had more reported physical activity and alcohol intake and had lower levels of fibrinogen [46]. A marked gender difference in the prevalence and severity of cardiovascular disease has been described in the MONICA Project, even after adjustment for traditional risk factors, which were more prevalent in males [47].

Gender difference in strength of association between risk factor and CVD: Risk factors may have a differential impact on the development of CHD in men and women. The extent to which cardiovascular risk factors can explain the gender difference in CHD risk has been investigated in the CARDIO2000 Study [48]. The contribution of certain coronary risk factors to the risk for CHD has been reported to be different for men and women: The presence of hypertension and depression had a significantly greater effect in women than men. Higher education level and the adoption of a Mediterranean diet had a more protective effect in women than men. The impact of other factors (i.e., smoking, diabetes, body mass index, physical activity, alcohol consumption, and financial status), on the coronary risk difference between genders was similar for men and women. Sex differences in susceptibility to several etiologic factors for peripheral atherosclerosis, has been reported: Plasma fibrinogen, plasma viscosity, and blood viscosity had stronger correlations with lower ABPI (ankle-brachial pressure index) in men than in women [46]. According to another report, women and men tend to have a similar dose‘ response for each CHD risk factor and a similar relative risk, but women's absolute risk of CHD is much lower for any given level of risk factor. The sex difference in incidence rates persists when stratified by level of risk factor. The investigators conclude that some other factors protect women against CHD. They suggest that the potential for women to reduce their risk of CHD by changing lifestyle may be less than for men [49].

Interrelation between several risk factors favors one of the sexes: Diabetes, low HDL cholesterol, and high triglycerides contribute more to the risk in women than men. These interrelated factors are part of the insulin resistance- associated metabolic syndrome. The effect of the metabolic syndrome, according to some studies, is stronger than of its' constituents, implying an effect of the interrelation beyond that of the individual risk factors. The metabolic syndrome will be discussed separately.

Risk Management: Given the effect of risk factor burden on lifetime risk of CVD [37, 40], the importance of preventing or delaying their appearance and treating them to target once they have appeared, cannot be overstressed. One aim of primary prevention is to reduce long-term r (>10 years) as well as short-term risk (10 years). LDL goals in primary prevention depend on a person's absolute risk for CHD (ie, the probability of having a CHD event in the short term or the long term): the higher the risk, the lower the goal. Lifestyle changes are the foundation of clinical primary prevention. Nonetheless, persons who are at higher risk are candidates for more aggressive management, including medications. The intensity of risk-reduction therapy should be adjusted to a person's absolute risk. The first step in risk management is risk assessment. Risk determinants include the presence or absence of CHD, other clinical forms of atherosclerotic disease, and the major risk factors. Secondary prevention aims at reducing total mortality, coronary mortality, major coronary events, coronary artery procedures, and stroke in persons with established CHD. The same goal should apply for persons with CHD risk equivalents which carry a risk for major coronary events equal to that of established CHD, ie, >20% per 10 years. These include other clinical forms of atherosclerotic disease (peripheral arterial disease, abdominal aortic aneurysm, and symptomatic carotid artery disease), diabetes, and the concomitance of multiple risk factors that confer a 10-year risk for CHD >20%.

Gender-related aspects of risk factor management: Recommendations for the primary and secondary prevention of CHD [50] relate to both genders. However, there are aspects of risk factor management that are unique to women. An emphasis on prevention of CHD in postmenopausal women is particularly important because the incidence of CHD rises with age. The use of estrogen replacement therapy, which has been extensively debated by the medical community, is beyond the scope of this chapter; nonetheless it is clear that special attention to the prevention and management of risk factors, using non-hormonal means, in this population is needed.

Other aspects of risk factor management are important in women: Diabetes is a more powerful risk factor in women than in men, therefore recommendations for management of diabetes should emphasize concomitant CVD risk factors control [50]. Low levels of HDL cholesterol are predictive of CHD in women and appear to be a stronger risk factor for women >65 years old than for men >65 [51], therefore more aggressive targets for HDL cholesterol and triglycerides should be considered in women.

Recommendations for aggressive risk factor management are based on the future probability of a cardiovascular event. This strategy allows high-risk patients who have not yet had an event to be considered for more intensive treatment [52]. Usually, aggressive risk factor management is applied in the setting of secondary prevention. Due to the increasing use of noninvasive tools to detect asymptomatic CHD, the line between primary and secondary prevention becomes less distinct. On the other side, first cardiovascular events are often fatal in women; therefore careful consideration should be given to individual risk factor management before the onset of clinical CHD in women. The importance of primary CHD prevention should be stressed in the general population, especially in women. The individual risk factors are discussed in more detail below.

Overweight and Obesity

Obesity, described by AHA as a major modifiable coronary risk factor, and overweight, were defined by the NHLBI and the National Institute of Diabetes and Digestive and Kidney Diseases (NIDDK) in 1998, as body mass index of $\geq$30 kg/m^2 and of 25 to 29.9 kg/m^2, respectively [53].

BMI: Body Mass Index (BMI), defined as a weight in kilograms divided by the square of the person's height in meters, correlates with body weight and fatness. It is a strong predictor of chronic disease, including CVD, hypertension and diabetes [54]. The association between overweight and coronary risk has been demonstrated by several longitudinal studies including the NHS [55] and the FHS [56]. A continuous increase in the prevalence of overweight and obesity has been observed [57]. BMI predicts body fat and health outcomes, but it's ability to measure adiposity is limited. It does not distinguish between fat mass and lean body mass, therefore in very muscular people it does not measure fatness. Although BMI provides a measure of overall adiposity, it does not indicate the location of the deposited fat which impacts on the related risk.

Fat distribution: Abdominal fat is more closely associated with more adverse metabolic and cardiovascular risk factors, as compared with gynecoid obesity, with fat accumulating in the thighs and hips [58]. Abdominal fat tissue in the waist, upper body and abdomen is metabolically more active than the adipose tissue in hip, thigh, or buttocks [59] It has been suggested that abdominal fat cells, by their heightened sensitivity to lipolytic agents, induce direct delivery of free fatty acids and glycerol to the liver, leading to insulin resistance [60]. The location of the fat has metabolic significance, therefore additional measures of fat distribution have been defined. Abdominal fat deposition is a central component in obesity [61]. Some studies have shown that it may be a better predictor than overall obesity for disease risks and all-cause mortality [62, 63].

Waist circumference and waist-hip ratio: Waist circumference and waist-hip ratio, which are widely used to evaluate abdominal and central obesity in epidemiological studies, can predict CVD and diabetes [64, 65].The waist-hip ratio also reflects the gluteo-femoral muscle mass, therefore it seems that waist circumference (WC) is simpler to interpret and is the most practical measure of fat distribution [66]. WC is a key component of the metabolic syndrome [67], and is associated with future risk of type 2 diabetes, cardiovascular disease, and all-cause mortality [68]. Abdominal adiposity increases mortality in obese people [69] and is an independent predictor of mortality risk for non-obese women [70].

The cutoff points for WC help to identify subjects who are at increased health risk within the various body mass index categories [71]. Abdominal obesity, defined as a waist circumference $\geq$102 cm ($\geq$40 inches) in men and $\geq$88 cm ($\geq$35 inches) in women, is particularly associated with several of the components of the metabolic syndrome. For this reason, ATP III recommended that abdominal obesity be considered one of the risk factors for the metabolic syndrome. Individuals can have the metabolic syndrome with a lesser degree of or no abdominal obesity if 3 of the remaining components are found. Only the International Diabetes Federation (IDF) definition has waist circumference as a mandatory component [72].

The Influence of Age

In developed countries, BMI gradually rises during most of adult life, peaks during late middle age, and then declines. Although the prevalence of obesity decreases somewhat after age 70, it is still greater than in young adults. In contrast, body fat increases through most of adulthood. The age-related increase in obesity is associated with an increase in age-related adiposity: Loss of muscle mass begins from 30 to 40 years of age and continues into advanced old age. Because fat replaces fat free mass with increasing age, older subjects tend to have a greater proportion of fat than younger individuals with the same BMI especially in men. They also have an increase in the proportion of visceral and abdominal fat, even when the total amount of fat is the same. An increase in intra-abdominal fat is associated with greater mortality, independent of overall adiposity [73].

Aging is associated with loss of lean body mass, therefore the validity of BMI as a measure of adiposity in the elderly is not clear. This may explain the weaker association between BMI and mortality found in older compared to young, adults. Although the BMI provides a measure of overall adiposity, the location of fat affects the related disease risk.

When the effect of age on the distribution of body fat was examined, a trend to increased central adiposity and fat distribution with increasing age, independent of BMI, was described [74]. In general, there is a progressive trend toward increasing upper and central body fat deposition [75] and an increase in waist circumference with age [62, 76, 77]. When age-associated changes in an older Chinese population were examined, the trend toward increasing abdominal adiposity persisted to very old age, despite a decrease in body weight and BMI after middle age [78]. Visceral fat shows an increase with advancing age, whereas a decrease in insulin sensitivity was has been noted only in older women. Unfavorable changes in plasma lipids were strongly associated with the age-related increase in visceral abdominal adipose tissue [79]. A prospective study of older persons showed association between waist-hip ratio and circulatory mortality for men and women, while BMI was not associated in men, and was negatively associated in women, with circulatory mortality [80]. All these data imply that waist-hip ratio is better indicator, especially in older persons, of overall and circulatory mortality.

Gender-Related Aspects of Obesity

Men and women differ in the regional fatty acids storage, mobilization and oxidation [81]. Women generally have a higher percentage of body fat than men, and there are indications that basal fat oxidation is lower in females as compared to men, thereby contributing to a higher fat storage in women [82].

Weight gain pattern – gender differences: Weight gain occurs differently in men and women. The greatest weight gain in men occurs in those with the highest BMI and in the older age groups. Compared with women, men become obese later in life. In women, the greatest weight gain is at a younger age. Recent epidemiological studies have shown that in women, weight loss is also accompanied by bone loss. Another difference in weight gain between men and women is that as women's educational level rises, obesity decreases, for both white and black women, whereas in men, educational level appears not to be related to obesity [83].

Lipid accumulation pattern – gender differences: The pattern of fat deposition differs between the sexes. Women are prone to develop peripheral adiposity, with accumulation of fat in the thighs and gluteal region, whereas men have a tendency towards central (android) adiposity [84]. When abdominal adiposity occurs in women, it has stronger association with CHD than in men [84, 85]. Upper and central body fat deposition increases with age; in women this trend accelerates postmenopausally. After menopause, fat distribution in women shift towards the male pattern. In both sexes, a tendency towards central obesity is observed in advanced age and after gonadectomy, related to a differential distribution of sex hormone receptors in visceral and subcutaneous fat [86].

Significant changes in body composition and fat distribution, dependent on gender and independent of physical activity, hormones or serum albumin, were found in a 2 years long, prospective study conducted in independently living, weight-stable elderly men and women Significant increases occurred in BMI and hip circumference, whereas height decreased significantly in both men and women. Significant increases in total body fat and percent body fat were observed in women but not in men. Lean body mass did not change significantly throughout the study in either sex [87]. In another prospective, 10 year study of older people, WC increased significantly in the women but not in the men, whereas hip circumference decreased significantly in the men. There was no significant change in calf circumference in the men, but there was an increase at that site in the women. Waist-to-thigh and waist-to-arm ratios increased in both sexes over time; however, the waist-to-hip ratio increased significantly only in the women [88].

It has been shown that gender affects the relationships between BMI, WHR and incidence of cardiovascular disease. The impact of waist-hip ratio on incidence of CVD is modified by the overall body weight and by gender. Waist-hip ratio adds prognostic information on the cardiovascular risk in women at all levels of BMI, and in men with normal weight [89]. Increased thigh and hip circumference in women reduces the CVD risk [90].

Sex differences in the relation between energy expenditure and body composition: Aging affects body composition and fuel metabolism differently in men and women, leading to reduced fat oxidation and accumulation of upper-body fat with loss of striated muscle in men, and to an increased ratio of upper- to lower-body fat and bone loss in women, the latter depending on fat mass [91]. The sexes differ also in the relation between energy expenditure and body composition, and in the impact of food intake on this relation. It has been observed that the percentage body fat (%BF) of active men tends to be lower than that of less active men, but this relation was not reported on women [92]. Physical activity energy expenditure is more strongly associated with %BF in men than in women. Macronutrient composition seems to have stronger influence on %BF in women than in men [93].

Sex differences in appetite control: Women show lower serotonin response to weight increase, than men do. Serotonin contributes to food intake regulation: its' synthesis decreases as the BMI increases. The reduction in serotonin synthesis occurs in women at a higher BMI than in men [94], implying a need for a different dietary approach to serotonin management, i.e. combination of high tryptophan protein and low glycemic-index carbohydrate in women. Another contributor to appetite control, leptin, a molecule produced by fat cells which is an important signal in the regulation of appetite and energy expenditure, and is thought to play a key role in the control of body weight, is most tightly correlated to subcutaneous fat. Women have higher circulating leptin levels than men: This gender difference can be explained by higher proportion of adipose tissue and by increased production rate of leptin in women [95].

Because of the nature of female adiposity (subcutaneous), leptin level correlates better to metabolic regulation in women than in men, whereas in men, insulin may be more dominant in driving adiposity signaling. The level of leptin in the blood is correlated with BMI, and is far higher in women than men at every BMI level [95, 96]. Testosterone appears to play a role in the regulation of leptin levels in the blood [97], while in women ovarian hormones may modulate the sensitivity of the brain to leptin and insulin [98]. Animal studies indicate that estrogen acts within the brain to increase leptin sensitivity, decrease insulin sensitivity, and favor subcutaneous over visceral fat [99].

Insulin Resistance, the Metabolic Syndrome and Type 2 Diabetes

Insulin Resistance

Insulin resistance is a generalized metabolic disorder in which the normal actions of insulin, i.e. increasing uptake, oxidation and storage of glucose in tissues, are impaired. Excess body fat (particularly abdominal obesity) and physical inactivity promote the development of insulin resistance, but some individuals also are genetically predisposed. Insulin resistance is the most accepted hypothesis for explaining the development of the metabolic syndrome and type 2 diabetes, two closely related conditions, sharing insulin resistance as a common denominator. Insulin resistance can be detected long before glucose tolerance decreases. In the presence of environmental stress, such as excess body weight, this genetic trait may present as the metabolic syndrome. An important contributor to the development of insulin resistance is an abundance of circulating fatty acids, derived from triglycerides, originating from the adipose tissue and from lipoproteins in the tissues. In insulin-sensitive tissues, excessive fatty acids modify downstream signaling, causing insulin resistance. Consequently lipolysis is increased in adipose tissue, leading to further inhibition of insulin activity, additional lipolysis and adverse effect on insulin-mediated glucose metabolism [100]. Insulin resistance increases the risk of developing diabetes or CVD [101, 102]. When insulin resistance worsens, the compensatory increase in insulin secretion fails and frank diabetes appears. Women with insulin resistance are prone to develop gestational diabetes during pregnancy; men and women with insulin resistance can progress to type 2 diabetes, especially in the presence of increased body weight, decreased physical activity, and older age [103]. Obesity [104] and insulin resistance [103] predict the development of diabetes in many populations. The prevalence of insulin resistance increases with age [105].

Metabolic Syndrome

The metabolic syndrome (MetS) is a common disorder that is related to the increasing prevalence of obesity, and is defined as a cluster of risk factors that identifies individuals at risk for cardiovascular disease and type 2 diabetes. The syndrome is defined by a constellation of cardiac risk factors that include obesity, atherogenic dyslipidemia, hypertension, and insulin resistance. Insulin resistance and central obesity are the main risk conditions underlying the metabolic syndrome. Criteria for defining the syndrome have been defined differently by various professional organizations, however the components are similar and include glucose intolerance, (type 2 diabetes, impaired glucose tolerance, or impaired fasting glycaemia), obesity, particularly central obesity, above normal blood pressure, and atherogenic dyslipidemia with low HDL cholesterol and elevated triglycerides. The metabolic conditions which are included are associated with high blood insulin levels. It is believed that the fundamental defect in the metabolic syndrome is insulin resistance, caused by excessive FFA and fat-derived inflammatory cytokines [100]. Interleukin-6 and TNF-α secreted from fat enhance insulin resistance and lipolysis, increase hepatic glucose and VLDL production, muscle insulin resistance, and induce a prothrombotic state by increasing the production of fibrinogen and plasminogen activator-inhibitor-1 by the liver. An additional contributory effect to the metabolic syndrome has been ascribed to the reduced production of adiponectin, an anti-inflammatory and insulin-sensitizing cytokine [100].

Several definitions for the metabolic syndrome have been proposed by international or national organizations: World Health Organization (WHO) [106], the Third Adult Treatment Panel (ATP III) of the National Cholesterol Education Program (NCEP) [107, 108], European Group for the study of Insulin Resistance (EGIR) [109], International Diabetes Federation (IDF) [72], and the American Association of Clinical Endocrinology [110]. There is general consensus regarding the main components of the syndrome but different definitions require different cut points and have different mandatory inclusion criteria [111]. Although insulin resistance is considered the major pathophysiological mechanism, only the WHO and EGIR definitions include it amongst the diagnostic criteria and only the IDF definition has waist circumference as a mandatory component [112].

MetS Prevalence: The metabolic syndrome is highly prevalent: The unadjusted and age-adjusted reported prevalence of the metabolic syndrome is 21.8% and 23.7%, respectively in one report [113]. Prevalence within individual cohorts varies with the definition used [114] and ethnicity [112, 115]. Since the metabolic syndrome is a clustering of CVD risk factors secondary to insulin resistance, the patients are, by definition, at risk of developing both diabetes and CVD. According to data from the FHS, the MetS accounts for up to one third of CVD in men and approximately half of new type 2 diabetes [116]. It is common in elderly patients with strong relation to CHD and coronary events [117].

Prognostic impact of MetS: Several studies examined the prognostic impact of metabolic syndrome on CVD and diabetes by different definitions on CVD [167-171] and on diabetes [118-121]. The metabolic syndrome predicts diabetes independently of other factors [118], beyond glucose intolerance alone [119]. It increases the risk for diabetes regardless of insulin resistance, but the simultaneous presence of metabolic syndrome and insulin resistance identifies people who are at greater risk [120]. In women and men, respectively, the MetS was seen in 10 and 15% of subjects with normal glucose tolerance, 42 and 64% of those with impaired fasting glucose/impaired glucose tolerance, and 78 and 84% of those with type 2 diabetes. MetS defined by the inclusion of glucose intolerance or diabetes as one of the criteria, intensifies cardiovascular morbidity. The risk for coronary heart disease and stroke is increased threefold in subjects with the syndrome [121]. CVD and total mortality are significantly higher in adults with than in those without MetS and are better predicted by the metabolic syndrome than by its individual components [122, 123]. Even 1 to 2 MetS risk factors confer increased risk for mortality from CVD [122]. The metabolic syndrome is associated with increased risk of major coronary events in both, hypercholesterolemic patients with coronary heart disease and in those with low high-density lipoprotein cholesterol [124].

Evaluation of the relative contributions of the MetS and dysglycemia to the risk of CVD showed that the increased CVD risk in individuals with impaired fasting glucose or diabetes was largely driven by the coexistence of multiple metabolic disorders, rather than hyperglycemia per se [125].

The metabolic syndrome is also related to increased severity of atherosclerotic vascular lesions. When the extension and severity of coronary artery lesions during a first coronary angiography were observed and scored, and the relative contribution of different cardiovascular risk factors in coronary artery disease patients with and without metabolic syndrome was examined, metabolic syndrome was related to more extensive and more severe vascular lesions [126].

Etiology of the metabolic syndrome: Three potential etiologic categories for the metabolic syndrome have been postulated [107]: (1) obesity and disorders of adipose tissue, (2) insulin resistance, and (3) a constellation of independent factors (eg, molecules of hepatic, vascular, and immunologic origin) that mediate specific components of the syndrome. Both genetic and acquired causes are implicated in each and more than one mechanism may be operative. The adipose tissue contributes to the complexity of the interactions among obesity, body fat distribution, and cardiovascular risk factors. Adipose tissue is recognized as a source of several molecules that are potentially pathogenic: nonesterified fatty acids (NEFA), cytokines, plasminogen-activator inhibitor (PAI)-1, and adiponectin. A high plasma NEFA leads to overloading muscle and liver with lipid, thus enhancing insulin resistance. Cytokine excess, a biomarker of which is a raised C-reactive protein (CRP) level, correlates with a proinflammatory state, while elevated PAI-1 contributes to a prothrombotic state. The second pathogenic category, insulin resistance, is believed to be the essential mechanism underlying the metabolic syndrome. Finally, some data support the concept that insulin resistance or its associated hyperinsulinemia are independent risk factors for CVD, but this association has not yet been confirmed in controlled studies. Much of the heterogeneity in the manifestation of the metabolic syndrome may therefore be due to the fact that many of the component factors are regulated independently of insulin resistance. Lipoprotein metabolism is regulated by genetic factors as well as by diet composition, and both can worsen atherogenic dyslipidemia. Blood pressure regulation is affected by dietary factors, physical activity, and renal/adrenal function. Additionally not all people with obesity and/or insulin resistance develop type 2 diabetes; for diabetes to appear, an independent defects in beta-cell function must be present [107]. Cross-sectional relations between CRP, a marker of inflammation, and individual components of the MetS in patients with CHD [117], imply that inflammation is associated with the MetS, and that it plays a pathogenic role in diabetes [127].

The Influence of Age

The prevalence of the metabolic syndrome is highly age-dependent, independent of definition being used [112, 113]. The prevalence of this cluster of diet-modifiable risk factors, as well of CVD, increases in middle-aged and older people. According to data from NHANES III, the prevalence increased from 6.7% among participants aged 20 to 29 years to 43.5% and 42.0% for participants aged 60 to 69 and 70 years, respectively [112].

Investigations in middle-aged populations linked the presence of metabolic syndrome with the development of CVD [128-130]. A prospective assessment of the association between the metabolic syndrome and CVD in older people showed that women and men with metabolic syndrome, free of diabetes mellitus and CVD at baseline, followed for 11 years, were 20% to 30% more likely to experience any CVD event than subjects without metabolic syndrome [131].

Several age-related modifiers may influence the clinical expression of the metabolic syndrome in advancing age. Physical inactivity, associated with aging, promotes the development of obesity and modifies muscle insulin sensitivity. Aging is commonly accompanied by a loss of muscle mass and by an increase in body fat, particularlyintra-abdominal fat. Both these changes increase insulin resistance. Moreover, recent studies suggest that aging is accompanied by specific defects in fatty acid oxidation in muscle, which also enhancing insulin resistance [107].

Gender-Related Aspects of the Metabolic Syndrome

The available data suggest that the pathophysiology of the metabolic syndrome and its contribution to the relative risk of cardiovascular events and heart failure differ with gender. This gender difference is of potential relevance for prevention, diagnosis, and therapy of the syndrome. Insulin resistance and central obesity are the main risk conditions underlying the metabolic syndrome. In the last decade there has been a 74% increase in obesity in the US, mostly in women. As obesity rates increase worldwide, especially in women, there is a concomitant rise in the accompanying insulin resistance, dyslipidemia, diabetes and hypertension; that in turn contribute to increasing rates of cardiovascular morbidity and mortality. In the US there are 2 million more women then men categorized as obese, and the trend for developing obesity and diabetes is on the upsurge. This epidemic underscores the importance of defining the gender-specific characteristics in order to better prevent and manage the MetS [132].

Gender-related prevalence of MetS: The age-adjusted prevalence of Mets in US population according to ATP III was similar for men (24.0%) and women (23.4%). However, US African American and Mexican American women had significantly higher prevalence of metabolic syndrome than men [113]. The female preponderance exists also among Turkish adults [133].

Sex differences in the relative contribution of metabolic disorders to the MetS: Clustering of metabolic disorders occurs frequently in men and women. However, the contribution of several metabolic disorders to the metabolic syndrome in both genders is not the same. Sexes differ in the relative contribution of the components of the metabolic syndrome in diverse populations: In a non-diabetic cohort in Mauritius, women had higher body mass indices and more impaired glucose tolerance [134]. In the French MONICA study, the most significant contributors to the metabolic syndrome were elevated body weight, waist girth and low HDL cholesterol in women and systolic and diastolic blood pressure and apolipoprotein B in men [135]. Abundance of abdominal fat tissue, which is the source of free fatty acids and cytokines, is related to the early development of insulin resistance and atherogenic lipid profile in men. It seems that women, who have a more favorable distribution of fat, need a higher degree of adiposity to achieve the same measure of metabolic disturbance [136]. In the German KORA, men had more frequent undiagnosed diabetes, impaired glucose tolerance and elevated fasting glucose. Risk factors for undiagnosed diabetes differed in men and women: Predominant risk factors were hypertriglyceridemia, hypertension and family history of diabetes in men, and waist circumference, hypertension and family history in women [137]. Studies in a US population reported an association between the metabolic syndrome and physical inactivity in overweight men and in normal and overweight women, suggesting a protective effect of physical exercise in women [138]. The association of socioeconomic status with the metabolic syndrome differs by gender. Low income was related to the metabolic syndrome in women but not in men. Education was associated with all components of the metabolic syndrome in women, but only three components (abdominal obesity, hypertension and hyperglycemia) in men [139].

Sex differences in the pattern of fat accumulation and related CVD risk: Patterns of fat deposition differ between women and men [140]. Premenopausal women more frequently develop peripheral obesity with subcutaneous fat accumulation, whereas men and postmenopausal women are more prone to central or android obesity. Android obesity in particular, is associated with increased cardiovascular mortality and the development of type 2 diabetes. Visceral adipocytes differ from peripheral adipocytes in their lipolytic activity and their response to insulin, adrenergic and angiotensin stimulation and sex hormones. Free fatty acids and cytokines, originating in the visceral fat, reach via the portal vein to the liver, induce insulin resistance and lead to an atherogenic lipid profile. Inflammation increases cardiovascular risk particularly in women [140].

Gender-related impact of MetS on CHD/CVD risk: Women with MetS are in greater risk of developing CHD than men with MetS. The relative risk for CHD in middle-aged participants of the ARIC study was 2.46 for women and 1.86 for men. The prevalence of MetS - associated CHD in 4 different age-gender subpopulations of the NHANES III was examined. Metabolic syndrome-associated CHD prevalence in women aged 35-54 years was almost the same as in the control, whereas in women aged 55-74 and in men aged 35-54 or 55-74, this prevalence was nearly 2-fold greater than that of the control. These findings suggest a role for endogenous estrogen in suppressing the pro-atherosclerotic effects of MetS-related risk factors. The transition from pre- to postmenopausal women is associated with emergence of a profile of cardiovascular risk factors similar to that of the men [141]. Endogenous estrogen may play a role in suppressing the pro-atherosclerotic effects of metabolic syndrome - related risk factors. The transition from pre-to postmenopausal women is associated with emergence of a profile of cardiovascular risk factors like that of the men [141].

Despite the observation in some studies that women with the metabolic syndrome are at greater risk of developing CHD then men with the syndrome, the metabolic syndrome, using four different definitions of the syndrome, predicted CVD mortality in men, but the prediction was weak in women [142-144].

Sex differences in the impact of MetS constituents on CVD risk: Some of the MetS constituents -low HDL cholesterol, high triglycerides, and especially diabetes - exert a stronger effect on females than males. In women, HDL cholesterol is more closely related to cardiovascular disease than is LDL cholesterol [145]. Low HDL and high triglyceride levels also have a stronger effect on CHD risk in women than men [146]. The relative risk of CHD related to diabetes is approximately twice as high in women as in men [147]. In addition, the sex-specific effect of type 2 diabetes mellitus on the risk of fatal ischemic heart disease has been recurrently reported [148, 149].

The prevalence of small, dense LDL, which is generally increased in the metabolic syndrome, differs by both age and sex. It is more common in men than in women and increases with age [150]. Women appear to have a larger and less atherogenic LDL particle size than men [151]. Small, dense LDL particles stay longer in plasma, are more susceptible to oxidation because of decreased interaction with the LDL receptor, and enter the arterial wall more easily, where they are retained more readily. Small, dense LDL promotes endothelial dysfunction and enhanced production of procoagulants by the endothelial cells, therefore it is more atherogenic than normal LDL [152].

An independent association between hyperinsulinemia and ischemic heart disease has also been suggested to contribute to CHD pathogenesis with a possible effect on the observed gender gap in CHD incidence. Insulin-CHD association has been inconsistently reported in men [153, 154] but not in women [154, 155]. This association disappears with the advent of diabetes.

A gender difference in the pathogenesis of CVD has been hypothesized by investigators in Turkey. According to this group, men have greater susceptibility to visceral adiposity regardless of obesity and therefore tend to develop metabolic syndrome and CVD, independent of the diabetes component, whereas women, who are more prone to obesity, sustain CVD by the intermediary of diabetes mellitus [156].

Sex differences in vascular measures of atherosclerosis: The relation between early carotid atherosclerosis, indicated by the carotid intima-media thickness, as assessed on B-mode ultrasonography, and the metabolic syndrome has been recurrently investigated. The effect of MetS on early atherosclerosis is more pronounced in women than in men [157, 158]. Different components of MetS seem to contribute differentially to early atherosclerosis. Hypertension and dyslipidemia in men [157-159], and hypertension [157] and blood glucose [158] in women have the strongest effect on the carotid intima-media thickness. In a prospective study, HDL-C was protective against progression of carotid atherosclerosis, but the known anti-atherogenic effect of HDL in women diminished around the menopause [129].

Gender-related CVD mortality in MetS: Women with MetS are in greater risk of developing CHD than Men with MetS. The relative risk for CHD in middle-aged participants of the ARIC study was 2.46 for women and 1.86 for men [142]. Sex difference in the prediction of CVD mortality by the metabolic syndrome, using 4 definitions of MetS, was demonstrated data derived from an epidemiological study on diabetes, based on nine cohort studies in Europe [143]. Metabolic syndrome predicted CVD mortality in men by the four different definitions being used, but the prediction was weak in women [144].

Unique female gender-related features: There are several unique features of the metabolic syndrome in women. Polycystic ovarian syndrome (PCOS), a hormonal condition that often affects fertility, is associated with 11-fold increased occurrence of metabolic syndrome as compared to women without PCOS [160]. Studies in women with PCOS also show that the more overweight women are, the greater their risk of metabolic syndrome 161]. An insulin-resistant state associated with both polycystic ovarian syndrome and increased abdominal fat may contribute to the development of the metabolic syndrome and increase cardiovascular risk when present. Decline in circulating estrogen levels, secondary to menopause, may increase cardiovascular risk through effects on adiposity, lipid metabolism, and prothrombotic state [162].

Type 2 Diabetes:

Type 2 diabetes presents with insulin resistance and relative insulin deficiency, and progresses later to insulin resistance and frank failure of insulin secretion. Type 2 diabetes is characterized in most patients by insulin resistance with inadequate insulin response to maintain normal levels of blood glucose [163]. Because in early disease there is no absolute absence of insulin, type 2 diabetes may be undiagnosed for many years. High insulin levels, indicating insulin resistance, are typical of the early stage. As the disease progresses, insulin production declines and at the time of DM diagnosis, about 50% of insulin secreting capacity is lost.

The prevalence of diabetes changes, according to the criteria used and to examined population. Diabetes prevalence increases with age: diagnosed and undiagnosed diabetes affects almost one in every five people 65 years of age and older. An additional 23% of the elderly meet diagnostic criteria for impaired glucose tolerance [164].

Obesity and type 2 diabetes: Total body adiposity is an established risk factor for type 2 diabetes [165]. The obesity-related risk for type 2 diabetes is higher in younger individuals [166], increases with the severity of obesity [166] and with a sedentary lifestyle [167], and may be affected by lifestyle intervention, which includes physical activity [168]. The strongest predictors for the development of type 2 diabetes are elevated fasting insulin concentrations and low insulin secretion [169]. Lifestyle and dietary factors, especially, those which induce obesity, may contribute to the development of diabetes. Most of the people with type 2 diabetes are obese, and weight loss is essential in management. When different metabolic (BMI, triglycerides, HDL-cholesterol, glucose and blood pressure) and lifestyle factors (physical activity, smoking, saturated fat biomarker and socioeconomic status) predictors of insulin sensitivity were compared, all factors except triglycerides and smoking were significant predictors. BMI remained the strongest predictor, followed by physical activity, HDL-C, saturated fat and socioeconomic situation. BMI is the strongest predictor also in normal-weight subjects [170].

Insulin resistance, type 2 diabetes, and lipid metabolism: The most common pattern of dyslipidemia in insulin resistance includes increased TG levels and decreased HDL-C levels. Patients with insulin resistance and type 2 diabetes have smaller, denser LDL particles, which explain the increased atherogenicity in spite of lack of increase in LDL-C concentration. Since diabetes is considered a risk factor for CVD, the LDL-C concentration target is < 100 mg/dl [171].

Insulin resistance, Metabolic Syndrome and CVD risk: Insulin resistance and impaired glucose tolerance are associated with increased CVD risk [172]. Several pathophysiologic mechanisms increase CVD risk in individuals with insulin resistance: formation of advanced glycation end products, hypertension, pro-inflammatory and pro-thrombotic states, and dyslipidemia [173]. The increased flux of free fatty acids from adipose tissue to the liver promotes dyslipidemia.

Both insulin resistance and metabolic syndrome (MetS) are independent predictors of incident CVD. The MetS based on NCEP criteria was associated with a 50% increased risk of CVD. Insulin resistance was identified as an independent risk factor of CVD adjusted for the MetS, indicating that insulin resistance may indeed be a factor in the pathogenesis of CVD [174]. The metabolic abnormalities caused by diabetes induce vascular dysfunction, which predisposes these patients to atherosclerosis. Complications of atherosclerosis cause most of the morbidity and mortality in patients with diabetes mellitus [175].

DM and the prevalence, morbidity and mortality of CVD: Starting with the Framingham Study [176], epidemiological studies have shown that diabetes confers an increased risk for CHD and cardiac mortality [177-179]. CVD is the main cause of morbidity and mortality in diabetes. Diabetes worsens early and late outcomes in acute coronary syndromes. In addition to the enhanced heart disease risk seen in diabetes, the clinical course of CHD in diabetic patients is accelerated, as compared to normoglycemic persons. Elevated glucose levels are associated with heart failure in patients with cardiovascular risk [180]. Diabetes mellitus markedly increases the risk of myocardial infarction, stroke, amputation, and death. People with diabetes are 2- 4 times more likely to die from heart disease, 4 times more likely to have peripheral vascular disease, and 2 -4 times as likely to have stroke, compared to people without diabetes. Regardless of the severity of the clinical presentation, patients who have diabetes and coronary events experience increased rates of MI and death [179, 181]. DM increases general and CVD mortality: The risk of death among adults with diabetes was reported to be 2.6 times that of adults without diabetes [181].

Gender-Related Aspects of DM

Gender differences in the prevalence of DM: Gender difference in the prevalence of diabetes appears after age 65, becoming higher for men than for women. Despite this women constitute 55% of all people with diabetes. Differences in diabetes prevalence between men and women may reflect differences in the distribution of risk factors and longer life expectancy for women, however the pattern may differ according to the examined population.

Gender differences in CHD risk in DM: Diabetic women have higher risk of CHD [182] than diabetic men. Compared to diabetic men, who have 2-3-fold increased risk of CHD, diabetic women are reported to have a 3-fold to 7-fold increased risk [183 - 185], thus eliminating the premenopausal advantage of women in the prevalence of CHD [1386]. The reasons for the excessive relative CHD risk in diabetic women compared with diabetic men are not completely understood. The stronger effect of type 2 diabetes on the risk of CHD in women compared with men can be in part explained by a heavier risk factor burden in diabetic women [187, 188].

Men and women differ in the predictors of CHD appearance: When CVD-free patients with type 2 diabetes patients were followed up for 4 years, following initial assessment, patients with microvascular complications showed higher incidence rates of all outcomes in both sexes. In men, glycemic control and treated hypertension were additional independent risk factors, although geographic location of the patients affected this data. In women, higher triglycerides and lower HDL-cholesterol were additional risk factors. These factors, hyperglycemia and hypertension, especially in men, and diabetic dyslipidemia, particularly in women, are risk factors amenable to more aggressive treatment [189].

Gender differences in CVD morbidity and mortality in DM: Diabetes increases the incidence of MI, peripheral artery disease (PAD), and stroke in women more than in men, equalizing the age-adjusted rates [128, 190, 191]. Although women experience relative protection from cardiovascular disease compared with men in the general population, diabetes blunts the benefit of female sex. Mortality from myocardial infarction is higher in diabetic women than in non-diabetic women and in men with or without diabetes [192]. Meta-analysis of prospective cohort studies showed that the rate of fatal CHD was higher in patients with diabetes than without (5.4% vs. 1/6%). The relative risk for fatal CHD in patients with diabetes compared to patients without diabetes was 50% higher in women than in men [193]. The greater coronary risk in women can be explained by more adverse coronary risk profiles among diabetic women and by possible disparities in management. The combination of diabetes and prior CHD identifies particularly high-risk women [194]. It was also reported that in men, established CHD signifies a higher risk for CHD mortality than diabetes. This is reversed in women, with diabetes being associated with greater risk for CHD mortality [195].

DM-related CVD outcome and gender: Changes in outcomes in diabetic women don't mirror those of non-diabetic cohorts. In the First National Health and Nutrition Examination Survey (NHANES) and the NHANES Epidemiologic Follow-up Survey conducted 10 years later, age-adjusted heart disease mortality decreased in nondiabetic men and women, less so in diabetic men, but increased by 23% in diabetic women [196].

CVD mortality has declined over the past years and overall longevity increases, but the progress in reducing mortality rates among diabetes patients has been limited to men. The age-adjusted mortality rate of men with diabetes has decreased by 43%, similar to that of non-diabetic men. Women with diabetes did not experience a decrease in mortality-rate, and the difference in mortality between diabetic and non-diabetic women doubled [147].This disparity has been explained by sex differences in primary [197] and secondary preventive care including less than optimal control of serum cholesterol in women [198, 199]. Analysis of studies which provided sex-specific adjusted results for CHD mortality, nonfatal myocardial infarction and cardiovascular all-cause mortality, showed that the excess relative risk of CHD mortality in women vs. men with diabetes was absent after adjusting for classic CHD risk factors, but men had more CHD deaths attributable to diabetes than women [200].

Interaction of sex hormones and insulin: Interaction of sex hormones and insulin has been described in women: Female sex hormones are very likely to play a major role in preventing insulin resistance and development of diabetes, as incidence of related metabolic abnormalities increases abruptly with onset of menopause [201]. Hormone replacement therapy improves insulin resistance in type 2 diabetic women [202]. It is not clear whether the changes are actually related to the reduced level of female sex hormones or the increased level of testosterone after menopause. Hyperandrogenicity is well known to correlate with insulin resistance in women with polycystic ovarian syndrome and in nondiabetic women with abdominal obesity. In female rats, moderate increases of testosterone concentration are followed by a marked decrease in whole-body insulin sensitivity [203]. Development of insulin resistance in the female gender can be established after an early, even transient, hyperandrogenemia [204]. Imbalance of sex steroids may contribute to adverse cardiac effects in men also: it has been postulated that low testosterone, due to the effects on insulin resistance, vasodilatation, obesity, coagulation, inflammation, and endothelial dysfunction, is related to a greater incidence of CHD in men [205]. Clinical observations and experimental data suggest that low testosterone levels in men and high testosterone levels in women predicted insulin resistance and incident type 2 diabetes in older adults [206]. It has been suggested that the effects of testosterone may be indirect, via its effect on release of adiponectin. In accordance with this hypothesis are earlier observations of lower plasma adiponectin concentrations in men than women. Furthermore, high levels of plasma adiponectin were found in castrated mice, and testosterone treatment reduced plasma adiponectin concentration in both sham-operated and castrated mice [206a]. In women, plasma adiponectin concentrations are not different before and after menopause, and in mice ovariectomy does not alter plasma adiponectin levels. In view of this, adiponectin is a likely candidate for mediating sex differences in insulin sensitivity.

Dyslipidemia

Atherosclerosis is a systemic diffuse disease that may manifest as an angiographically localized coronary, cerebral, mesenteric, renal, and/or peripheral arterial stenosis, or as diffuse atherosclerosis [207]. It is a chronic inflammatory process which begins early and develops into later life, resulting from interaction between modified lipoproteins, monocyte-derived macrophages, T-cells and cellular elements of the arterial wall, and leading to the formation of plaques [208]. Dietary and endogenously produced lipids are transported by various lipoprotein particles; since LDL has the essential role of carrying cholesterol to peripheral tissues, increased LDL-cholesterol levels are associated with increased risk of CVD. Oxidative modifications in the lipid- and apolipoprotein B- (apo B) components of LDL are involved in the initial formation of fatty streaks underlying the vascular endothelium, contributing to plaque formation with subsequent inflammation, altered thrombosis, altered vessel tone, and biochemical interactions. Plaque rupture and thrombosis result in acute complications of CVD [207]. Therefore, cholesterol and lipoproteins play a crucial role in the atherosclerotic process.

Total cholesterol and low-density lipoprotein cholesterol (LDL-C): Epidemiological surveys have shown that serum total cholesterol levels are continuously correlated with CHD risk [209, 210], and reduction of serum cholesterol reduces CHD risk and mortality [211, 212]. Serum LDL-C levels correlate highly with total cholesterol in populations, and the same relation exists between LDL-C concentrations and CHD risk. In addition, clinical trials show that LDL-lowering therapy reduces risk for CHD events and mortality [213]. The risk of developing CVD increases parallel to the increase of the LDL-C levels, the higher the LDL-C level, the greater the CHD risk is [210]. Therefore, the NCEP has identified serum LDL-C as a primary target of cholesterol-lowering therapy. The primary goals of therapy and the cut-points for initiating treatment are stated in terms of LDL. LDL levels are classified as follows: optimal, <100 mg/dL; near or above optimal, 100 to 129 mg/dL; borderline high, 130 to 159 mg/dL; high, 160 to 189 mg/dL; and very high, ≥190 mg/dL [214]. Although the association between LDL-C levels and CHD risk is continuous, it is not linear; risk rises more steeply with increasing LDL-C concentrations [215]. Clinical trials of LDL-lowering therapy suggest that for every 30-mg/dL change in LDL-C, the relative risk for CHD is changed in proportion by about 30% [215].

Triglycerides (TG): Evidence that elevated serum triglyceride levels [216], fasting [217] and non-fasting [217-219] are associated with increased risk for atherosclerotic events, is increasing. Elevated TG level is a component of the atherogenic dyslipidemia, commonly found in patients with excess adiposity, the metabolic syndrome and type 2 diabetes mellitus [220], although secondary (medications) or genetic factors can heighten triglyceride levels. Serum triglycerides have been classified as follows: Normal triglycerides: <150 mg/dL, borderline-high triglycerides 150-199 mg/dL, high triglycerides 200-499 mg/dL and very high triglycerides ≥500 mg/dL [214]. There are a number of underlying causes of elevated serum TGs: genetic predisposition, overweight and obesity, physical inactivity, cigarette smoking, excess alcohol consumption, high-carbohydrate diets (>60% of total energy) and diseases such as type 2 diabetes mellitus, chronic renal failure, and nephrotic syndrome.

High-density lipoprotein cholesterol (HDL-C): Low HDL cholesterol, defined in ATP III as a level <40 mg/dL in men and <50 mg/dL in women is a strong independent predictor of CHD. Low HDL cholesterol both modifies the goal for LDL-lowering therapy and is used as a risk factor to estimate 10-year risk for CHD. The levels of HDL-C are inversely related to those of triglycerides [221] and to the risk of developing CVD [214]. This association is mediated by a constellation of events collectively referred to as reverse cholesterol transport—the transport of cholesterol from peripheral tissues to the liver for subsequent metabolism or excretion. HDL directly protects against the development of atherosclerosis. In addition, in the presence of high serum levels of triglycerides, LDL-C and HDL-C become small and dense, creating a highly atherogenic state [222]. The major nongenetic determinants of low HDL cholesterol levels are hyperglycemia, diabetes, hypertriglyceridemia, very low-fat diets (<15% energy as fat), and excess body weight. Determinants of high triglycerides are mainly the same as those of low HDL cholesterol [223].

Lipoprotein(a) [Lp(a)]: Lipoprotein(a) is an atherogenic lipoprotein, which has a potential role in atherothrombogenesis [224]. It is a modified form of LDL, in which a large glycoprotein, apolipoprotein (a), is covalently bound to apo B by a disulfide bridge. Because of the resemblance of the apo(a) chains to plasminogen, it is hypothesized that Lp(a) interferes with fibrinolysis by competing with plasminogen binding to molecules and cells [225]. Lp(a) is present in atherosclerotic plaques in the vascular tree. There is a conflicting evidence as to whether Lp(a) is an independent risk factor for CHD. Many retrospective studies exhibited positive association between Lp(a) and CHD, but data in prospective studies are inconsistent. Some prospective observational studies have identified Lp(a) as a predictor of cardiovascular events [226, 227]. However, other studies demonstrated no association between levels of Lp(a) and adverse cardiovascular outcomes [228, 229]. The apo-B:A-1 ratio has been suggested as a strong marker of coronary heart disease risk [230].

Serum Lipids – Gender Perspective

Recent studies confirm the strong relationship between lipoproteins and coronary heart disease development among women and extend these observations to more diverse populations. LDL-cholesterol, non-HDL-cholesterol, and triglycerides, are associated with increased risk of CHD in both sexes, while triglycerides, non-HDL-cholesterol and HDL-cholesterol appear to be a stronger predictor of CHD in women than in men [231, 232].

Gender differences in the change in lipid levels with age: Several large epidemiological studies examined the lipoprotein levels change with age in the US [233, 234] and in France [235]. According to these reports, levels of TC and LDL-C were higher in men than in women and increased with age [233-235]. The sex differences decreased with age [235], disappeared in the French cohort after age of 55 [234], or were reversed. In the US, women aged 70 years or older had higher mean LDL cholesterol levels than men of the same age [233]. HDL-C was higher in women at all age ranges [233-235]. Serum triglyceride levels were lower in women than men [233-235], excluding Mexican American adults in the US cohort [233], and were reported to be higher in whites than blacks [234]. TG levels increased with age in women, but remained stable in men [234]. Apoprotein A-I and B levels followed the same trends as HDL cholesterol and LDL cholesterol levels, respectively. Lp(a) levels were twice as high in blacks than in whites, and women's Lp(a) levels were higher than those in men in both race. Menopause was associated with elevated total cholesterol, LDL cholesterol, apoprotein B and Lp(a) levels. Hormone replacement medication in postmenopausal women was associated with higher HDL cholesterol, triglyceride, and apoprotein A-I levels and lower LDL cholesterol, apoprotein B, and Lp(a) levels [234].

Gender-related differences in lipid metabolism: Research data have demonstrated the presence of sexual dimorphism in lipid metabolism [236-237], not consistently accounted for by body composition, i.e. regional fat distribution [237]. Gender differences in substrate kinetics include a greater rate of lipolysis in women leading to greater basal rate of fatty acid appearance in the bloodstream, potentially influenced by female sex hormones, a slower resting energy expenditure rate, and higher percent body fat than in men, as well as higher levels of circulating insulin and response to its lipolytic effects [237, 238]. Increased plasma clearance of VLDL-TG and VLDL-apoB-100, described in women, accounts for lower concentrations of these particles in women than men. Further, the type of VLDL produced by women was shown to be richer in triglycerides, and therefore more atherogenic, than those in men [239].

TC and LDL-C - the gender aspect: Total cholesterol and LDL levels in women rise following the menopause [240]. In the presence of low endogenous estrogen levels, LDL receptor activity is reduced. This leads to the elevated LDL concentration observed in postmenopausal women. HRT modifies the activity of the LDL receptor [241]. It has also been suggested, based on animal trials, that estrogen affects the LDL-C oxidative processes [239]. Women respond as well as men to cholesterol lowering therapy given for primary [242] and secondary prevention of CHD [243, 244].

HDL-C – the gender aspect: Starting at a young age, HDL levels are higher in women than in men [234, 235]. Some studies [245, 246] have described a decrease in HDL levels following the menopause. In other studies a modest decline in HDL-C levels after menopause was accompanied by a rise in apoA-I levels, implying a change in HDL composition [247]. Low levels of HDL cholesterol are predictive of CHD in women and appear to be a stronger risk factor for women >65 years old than for men >65 [248]. It might be appropriate to apply a gender specific approach in interpreting HDL levels because of the higher absolute levels and possible greater impact of HDL in women.

Triglycerides – the gender aspect: A meta-analysis based on 17 published reports of population-based, prospective studies examined the association between fasting triglyceride levels and incident cardiovascular endpoints. A 1-mmol/L increase in triglyceride was associated with a 32% increase in disease risk in men and 76% increase in disease risk in women. After adjustment for high-density lipoprotein cholesterol and other risk factors, these risks were decreased to 14% in men and 37% in women, but remained statistically significant [249]. Increased mortality from coronary heart disease, cardiovascular disease, and all- cause mortality among middle aged women, in contrast to men, has been described in association with elevated non-fasting concentration of triglyceride, which is defined as an independent risk factor [250]. Whether the magnitude of postprandial TG concentrations is related to endogenous estrogen changes secondary to the menopause [251] or dependent on age [252], is not yet clear.

Lipoprotein(a) – the gender aspect: Lp(a) levels are independent of other lipid parameters [253]. Emerging evidence suggests that the atherogenic effects of Lp(a) may be age- and sex-specific [254]. In women, circulating Lp(a) levels increase after the menopause in parallel with the other lipid parameters (triglycerides, LDL and total cholesterol) [255]. Other data indicate that Lp(a) is not as strong a risk factor for CHD in women as in men [256, 257]. Most of the studies were conducted in middle-aged men. In a study of older subjects, Lp(a) was shown to predict CVD mortality in older men, but not women [258]. More data are necessary to determine whether gender-related differences are clinically relevant.

Novel Markers of CVD

The classic, conventional risk factors are related to perceiving CVD as a metabolic disease, tightly related to the lipid-diet connection. However, although the cardiovascular disease risk issue is composed of many components, of which lipids represent a big part, the diet-lipid-heart hypothesis excludes many effects of diet on old and new risk factors, including blood pressure, endothelial function, vascular inflammation, insulin sensitivity, and oxidative stress. Novel biomarkers which have joined the traditional, known since half of a century, primarily originating in the FHS data classical risk factors, through associations with CHD imply the existence of more complex mechanisms. They include markers for inflammation (CRP, fibrinogen), markers for oxidative stress (homocysteine), markers for endothelial function (plasminogen activator inhibitor type 1), and markers for thrombosis (fibrinogen, D-dimer). These markers extended the understanding of the atherosclerotic process beyond the diet-lipids-heart association and reinforce the involvement of additional mechanisms, which integrate into the development of the atherosclerotic process - inflammation and endothelial dysfunction. Inflammation, parallel to its contribution to the establishment of the atherosclerotic plaque, takes a crucial part in the development of insulin resistance, as previously described, and contributes to the development of the metabolic syndrome. These mechanisms, their gender-related aspect and their nutritional applications, will be discussed hereby.

Vascular Inflammation and Endothelial Dysfunction

Atherosclerosis as an inflammatory process: Inflammation has gained widespread attention for its role in the initiation and progression of CVD [259]. Strong associations between biochemical markers of systemic inflammation and both the presence of and future risk for symptomatic CVD have been repeatedly documented [260]. The concept that atherosclerosis is a specific form of chronic inflammatory process resulting from interactions between plasma lipoproteins, cellular components (monocyte/macrophages, T lymphocytes, endothelial cells and smooth muscle cells) and the extracellular matrix of the arterial wall, is now well accepted. Histologically, atherosclerotic lesions from the early-stage (fatty streak) to more complicated lesions possess all the features of chronic inflammation. It has been demonstrated that atherogenic lipoproteins such as oxidized low density lipoprotein (LDL), remnant lipoprotein (beta-VLDL) and lipoprotein Lp(a) play a critical role in the pro-inflammatory reaction, whereas high density lipoprotein (HDL), anti-atherogenic lipoproteins, exert anti-inflammatory functions [260, 261].

In cholesterol-fed animals, the earliest events in the arterial wall during atherogenesis are the adhesion of monocytes and lymphocytes to endothelial cells followed by the migration of these cells into the intima. These early events in atherosclerosis are triggered by the presence of high levels of atherogenic lipoproteins in the plasma and are mediated by inflammatory factors such as cytokines and adhesion molecules [262]. Lipoprotein particles such as LDL, very low–density lipoprotein (VLDL) and intermediate-density lipoprotein have an atherogenic potential: After undergoing oxidative modification in the intima, modified lipids can induce the expression of adhesion molecules, chemokines, proinflammatory cytokines, thus promoting endothelial dysfunction [263] and atherogenesis [264]. Oxidative stress, platelets, the CD40/CD40L signaling system, and angiotensin II are also involved in the initiation and perpetuation of inflammation in CVD [265,266]. The early stage of atherogenesis and atheroma formation includes recruitment of leukocytes and elaboration of pro-inflammatory cytokines. Later, inflammatory pathways promote thrombosis, a late complication of atherosclerosis. Advancement of the atherosclerosis lesion is characterized by both inflammation and release of fibrogenic mediators, and later thrombosis.

Adipose tissue and inflammation: Adipose tissue has an important role in inflammation process. Visceral fat in particular acts as an endocrine organ, producing adipokines – proinflammatory proteins which may induce low-grade chronic inflammatory state, which contribute to the development of the metabolic syndrome, diabetes and atherosclerosis, through both insulin resistance and endothelial dysfunction [267].

Another factor which underlies the atherosclerotic process is endothelial dysfunction. It includes imbalance of endothel-dependent vasodilation, coagulant activity and inflammatory processes, related to oxidative stress, which plays role in the pathogenesis of atherosclerosis [268].

Inflammatory biomarkers: Clinical information supports the use of markers of inflammation, oxidation, and endothelial function as prognostic and predictive instruments for predicting risk for various complications of atherosclerosis, including CHD. Inflammatory biomarkers in the plasma correlate with risk for acute coronary syndromes; the most prominent of them is C-reactive protein (CRP).

Several studies have demonstrated that elevated concentrations of CRP are predictive of cardiovascular events [269, 270] and may be precursors of type 2 diabetes and MetS [271]. Prospective epidemiological studies have found increased vascular risk in association with increased basal levels of cytokines such as in interleukin-6 (IL-6) and tumor necrosis factor-α (TNF-α) [272], cell adhesion molecules, such as soluble ICAM-1, P selectin, and E selectin [273]; and acute-phase reactants such as CRP, fibrinogen, and serum amyloid A [274]. For clinical purposes, the most useful inflammatory biomarker is CRP, which has a long half-life and stable level without circadian variation. CRP measurements may provide information for global risk assessment for coronary heart disease beyond that obtained from established risk factors [275].

Homocysteine: Homocysteine is an independent risk marker for coronary and peripheral vascular artery disease [276] and is related to oxidative stress [277] and endothelial dysfunction [278, 279]. Several studies have investigated the role of homocysteine in promoting oxidative stress and have obtained conflicting results, possibly due to study population characteristics [280]. Plasma homocysteine can often be lowered by oral administration of folic acid or combinations of B vitamins, raising the potential for prevention of CVD and its complications [281, 282].

Inflammation, Endothelial Dysfunction, and Gender

Inflammation and gender: CRP level reflects inflammation and predicts CVD events in healthy middle aged and elderly men and women [283-286]. In several studies the findings implied sex differences: Chronic inflammation, as indicated by elevated CRP concentration, seems to have greater effect on insulin resistance and on the development of MetS in women than in men [271]. Greater increase in CRP concentrations with an increased number of MetS components was observed in women than in men. Stronger association between CRP concentration and BMI in women than in men, and more pronounced increase in CRP concentration with obesity and MetS, imply that in women cytokines derived from adipose tissue may increase the inflammatory process, thus increasing the contribution of obesity [287, 288]. In a study which presented CRP as the most significant risk factor for CVD in healthy middle-aged women, the investigators suggested to add CRP measurements to standard lipid screening [272]. It seems that CRP as a marker for future CVD is more remarkable for women.

When serum fatty acid composition and circulating inflammatory markers were studied, the following gender differences were identified: in overweight men, the ratio of SFA:n-3 PUFA was independently associated with increased IL-6, and serum CRP was significantly associated with n-6 PUFA linoleic acid and n-3 LCPUFA eicosapentaenoic acid in nonsmoking men and with n-3 LCPUFA docosahexaenoic acid in nonsmoking women [289].

During the reproductive years, women have significantly greater capacity for transformation from ALA to LCPUFA than do men, suggested to be related to estrogen activity [290]. Thus, a decrease in this capacity with estrogen loss, combined with a general age-related decline in delta-6-desaturase [291], may be relevant to postmenopausal acceleration of the CVD process.

Homocysteine and gender: A gender difference exists also for homocysteine metabolism . Homocysteine tend to be higher in men than in women and in older subjects versus younger. In women, postmenopausal levels tend to exceed premenopausal [292].

The impact of homocysteine on cardiovascular disease can be more detrimental in women than in men. Women with high homocysteine levels have shown the worst all-cause and CVD survival, unrelated to atherosclerotic burden [293].

Gender-related factors in endothelial function: The main mechanism of possible cardioprotection by estrogens appears to be a direct effect on the vasculature, resulting in an improvement of endothelial function and inhibition of atherogenesis.

Numerous observational and experimental studies have demonstrated a positive correlation between estrogens and markers surrogating direct vascular effects. The few data available on the direct effects of androgens on the vascular wall indicate a less favorable action of androgens on biochemical markers than of estrogens [294]. The practical relevance of marker measurements is currently under discussion

Management of the CVD Risk Factors

Awareness of the importance of lifestyle changes in the prevention of CVD has evolved concomitantly with the expanding knowledge of various aspects in the pathogenesis of CVD and CVD risk factors. Lifestyle modifications can effectively control CVD risk factors and lower CVD risk. In order to do so, individuals should aim for a desirable body weight, be physically active, avoid tobacco exposure, and follow a diet and lifestyle consistent with current dietary recommendations. The proven effect of several aspects of diet in the pathogenesis of CVD and its risk factors point to the importance of dietary management of CVD risk and make medical nutritional therapy (MNT) part and parcel of the treatment regimen in people with or at high risk for CVD. The effect of specific nutrients, of dietary patterns, and the interrelation between risk factors should be taken into consideration when planning MNT. Since many aspects of CVD risk and overt CVD, as well as the effects of diet are gender-related, gender should be taken into consideration when discussing nutritional management for CVD.

Answers to the following are summarized:

1) What are the dietary determinants of the different components of the atherosclerotic process?
2) How do different nutrients and foods affect CVD risk factors?
3) What is the effect of dietary clusters and specific dietary patterns on CVD risk and CVD risk factors?
4) What are the nutritional recommendations for CVD risk management?
5) What is the impact of gender on the nutrition-CVD interrelation?

Dietary Determinants of CVD Risk Factors

Dietary Determinants of Serum Lipids

Since the first report in 1957 [295], evidence for the effect of diet on serum lipids profile has been accumulating. Animal model studies [296] and clinical studies show that serum cholesterol levels can be manipulated by dietary changes [297, 298], and that this intervention affects CVD incidence and mortality [299, 300]. Accumulating data have led to the development of equations which predict the relative effect of the various classes of fatty acids and cholesterol in the diet on serum cholesterol [297, 301, 302]. The major determinant of LDL cholesterol concentrations is saturated fat [303, 304]. Saturated fatty acids increase LDL and HDL cholesterol, PUFA decrease LDL and HDL cholesterol. MUFA decrease LDL and HDL cholesterol concentrations to a lesser extent than PUFA. The total cholesterol-to-HDL cholesterol ratio is similar and more favorable for polyunsaturated and monounsaturated fatty acids than for saturated fatty acids [348]. Dietary cholesterol has been positively associated with CVD risk and both LDL and HDL cholesterol concentrations [305, 306]. In contradistinction, findings of a non-significant association of dietary cholesterol with CHD risk [307-310], and with plasma total or LDL-cholesterol [311, 312], were reported. Over the years there has been considerable debate whether eggs in the diet contribute to elevated plasma cholesterol levels and heart disease risk. No significant relationship between egg consumption and plasma lipid levels, nor between egg intake and coronary heart disease incidence, was demonstrated [313-315]. It is possible that dietary fat, not egg consumption, remains the key dietary focus for most patients [316]. A meta-analysis of 17 studies showed that dietary cholesterol significantly increased the ratio of total to HDL-cholesterol levels. This suggests that the favorable increase in HDL cholesterol with increased dietary cholesterol intake fails to compensate for the adverse rise in total and LDL concentrations. Therefore, the increased intake of dietary cholesterol may raise the risk of coronary heart disease [317]. Estimating the absolute effect of dietary cholesterol on plasma lipoprotein concentrations has been difficult because of the high degree of variability in response among individuals [318]. In controlled studies in young males and females, it was demonstrated that for every additional 100 mg of dietary cholesterol, fasting plasma total cholesterol concentrations increased by 1.47 and 0.73 mg/dl, respectively, with parallel increases in LDL cholesterol and apoprotein B concentrations [319, 320]. Subsequent to the evidence that diets low in cholesterol and fat reduce the risk of CVD, and that serum cholesterol levels can be manipulated by dietary changes, patients have been advised to limit the intake of saturated fat and cholesterol.

Dietary Determinants of Inflammation

Diet-related inflammatory risk: One of possible mechanisms underlying association between a diet, high in refined starches, sugar, and lipids, and poor in natural antioxidants and fiber, and metabolic disorders and CVD, is the generation of a pro-inflammatory milieu [321]. Clinical data suggest that post-prandial hyperglycaemia [322] and hypertriglyceridaemia [323] are a risk factor for cardiovascular disease and may be a predictor of carotid intima-media thickness in type 2 diabetic patients [323]. Post-prandial hyperlipidaemia and hyperglycaemia are simultaneously present in the post-absorptive phase, particularly in diabetic patients and in subjects with impaired glucose tolerance. Both post-prandial hyperglycaemia and hypertriglyceridaemia may cause endothelial dysfunction, which is considered an early marker of atherosclerosis. The level of triglycerides after a high-fat (saturated) meal is inversely associated with endothelial function. Meals rich in carbohydrates or saturated fats are associated with impairment of endothelial function [266], with inverse relation between the TG level and endothelial impairment. Maximal impairment occurs at the time of the simultaneous presence of post-prandial hyperglycaemia and hypertriglyceridaemia.. Oral or intravenous glucose increases generation of ROS (reactive oxygen species). A high fat diet is associated with raised levels of circulating inflammatory cytokines that induce endothelial dysfunction, by increasing the concentrations of the adhesion molecules VCAM-1 (vascular cell adhesion molecule-1) and ICAM-1 (intercellular adhesion molecule-1), and plasma concentrations of IL-6 and TNF-α [324]. Ingestion of particular macronutrients causes a shift towards oxidative stress and inflammation, which in turn may reduce insulin sensitivity [325, 326], and promote atherogenesis.

The Effect of Different Dietary Constituents on CVD Risk

Dietary Fatty Acids

Effect of dietary fatty acids on CVD risk: Strong positive correlations between saturated fat intake and risk of CHD have been found in epidemiological [327, 328] and prospective [329, 330] studies. Higher intakes of *trans*-fat and, to a smaller extent, saturated fat were associated with increased risk, whereas higher intakes of nonhydrogenated polyunsaturated and monounsaturated fats were associated with decreased risk [307].

Effect of dietary fatty acids on plasma lipids: LDL: The strongest dietary determinants of elevated LDL cholesterol concentrations are dietary saturated fatty acid and *trans* fatty acid intakes. Saturated fatty acids increase the level of LDL slightly more than *trans* fatty acids, but they also increase HDL cholesterol concentrations, whereas *trans* fatty acids do not [331, 347]. To a lesser extent, dietary cholesterol and excess body weight are positively related to levels of LDL cholesterol [214]. LDL-C oxidation, considered to be a CVD risk factor independent of LDL-cholesterol levels, has been observed to be sensitive to degree of saturation in fatty acids and to antioxidant status [332]. Hydrogenated fat intake in hypercholesterolemic postmenopausal women seems to contribute to decreased HDL-C and apo B-100 and increased LDL-C and apo-AI concentrations. The mechanism for the adverse lipoprotein profile observed with hydrogenated fat intake can be attributed in part to increased apoA-I and decreased apoB-100 catabolism [333].

HDL: Fatty acid composition of the diet affects HDL and TG levels. Because dietary fatty acids have major effects on LDL-C and HDL-C, it is necessary to evaluate these effects in order to more accurately assess the potential impact of HDL change on coronary disease risk. Increased weight is a determinant of low HDL-C levels [82]; therefore weight loss has favorable effects on HDL-C levels [82, 334].

TG: A moderate inverse relationship exists between triglyceride and HDL cholesterol concentrations, and determinants of high triglycerides are mainly the same as those of low HDL cholesterol [223]. Diet and body weight can affect HDL cholesterol (HDL-C) and triglycerides (TG) [335]. When investigated in pre- and post- menopausal women who took part in the Framingham Offspring Study, TG levels were inversely related to polyunsaturated fat and directly related to saturated fat and oleic acid in. take. Dietary fat was directly related to HDL cholesterol in postmenopausal women only. Plasma total and LDL cholesterol levels were related to the amount of ingested saturated fat, but not cholesterol [336, 337].

PUFA: N-3 PUFA are believed to play a protective role in CVD risk, partially through actions on the inflammation and coagulation pathways. Flax seed oil consumption (20 g/d, 1 month) has been reported to improve arterial compliance despite increased LDL oxidation. In addition, fish oil supplements (3 to 10 g/d) consistently aim EDV (endothelium-dependent vasodilation) [338]. This beneficial effect of marine n-3 PUFA might be mediated by increased membrane fluidity of endothelial cells and promotion of synthesis and/or release of nitric oxide [339]. Moreover, a moderate intake of n-3 PUFA was found to reduce endothelial expression of vascular cell adhesion molecule 1 (VCAM-1), E-selectin, intercellular adhesion molecule 1 (ICAM-1), interleukin 6 (IL-6), and IL-8 in response to IL-1, IL-4, tumor necrosis factor, or bacterial endotoxins. The effect paralleled n-3 incorporation into cellular phospholipids, and a reduction in VCAM-1 messenger RNA, indicating a pretranslational effect [340]. In overweight women with an inflammatory phenotype, n-3 PUFA supplementation was observed to result in declines of CRP and IL-6 [341]. A cross-sectional study of 727 healthy middle-aged women (43-69 years) from the Nurses' Health Study I cohort found that dietary n-3 PUFA were associated with reduced biomarkers for inflammation and endothelial activation – specifically, CRP, IL-6, E-selectin, sICAM-1, and sVCAM-1 (the latter two specifically related to n-3 PUFA intake). These had not been responsive to hormone replacement therapy or other dietary components, such as fiber or vitamin E alone [342]. A previous study had shown similar results with n-3 PUFA supplementation in postmenopausal women [343].

Effects of dietary manipulations of fatty acids: Many studies of the effects of different dietary fatty acids on serum cholesterol levels reported that saturated fatty acids (SFA) increase and polyunsaturated fatty acids (PUFA) decrease total and LDL cholesterol. Two dietary approaches were tested: replacing saturated fat with polyunsaturated fat, without changing total fat, and lowering total fat. The high-polyunsaturated-fat trials demonstrate reduction of the serum cholesterol level [298, 344, 345], although the rate of cardiovascular events was not significantly reduced [345]. Two secondary prevention trials testing the approach of total fat reduction did not find a significant reduction in serum cholesterol or CHD events [346]. All 3 classes of fatty acids (saturated, monounsaturated, and polyunsaturated) elevate high-density lipoprotein cholesterol (HDL-C) when they replace carbohydrates in the diet; this effect is slightly greater with saturated fatty acids and decreases with increasing desaturation of the fatty acids [297].

Replacement of carbohydrates by fatty acids also decreases triglyceride levels [297]. When displacing carbohydrate from the diet, SFA increase total cholesterol, PUFA decrease total cholesterol, and monounsaturated fatty acids (MUFA) have a neutral effect. It is estimated that the total cholesterol-increasing effect of SFA is approximately twice the cholesterol-decreasing effect of PUFA, resulting in recommendations to reduce dietary saturated fat [348].

When saturated fat is replaced with carbohydrates, both LDL-C and HDL-C will be reduced, with no significant effect on the LDL-HDL ratio. This change in diet would be expected to have minimal benefit on CHD risk. However, when monounsaturated or polyunsaturated fats replace saturated fat, LDL-C decreases and HDL-C changes only slightly. Moreover, substituting polyunsaturated fat for saturated fat may have beneficial effects on insulin sensitivity and type 2 diabetes [349].

ω -3 Fatty Acids

The effects of dietary unsaturated fatty acids on plasma lipoprotein patterns and on the CVD risk are related to their structure. ω -3 fatty acids which are important in human nutrition, being capable to afford some degree of protection against CHD are: α-linolenic acid (ALA), eicosapentaenoic acid (EPA), and docosahexaenoic acid (DHA). The physiological potency of EPA and DHA is much greater than that for α-linolenic acid. The major dietary source of EPA and DHA is oily fish. ALA, a plant source of ω-fatty acids, which appears in canola and soybean oils, can be converted to EPA at very low rate [350].

Interest in the protective effect of the ω-3 fatty acids have been supported by observational [351-353] and interventional [354, 355] studies. The inverse relationship between ω-3 fatty acid intake and CVD events has been demonstrated by several reviews and meta-analyses: Some of these studies concluded that this relationship is significant for EPA and DHA but not for α-linolenic acid (ALA) [356-358]. ω-3 fatty acids may reduce risk of CHD by preventing cardiac arrhythmia, lowering serum triglyceride levels, decreasing thrombotic tendency, and improving endothelial dysfunction [359-361]. A decrease in the thickness of the carotid arteries along with improvement in blood flow by administration of purified EPA to patients with type 2 diabetes has been reported [362]. In individuals with increased triglyceride levels, ω- fatty acids decrease plasma concentrations by decreasing hepatic production rates of VLDL, with little effect on fractional catabolic rates [348].

Trans Fatty Acids

Trans fatty acids are monounsaturated or polyunsaturated fatty acids which contain at least one double bond in the *trans* configuration. Their effect on plasma lipid and lipoprotein concentrations arouses considerable interest [363, 364]. The major source of dietary *trans* fatty acids is partially hydrogenated fats and products formulated with these fats, such as commercially prepared baked and fried foods. A smaller proportion of dietary *trans* fatty acids comes from ruminant animal fats found primarily in meat and full fat dairy products. As do saturated fatty acids, *trans* fatty acids increase LDL cholesterol concentrations. In contrast to saturated fatty acids, they do not increase HDL cholesterol concentrations. Relative to unsaturated fat, both saturated fat and partially hydrogenated fat result in higher LDL cholesterol concentrations attributable to lower fractional catabolic rates, with little change in production rates. In a similar manner, partially hydrogenated fat results in lower HDL cholesterol concentrations. Collectively, these changes result in a less favorable total cholesterol or LDL cholesterol-to-HDL cholesterol ratio [347, 349].

Fruits and Vegetables

Consumption of fruits and vegetables is associated with a reduced risk for CVD [365, 366]. Studies which examined diets supplemented with fruits and vegetables taken as a whole rather than a source of particular nutrients, showed association of these diets with a lowering of blood pressure and plasma cholesterol [367, 368]. The mechanisms through which vegetables and fruits protect against CVD are likely to be multiple. Beneficial effects of various constituents, including antioxidant vitamins, folate, fiber, and potassium, can contribute to this relationship. Folate and vitamin B_6 are assumed to reduce CHD risk by decreasing homocysteine levels [369]. Intake of vitamin E from supplements [370, 371] and diet [372] may also have a protective effect. Many studies showed association of fiber intake with lower risk for CHD [373]. A diet that is higher in vegetables and fruits can increase the antioxidant capacity of serum and protect against lipid peroxidation [374]. Other compounds such as flavonoids [375] and other phytochemicals may also have protective effects in reducing CHD risk. Confounders, both nutritional (i.e. intake of protein, cereal fiber, saturated and polyunsaturated fat, cholesterol) and non-nutritional (i.e. smoking, physical activity) should be taken into consideration, when analyzing these associations.

Dietary Fiber

Dietary fiber, comprising nondigestible polysaccharides in plants, has been associated with reduced incidence of ischemic heart disease (IHD) and stroke in predominantly middle-aged [376, 377] and older [378] populations. An analysis of data pooled from 10 prospective cohort studies demonstrated inverse association between consumption of dietary fiber from cereals and fruits with risk of coronary heart disease. Results were similar for men and women

[379]. Potential cardiovascular benefits of dietary fiber include favorable effects on serum lipid levels [380], insulin sensitivity [381], and blood pressure [382], which may slow the development of atherosclerosis. Soluble fibers appear to have a greater potential to alter serum lipid levels than do insoluble fibers [383].

Whole Grain

A protective effect of whole grain with decreased risk of CHD has been demonstrated in epidemiological studies [384, 385]. The lower risk associated with higher whole-grain intake was not sufficiently explained by it's contribution to increased intake of dietary fiber. Although whole grain are a good source of dietary fiber, their protective effect against CHD extends beyond that of dietary fiber, and include folate, vitamins B6 and E, and various phytochemicals [386]. The influence of whole grains on cardiovascular disease risk may be mediated through multiple pathways, eg, a reduction in blood lipids and blood pressure, an enhancement of insulin sensitivity, and an improvement in blood glucose control. In the Framingham Offspring Study cohort, whole-grain intake was inversely associated with body mass index, waist-to-hip, total cholesterol, LDL cholesterol, and fasting insulin. The inverse association between whole-grain intake and fasting insulin was most striking among overweight participants [387].

Nuts

Beneficial effects of nut consumption on CHD [389, 390] and on blood lipids [391] have been observed. Most fats in nuts are mono- and polyunsaturated fats, which lower LDL-cholesterol level. Based on the data from the Nurses' Health Study, it has been estimated that substitution of the fat from 1 ounce of nuts for equivalent energy from carbohydrate in an average diet was associated with a 30% reduction in CHD risk and the substitution of nut fat for saturated fat was associated with 45% reduction in risk [392]. Walnuts have a special advantage, as compared to other nuts, because of the abundance of n-6 (linoleate) and n-3 (linolenate) polyunsaturated fatty acids (PUFAs), while other nuts contain monounsaturated fatty acids (MUFAs).In addition, walnuts contain also high levels of fiber, folate, arginine, tannins, and polyphenols. Walnut supplementation, as a way of enriching serum lipids with LA and ALA, was shown to have a favorable effect on plasma lipids and lipoproteins [393, 394]. Walnuts are a rich source of both, antioxidants and alpha-linolenic acid, a plant n-3 fatty acid, which may improve CHD-associated endothelial dysfunction [395], therefore their cardioprotective effect extends beyond cholesterol lowering.

Legumes

A population study, using data from the NHANES I, implied an association between consumption of legumes and reduced risk of CHD and CVD [396]. Reduced CHD risk was explained by the lowering effect on plasma cholesterol levels, ascribed to high content of soluble fiber, shown to reduce total and LDL-cholesterol levels [383], and to the effect of substituting protein from vegetable sources, for protein from animal sources, shown to reduce serum cholesterol levels [397].The increased consumption of legumes may displace foods relatively high in saturated fat and cholesterol from the diet and exert an indirect blood cholesterol-lowering effect [398]. Legumes are also generally low in sodium - low dietary intake of sodium has been associated with a reduced risk of cardiovascular disease (CVD). The most prominent legume in the domain of CVD prevention is soybean [399] A meta-analysis indicated a 13% reduction in LDL-cholesterol concentration, related to a mean intake of 47gr/day soy protein [397]. The hypocholesterolemic effect was even more prominent among persons with higher basal cholesterol levels. The hypocholesterolemic effect of soy products may be secondary to estrogenic activities of soy isoflavones. However, this influence is subjected to controversy [400]. Daily consumption of soy isoflavones has been shown to result in positive effect on inflammation, independent of lipid and antioxidant effects in postmenopausal women, both healthy [401] and hyperlipidemic [402], and reduction of adhesion molecules [403].

Although the mechanisms by which soy modulates blood cholesterol and lipoprotein levels need further research, daily consumption of 25 g of soy protein with its associated phytochemicals intact can improve lipid profiles in hypercholesterolemic humans.

Carbohydrates

A high intake of complex carbohydrates, mainly starch, and avoidance of simple sugars has been recommended [405]. However, many starchy foods, such as baked potatoes, are rapidly digested to glucose and produce even higher glycemic and insulinemic responses than sucrose. Foods with a low degree of starch gelatinization such as spaghetti and oatmeal, and a high level of viscose soluble fiber, such as barley, oats, and rye, tend to have a slower rate of digestion and, thus, lower GI (glycemic index - the incremental area under the curve for blood glucose levels – values). Feeding low-GI meals may improve the glycemic control and lipid profile in diabetic patients [406].

Glycemic load (GL - the product of the GI value of a food and its carbohydrate content) has been used to represent both the quality and quantity of the carbohydrates consumed [407]. Dietary GL, more strongly than GI, is associated with higher fasting triglycerides and lower HDL-C levels [408]. A strong positive association between GL and risk of CHD has been observed [409]. The increased risk was more pronounced among overweight and obese women, indicating that the adverse effects of a high GL diet are exacerbated by underlying insulin resistance [410]. Thus, carbohydrate-containing foods should not be evaluated by their GI values only; the amount of carbohydrates, fiber, and other nutrients are also important.

Another way to classify dietary carbohydrates is to subdivide cereal grains into whole and refined grains. Most cereal grains are highly processed before they are consumed. Refined grain products contain more starch but substantially lower amounts of dietary fiber, essential fatty acids, and phytochemicals and are therefore less recommended. Dietary fiber and whole grain have been discussed separately.

Antioxidants

Antioxidants for improved endothelial function: Dietary antioxidants – including vitamins and botanical polyphenols, i.e. from red wine, green and black tea, and chocolate – improve endothelial dysfunction under experimental conditions of increased ROS [411].

Antioxidants for reduced LDL oxidation: The oxidizability of the lipoprotein particles is highly dependent on d effietary and endogenous antioxidants. High amounts of vitamin E (400 mg/day) have been shown to significantly reduce LDL oxidative susceptibility [412]. Moreover, moderate amounts of vitamin E, together with carotenoids, may significantly increase the LDL total antioxidant capacity and reduced their lag time to oxidation [413]. A significant and progressive decrease in tocopherols and carotenoids such as lutein, zeaxanthin, beta-cryptoxanthin, beta-carotene, and lycopene was found with increased LDL density, from light to dense LDL (from LDL1 to LDL5) subspecies, which could underlie the increased oxidizability of small dense LDL [414]. However a beneficial effect on cardiovascular outcome by the addition of vitamin E could not be demonstrated in controlled trials [415].

The Effect of Specific Dietary Patterns on CVD Risk and CVD Risk Factors

Dietary Patterns: In spite of the abundance of information related to individual nutrients and risk of CHD, little is known about the role of overall eating pattern. Traditionally, nutritional research has largely focused on the effects of single nutrients or foods on disease outcomes. However, because nutrients and foods are consumed in combination, their joint effects may be best investigated by considering the entire eating pattern. A concept of specifying clusters of dietary habits and identifying dietary patterns characteristic of specific populations has been developed. Analyzing food consumption in the form of dietary patterns offers a perspective different from the traditional single-nutrient focus and may provide a comprehensive approach to disease prevention or treatment. On the other hand, because there are many potential differences in nutrients between dietary patterns, this approach cannot be specific about the particular nutrients responsible for the observed differences in disease risk, and thus it may not be very informative about biological relations between dietary components and disease risk. Dietary patterns are likely to vary by sex, socioeconomic status, ethnic group, and culture.

Different dietary pattern clusters: A population based study, based on nutritional data from the Framingham Study, has established, by the use of dietary pattern analysis, the concept of 5 dietary pattern clusters, while using dietary pattern analysis: Heart Healthy, Light Eating, Wine and Moderate Eating, High Fat, and Empty Calorie. Dietary patterns differ substantially in terms of individual nutrient intakes, overall dietary risk, heart disease risk factors, and predicted heart disease risk. Women in the Heart Healthy cluster had the most nutrient dense eating pattern, the lowest level of dietary risk, more favorable risk factor levels, and the lowest probability of developing heart disease. Those in the Empty Calorie cluster had a less nutritious dietary pattern, the greatest level of dietary risk, a heavier burden of heart disease risk factors, and a relatively higher probability of developing heart disease [416]. The predictive ability of these 5 dietary patterns was examined in a prospective study of healthy female participants of the FOS (the Framingham Offspring-Spouse) study, which demonstrated the highest occurrence of MetS in the participants with the Empty Calorie pattern [417]. Women with a higher nutritional risk profile consumed more dietary lipids (total, saturated, and monounsaturated fats) and alcohol, and less fiber and micronutrients. They had higher cigarette use and waist circumferences. Compared with women with the lowest nutritional risk, those in the highest tertile had a 2- to 3-fold risk of development of abdominal obesity and MetS during the follow-up period [418].

In a study conducted in Tehran 3 major dietary patterns had been identified by factor analysis: The healthy dietary pattern (high in fruits, tomatoes, poultry, legumes, cruciferous and green leafy vegetables, other vegetables, tea, fruit juices, and whole grains), the Western dietary pattern (high in refined grains, red meat, butter, processed meat, high-fat dairy products, sweets and deserts, pizza, eggs, hydrogenated fats, and soft drinks, and low in vegetables and low-fat dairy products) and the traditional dietary pattern (high in refined grains, potatoes, tea, whole grains, hydrogenated fats, legumes and broth). The healthy dietary pattern was associated with the lowest odds ratio for the metabolic syndrome [419].

Prudent pattern vs. Western pattern: When factor analysis was applied to dietary information derived from 2 large prospective cohort studies, the Nurses' Health Study and the Professionals' Follow-up Study two major dietary patterns were observed: The prudent pattern was characterized by higher intakes of fruits, vegetables, legumes, fish, poultry, and whole grains. On the other hand, the Western pattern was characterized by higher intakes of red and processed meats, sweets and desserts, French fries, and refined grains. A significant inverse association between the prudent pattern and the risk of total CHD and a positive association between the Western pattern and the risk of CHD were found in both men and women [420].

These major dietary patterns may predict the risk of CHD, even after adjustment for potential beneficial nutrients such as folate and cereal fiber and for potential deleterious nutrients such as saturated fat, trans fat, and cholesterol. The associations persisted also in subgroup analyses according to cigarette smoking, body mass index, and parental history of myocardial infarction, suggesting that major dietary patterns predict risk of CHD, independent of other lifestyle variables [421]. A diet high in fruits, vegetables, legumes, whole grains, poultry and fish, and low in red and processed meats and refined grain products may lower risk of CHD in men and women.

Mediterranean Diet: Distinct eating patterns, reflecting different dietary traditions, have been related to disease rates in different countries [422]. The prudent diet pattern is comparable with the geographically based Mediterranean-style diet. The food pattern that is characteristic of Mediterranean-style diets is high in fruits, vegetables, whole-grain products, potatoes, beans, nuts, and fish and low intakes of red meat, high-fat dairy products, and other animal products. It includes olive oil as an important fat source; eggs are consumed zero to 4 times weekly. In addition, wine is consumed in low to moderate amounts. Mediterranean and Asian populations have very low rates of CHD compared with Western populations, which may in part result from their respective dietary patterns [423, 424]. Among 70- to 90-year-olds, adherence to a Mediterranean diet and healthful lifestyle is associated with a more than 50% lower rate of all-cause and cause-specific mortality [424]. The Lyon Diet Heart Study demonstrated the efficiency of the Mediterranean-type diet in secondary prevention of CHD, implying that a cardioprotective diet should be included along with other means aimed at reducing modifiable risk [425, 426].

Effect of specific dietary patterns on inflammation: Specific dietary patterns may reduce or enhance inflammation: The raised flux of nutrients in the post-prandial state is associated with an increase in circulating levels of pro-inflammatory cytokines, recruitment of neutrophils, and oxidative stress. Dietary patterns high in refined starches, sugar, and lipids and poor in natural antioxidants and fiber may produce an inflammatory milieu. Visceral obesity, which may also be promoted by 'Western' dietary patterns, contributes to inflammation.

An inverse correlation between adherence to a Mediterranean-style diet and death, both total and due to CHD [423, 424], and beneficial effect of this diet on patients with metabolic syndrome (decrease in the incidence of metabolic syndrome, weight loss, lowering of CRP and pro-inflammatory cytokine levels) imply possible mechanisms for the beneficial effects of a Mediterranean-style diet [427]. Interventions aimed at weight reduction and adherence to a Mediterranean-type diet lead to reduced inflammation and the associated metabolic and cardiovascular risk [267]. Higher consumption of fruits and cereals was associated with lower concentrations of IL-6. Subjects with the highest consumption of nuts and virgin olive oil showed the lowest concentrations of VCAM-1, ICAM-1, IL-6 and CRP [428]. Whole-grain intake in healthy postmenopausal women showed a reduction in mortality larger than that previously reported for coronary heart disease and diabetes. Because a variety of phytochemicals are found in whole grains that may directly or indirectly inhibit oxidative stress, and because oxidative stress is an inevitable consequence of inflammation, it was suggested that oxidative stress reduction by constituents of whole grain is a likely mechanism for the protective effect [429].

Nutrients associated with specific dietary patterns: Since there are many potential differences in nutrients between dietary patterns, this "pattern" approach cannot be specific about the particular nutrients responsible for the differences in disease risk observed. However, the dietary patterns which have been specified are consistent with associations between intakes of nutrients and foods identified in previous epidemiologic studies. Intakes of nutrients that are directly correlated with the prudent diet pattern include constituents which, as previously detailed, are protective against CHD (fruit and vegetable, fish, whole-grain products), folate and vitamin E. On the other hand, red meat consumption was associated with increased CHD risk [370]. Carbohydrate-containing foods with a high glycemic index, such as white bread and mashed potatoes, have been associated with an increased risk of type 2 diabetes [430] and CHD [415]. When the association between food groups and indices of glycemic control in adults with type 2 diabetes and CVD were investigated in a cross-sectional study, a higher consumption of red meat was positively associated with hyperglycemia, hyperinsulinemia, and insulin resistance. Since higher consumption of red meat may aggravate hyperinsulinemia and insulin resistance in non-diabetic people, quantities consumed in a diet of persons at risk should be markedly reduced.

Epidemiologic and intervention studies have demonstrated the efficiency of the Mediterranean diet in primary and secondary prevention of CHD. It has a characteristic pattern, rich in oleic acid, poor in saturated fats and low in omega-6 fatty acids- therefore it should be used with fatty-acids supplements: Even small doses of omega-3 fatty acids (about 1g EPA + DHA in the form of fish oil capsules or 2 g alpha-linoleic acid in canola oil and margarine) might be very protective. The intake of linoleic acid should not exceed 7 g per day [431].

Low-fat diet: A low-fat diet is a diet in which ≈30% total energy is derived from fat. Various scientific bodies [432, 433] have recommended reductions in dietary fat intake to treat or prevent coronary disease. The suggested daily intake of dietary fat is 30% or less of total energy intake. The dietary level of saturated fat should be reduced to 6 to 8 percent of energy intake, along with a reduction in dietary cholesterol. Most recommendations have specified that the saturated fat eliminated from the diet should be replaced by carbohydrates from grains, vegetables, legumes, and fruits – thus turning the diet to be "low-fat, high-carbohydrate diet" while adding protective constituents from plant sources. Low-fat diets are recommended for weight reduction, to lower the risk of coronary heart disease, and certain forms of cancer. Since low-fat, high –complex carbohydrate diets reduce total energy intake, increase satiation, and are metabolized with less energetic efficiency then high fat diets, they have been advocated to prevent obesity and promote weight loss in overweight persons [434]. It has been reported that the low-fat, high carbohydrate diet, doesn't result in weight gain in post-menopausal women [435, 436], nor in older (aged 55 to 80 years) men [436].

The effectiveness of low fat dietary pattern in prevention of CHD has been inconsistent. When examined in intervention trials, the Women's Health Initiative (WHI) Dietary Modification Trial [437] and the NIH-funded Multiple Risk Factor Intervention Trial (MRFIT) [438], aiming at primary prevention of CHD, it did not significantly reduce the CVD risk. The effect of the low-fat dietary pattern on secondary prevention was examined in the Diet And Reinfarction Trial (DART). The advice on decreased fat intake and increased fiber intake appeared not to affect mortality or cardiac events. Advice to eat more fish did demonstrate improved survival [346].

DASH diet: Another example of a low-fat whole-diet approach is the DASH (Dietary Approaches to Stop Hypertension) diet, a dietary modification which calls for eating foods low in saturated and total fats along with increasing consumption of fruits and vegetables. It is a carbohydrate-rich diet that emphasizes fruits, vegetables, and low-fat dairy products. It comprises of whole grains, poultry, fish, and nuts; and is reduced in fats, red meat, sweets, and sugar-containing beverages. The DASH diet is aimed at reducing blood pressure by reducing salt intake, weight loss through caloric deficit, and moderation of alcohol consumption, among those who drink [439].

Low-Carbohydrate diet: Carbohydrate-restricted diets remain controversial, partly due to inconsistency of the term "carbohydrate-restricted diet". A very low-carbohydrate, moderate-protein, high-fat diet, with a carbohydrate: protein: fat ratio of approximately 10:25:65, is commonly referred to as the Atkins diet [440]. A moderate-carbohydrate, high-protein, low-fat diet (40:30:30), usually referred to as the Zone diet [441], adds protein to replace carbohydrate while maintaining a low-fat content of about 30% of total calories in a diet with moderate-carbohydrate restriction. Different carbohydrate-related diets represent a spectrum of carbohydrate intake: Atkins diet – very low in carbohydrate, Zone – low in carbohydrate, LEARN (Life style, Exercise, Attitudes, Relationships, and Nutrition [442] – based on the US national guidelines, low in fat, high in carbohydrate diet, and Ornish [443] – very high carbohydrate diet. In a prospective, intervention study which compared these 4 diets for effects on weight loss and related metabolic variables (lipid profile, percentage of body fat, waist-hip ratio, fasting insulin and glucose levels, and blood pressure) premenopausal, overweight women assigned to the diet with the lowest carbohydrate content (Atkins Diet) had more weight loss and more favorable changes in related metabolic risk factors than women assigned to the other 3 diets.

The carbohydrate-restricted diets can be compared with the standard high-carbohydrate, low-protein, low-fat (55:15:30) diet. In the WHI, a low-fat dietary pattern was not associated with a reduced risk of coronary heart disease during an 8-year follow-up [444], therefore the increase in total fat that is common among women who follow low-carbohydrate diets would not be expected to increase the risk of coronary heart disease.

In a meta-analysis of five randomized trials comparing a low-carbohydrate diet with a low-fat diet for at least 6 months, the low-carbohydrate diet was found to have a beneficial effect on HDL cholesterol and triglyceride levels but an adverse effect on total cholesterol and LDL cholesterol levels [445]. Some data indicate that carbohydrate-restricted diets work significantly better in persons with existing insulin resistance, implying that the metabolic state of the individual may determine the most appropriate diet for weight loss [446].

A review of 107 articles, reporting data of 3268 patients who participated in 94 dietary interventions, evaluated the efficacy and safety of low-carbohydrate diets. The conclusion was that the evidence is still insufficient to make recommendations for or against the low-carbohydrates, particularly for participants older than age 50 years, for use longer than 90 days, or for diets of 20g/d or less of carbohydrates. Among the published studies, weight loss was associated with decreased caloric intake and increased diet duration, but not with reduced carbohydrate content [447].

In conclusion, diets for prevention of CHD are based on accumulating evidence of epidemiologic studies, which have examined the contribution of specific constituents of the diet to the risk of CHD, and on the outcomes of interventional diets. Identifying dietary patterns, based on analyzing dietary information from large cohorts, or on observation of dietary habits of specific populations, related to the occurrence of CVD in these populations, support the clinical utility of a whole-diet approach in the prevention of cardiovascular disease.

Nutrition Recommendations for the Management of CVD Risk

The intensity of risk-reduction therapy should be adjusted to a person's absolute risk. Risk determinants include LDL cholesterol, the presence or absence of CHD, other clinical forms of atherosclerotic disease, and the major risk factors other than LDL. Current recommendations for CVD prevention relate to the 10-year risk of developing CVD and the presence of CVD-related risk factors. One aim of primary prevention is to reduce long-term risk (>10 years) as well as short-term risk (10 years). LDL goals in primary prevention depend on a person's absolute risk for CHD – the higher the risk, the lower the goal. Therapeutic lifestyle changes are the basis of clinical primary prevention. Dietary changes are recommended for all individuals; for those at moderate or high risk because of high or very high LDL cholesterol levels or because of multiple risk factors, LDL- lowering drug therapy is often prescribed.

Secondary prevention aims at reducing total mortality, coronary mortality, major coronary events, coronary artery procedures, and stroke in persons with established CHD. The same goal should apply for persons with CHD risk equivalents. CHD risk equivalents, which carry a risk for major coronary events equal to that of established CHD, ie, >20% per 10 years, comprise other clinical forms of atherosclerotic disease (peripheral arterial disease, abdominal aortic aneurysm, and symptomatic carotid artery disease), diabetes , and multiple risk factors that confer a 10-year risk for CHD >20%.

The 2 major modalities of LDL-lowering therapy are therapeutic lifestyle changes (weight reduction, increased physical activity, abstaining from smoking, and diet modification) and drug therapy whenever needed according to recommendations. Two main objectives of the nutritional approach are weight reduction and the management of lipid profile, aiming at the classic risk factors, although due to the overlap between the risk factors and their complex interrelations, weight loss affects the related metabolic variables, including lipid profile, percentage of body fat, waist-hip ratio, fasting insulin and glucose levels, and blood pressure.

Nutritional Management of Body Weight

Dietary fat, carbohydrate, and protein are the primary energy-containing macronutrients consumed on a routine basis by humans. In general, under conditions of fixed weight, different types of dietary protein or individual amino acids have little effect on lipoprotein patterns. When carbohydrate replaces fat, plasma triglyceride concentrations increase, and HDL cholesterol level decreases. Various types of carbohydrate may have different, but difficult to asses, effects, because of differences in rates of absorption and confounding of dietary fiber. Saturated fatty acids (SFA) increase LDL and HDL cholesterol, whereas *trans* fatty acids increase LDL but not HDL cholesterol [347, 348]. Unsaturated fatty acids (UFA) decrease LDL and HDL cholesterol, the effect of polyunsaturated been more prominent than of monounsaturated [348].

To maintain a stable body weight, if the intake of one macronutrient is increased or decreased, a compensatory adjustment in one or both of the other macronutrients is needed; therefore, the effect on plasma lipoprotein patterns can be attributable to either the addition of one macronutrient or the reduction of the other(s). If a single macronutrient is increased or decreased without compensatory adjustments in the amount of the other macronutrients, body weight will change and any effect on plasma lipoprotein patterns will result from changes induced by weight loss or gain, a shift in the relative energy distribution of each macronutrient, or some combination of these factors. The interrelation between changing dietary macronutrients, lipoprotein patterns and weight loss has been subject to many studies and debates. Short-term data favor substituting protein and fat for carbohydrate, whereas long-term data have failed to show a benefit for weight loss. During an active weight loss period low-carbohydrate diets more favorably affect triglyceride and HDL and less favorably affect LDL cholesterol concentrations. [348]. Very low-fat diets tend to increase TG levels and decrease HDL-C levels in the short term, therefore caution is indicated when elevated TG or depressed HDL-C cholesterol levels are present, as well as in persons with hyperinsulinemia, due to the potential for elevated TG and decreased HDL-C levels [448].

Nutritional Management of Lipids

The TLC Diet stresses reductions in saturated fat and cholesterol intakes. When the metabolic syndrome or its associated lipid risk factors (elevated triglyceride or low HDL cholesterol) are present, TLC also stresses weight reduction and increased physical activity. Diet stresses reduction in saturated fat and cholesterol intakes. If the metabolic syndrome or its associated lipid risk factors (elevated triglyceride or low HDL cholesterol), weight reduction and increased physical activity should be stressed. It is difficult to isolate the independent effects of dietary fat, carbohydrate, and protein on plasma lipoprotein profiles. The effects of fatty acid subclasses on plasma lipoprotein patterns and the metabolic basis for these effects are known, but the available data are confounded by changes in body weight, by combined intake of two or more macronutrients and by variability in response among individuals. The variability in response underscores the need for specific recommendations for dietary fat, carbohydrate, and protein to optimize plasma lipoprotein patterns on a case-by-case basis, taking into consideration the anticipated level of compliance.

A growing number of diet-based treatment options can be applied selectively to individualized diet therapy for both primary and secondary prevention of coronary disease. The collaborative approach guidelines for managing abnormal blood lipids [449] include detailed recommendations for dietary management.

LDL-C: The strongest dietary determinants of elevated LDL cholesterol concentrations are dietary SFA and *trans* fatty acid intakes. *Trans* fatty acids are found in stick margarine, vegetable shortenings, commercial bakery and deep-fried foods. Both should be replaced with dietary carbohydrate and/or UFA. The reductions in LDL-C that may be expected with the adoption of diets that are low in saturated fat are 8% to 10% and an additional 3% to 5% when dietary cholesterol is reduced (<200 mg/day). Thus, implementation of a diet low in saturated fat and cholesterol would be expected to lower LDL-C by ≈11% to 15% and possibly by as much as 20%. Intake of foods rich in oat (soluble) fiber is been associated with lower TC and LDL-C concentrations [480]. An increase in viscous fiber of as little as 5 to 10 g/day is expected to reduce LDL-C by 3% to 5%. Inclusion of 2 g/day of plant stanols/sterols would be expected to reduce LDL-C by 6% to 15%. Therefore, increasing viscous (soluble) fiber (10 to 25 g/day) and plant stanols/sterols (2 g/day) to enhance lowering of LDL-C is recommended. In addition, weight management and increased physical activity are recommended. A 10-lb weight loss can lead to LDL-C decrease by 5% to 8%. In conjunction with reductions in saturated fat and cholesterol, according to the therapeutic diet above (including weight loss) is expected to decrease LDL-C by 20% to 30% [449]. Additional dietary modifications, such as including soy protein and nuts can increase the LDL-C reduction.

A higher intake of some nutrients and specific food compounds, such as MUFA, PUFA, flavonoids, is recommended due to their effect on CVD risk. N-3 PUFA, particularly n-3 LCPUFA (docosahexaenoic acid, DHA, and eicosapentaenoic acid, EPA) are believed to play a protective role in CVD risk. The majority of n-3 PUFA in the modern diet is obtained as essential alpha-linolenic acid (ALA 18:3), which must be converted to LCPUFA endogenously. Findings from NHANES III suggest the American diet meets only the minimum recommendation for ALA, and less than the minimum for LCPUFA [450]. Further, a general age-related decline has been noted in delta-6-desaturase, the enzyme required for conversion of ALA [291].

The Mediterranean diet (with MUFA-rich virgin olive) has a significant advantage on to a low-fat diet. The "portfolio" pattern – very low in saturated fat and high in plant sterols (1 g/1,000 kcal), soy protein (23 g/1,000 kcal), and viscous fibers (9 g/1,000 kcal) – has been associated with reduction in LDL-C similar to those achieved with statin therapy in hyperlipidemic postmenopausal women and age-matched men, and therefore is recommended as first-line intervention [452].

HDL-C: Although clinical trial results suggest that raising HDL will reduce CVD risk, the evidence is insufficient to specify a goal of therapy. In all persons with low HDL cholesterol, the primary target of therapy is LDL cholesterol; after the LDL goal has been reached, emphasis shifts to weight reduction and increased physical activity (when the metabolic syndrome is present) [214].

TG: The treatment strategy for elevated triglycerides depends on the causes of the elevation and its severity. Weight loss is a primary goal as a means to lower TG levels in individuals with atherognic dyslipidemia and metabolic syndrome [107, 405]. For all persons with borderline high or high triglycerides, the primary aim of therapy is to achieve the target goal for LDL cholesterol. When triglycerides are borderline high (150-199 mg/dL), emphasis should also be placed on weight reduction and increased physical activity. For high triglycerides (200-499 mg/dL), non-HDL cholesterol becomes a secondary target of therapy. Aside from weight reduction and increased physical activity, drug therapy can be considered in high-risk persons to achieve the non-HDL cholesterol goal [214, 215].

Dietary n-3 PUFA are believed to reduce plasma TG. Diets enriched in eicosapentaenoic acid (EPA) and docosahexaenoic acid (DHA) – with an n-6:n-3 of approximately 3:1 – were shown in men and postmenopausal women aged 45-70 years to lower fasting and postprandial TG concentrations and the proportion of small-dense LDL, independent of insulin sensitivity or lipase activities [453]. Beneficial influence of intake of omega-3 fatty acids has been discussed.

On the basis of the available data, the American Heart Association recommends that the general population consume at least two fish meals per week, individuals with established CVD consume 1 g of EPA plus DHA per day, and hypertriglyceridemic individuals consume 2–4 g of EPA plus DHA per day [355]. A perceived risk of fish oil ω-3 supplementation has been heavy metal poisoning - in particular mercury, lead, nickel, arsenic and cadmium. The FDA recommends that total dietary intake of omega-3 fatty acids from fish not exceed 3 grams per day, of which no more than 2g/day are from nutritional supplement [453a].

Fiber: Recognizing the protective effect of dietary fiber on CHD risk reduction, an intake of ≥25 g per day from different sources (vegetables, cereals, grains, and fruits) has been recommended.[405].

Nuts: On the basis of the nut intervention studies, it was recommend that normo- and hyperlipidemic individuals consume a variety of nuts (50–100 g) at least 5 times/wk [391].

Legumes: The Nutrition Committee of the AHA recommends including soy protein foods in a diet low in saturated fat and cholesterol to promote heart health [404].

Carbohydrates: Dietary carbohydrates are the major determinant of elevated TGs in atherogenic dyslipidemia. Sugars should be consumed in the form of complex carbohydrates to reduce the glyceridemic effect. The recommended level of dietary fat is 25% to 35% of calories. Within this range, complex carbohydrates and a high-fiber diet are advised to lower TG and to increase the levels of HDL-C and larger LDL particles [449].

What is the Impact of Gender on the Nutrition-CVD Interrelation

Nutrition affects CVD and CVD risk and constitutes one of the most important modifiable factors. Evidence is accumulating that sexes differ in the effects of nutrition on health components, and in the way nutrition may affect CVD risk. Since nutrition is an important element in cardiovascular health, and nutritional intervention is evolving into a crucial component of primary and secondary prevention of CVD, the effect of gender on these issues is of enormous importance. The evidence should be assembled and interpreted, and conclusions should be applied for improving the health outcomes of both sexes.

Gender Aspects of Weight Reduction

Exercise appears to reduce blood leptin concentrations in women but not in men [453] and fat loss during weight reduction to be primarily subcutaneous in women vs. abdominal in men. Because of this, men tend to experience greater declines in triglyceride levels and increases in HDL cholesterol levels compared to women losing the same amount of weight [454].

Metabolic risk factors reduction can be achieved by reduced calorie diets and by training, both aerobic and resistance exercise [455]. A 2-fold greater improvement in insulin action in response to a combination of diet and aerobic exercise as compared with diet alone was reported in men [456], but in women there was no difference in improvement across the treatment groups [457].

While traditional "sensible" weight loss strategies have included reduction of total fat and increases in protein and carbohydrates, cohort studies evaluating the impact on CVD risk have been somewhat inconsistent. Most studies have been performed in men, a few in premenopausal women, and fewer still in postmenopausal women, resulting in the establishment of relatively sparse response patterns. The existing evidence suggests that fat composition of diets may have different effects on CHD risk factors in men and women, and that the latter may be more sensitive to carbohydrates and specific classes of fats postmenopausally. Increased saturated fat intake prevented progression of atherosclerosis in primarily overweight postmenopausal women, particularly when replacing polyunsaturated fatty acids in the diet, while increasing HDL and lowering triglycerides in plasma [458]. This study corroborated previous findings that may suggest negative effects of low-fat and low-saturated fat diets in women, particularly compared to men.

Differences in response to weight-reducing diets: When 2 diets, resulting in the same extent of weight loss, but varying in diet composition, were applied, women lost much more total fat and abdominal fat on 30% protein diet than on 15% protein diet. In men, the protein content of the diet did not affect the fat tissue loss [459]. Reduction of the triglycerides concentration was equal in both sexes and HDL-D didn't change during weight loss. LDL-C and total cholesterol concentrations decreased, the reduction being greater on the higher protein diet, with no gender difference.

The above may imply that strategies for reducing body weight in males and females might differ, particularly with regard to how changes in dietary manipulation ultimately impact atherogenesis.

Gender Aspects of Plasma Lipids Management

Low levels of HDL cholesterol are predictive of CHD in women and appear to be a stronger risk factor for women >65 years old than for men >65 [460]. Women tend to have higher HDL-cholesterol levels than men, and triglyceride levels may be a significant risk factor in women, especially older women. The current NCEP guidelines suggest considering more aggressive targets for HDL cholesterol and triglycerides in women [461]. The NCEP also recommends the use of ERT before cholesterol-lowering drugs to reduce LDL cholesterol in postmenopausal women. In this statement, the recommendation has been modified to consider statins a first-line therapy in postmenopausal women on the basis of recent data, implying that women may have at least as much benefit from LDL-cholesterol reduction with statins as men [462].

Antioxidant treatment too has a gender aspect: Studies in humans have suggested benefits of antioxidants in healthy men [463], but to lesser extent in high-risk women, as in postmenopause [464-466]. Even high doses of the antioxidant vitamins C and E did not improve endothelial vasodilator function in postmenopausal women with established coronary artery disease [466]. However, a lack of definitive results in related studies in general, as well as a lack of investigation into gender differences in this specific area leave insufficient information to draw conclusions. Estrogens have a potent antioxidant effect on low-density lipoprotein (LDL) cholesterol in vitro and in vivo, and so a variety of compounds with antioxidant properties, such as vitamins and other hormones, have been recommended in clinical practice to prevent several diseases related to oxidation in postmenopausal women [467]. Vitamin E supplementation in postmenopoausal women has been associated with a significant decrease in LDL oxidation [468], but to a lesser degree than hormone replacement [467].

The influence of diet on the progression of atherosclerosis is not well established, particularly in postmenopausal women, who may have different risk factors than men. When the association between dietary macronutrients and progression of coronary atherosclerosis was investigated among postmenopausal women with relatively low total fat intake, a greater saturated fat intake was associated with greater progression. Polyunsaturated fatty acids have been associated with greater progression of atherosclerosis when replacing saturated fatty acids, the role of fatty acid oxidation in atherogenesis [458].

Gender Differences in the Effect of Diet Constituents

Saturated fatty acids: A diet restricted in saturated fat and cholesterol is recommended for subjects with elevated LDL cholesterol concentrations, with and without drug therapy [469]. Previously, diet, weight loss, and exercise were found to be less effective in altering lipoprotein levels in women than in men [247], with a high degree of variability in lipoprotein subspecies response to low-fat diets being related in part to gender. When low-fat, high in vegetables, fruits and whole grains diet, was applied to big cohort of postmenopausal women of diverse backgrounds and ethnicities, participating in the Women's Health Initiative Randomized Controlled Dietary Modification Trial, the dietary intervention did not significantly reduce the risk of CVD and had only minimal impact on risk factors. These findings point to the need for more focused lifestyle interventions to improve risk factors and reduce CVD risk [444].

Postprandial TG and LpAI:AII concentrations were reduced in men, but not in women. The observed decreases in LpAI concentrations and LDL and HDL particle size were similar in men and women, all independent of body weight. These data are consistent with the concept that middle aged/elderly men may have a more favorable lipoprotein response to a low fat, low cholesterol diet than postmenopausal women [469].

Carbohydrates: Dietary glycemic load is significantly and positively associated with plasma CRP levels in healthy middle-aged women, independent of conventional risk factors for ischemic heart disease. It has been suggested that the mechanism whereby a high intake of rapidly digested and absorbed carbohydrates increases the risk of ischemic heart disease is the exacerbation of a proinflammatory process, especially in overweight women prone to insulin resistance [470].

Replacing saturated fat with carbohydrate from grains, vegetables, legumes, and fruit has been shown to reduce TC and LDL-C in men, with a minor reduction in TG as well as HDL-C, but the latter not enough to limit improvement in LDL:HDL ratio [471]. A similar dietary pattern was not associated with significant effects on HDL-C or TG in nearly 50,000 postmenopausal women aged 50-79 years who took part in the WHI cohort, and the reduction in LDL-C – though statistically significant – was moderate. No significant changes in CVD composite outcome were observed [444]. An earlier trial, the Women's Healthy Lifestyle Project – which lowered total fat to 25% of calories, SFA to 7%, and cholesterol to 100 mg/day, consistent with the NCEP Step II diet – was found to only partially reduce the rise in LDL-C observed during the transition from perimenopause to postmenopause [472].

High carbohydrate intake may be associated with a more detrimental lipid profile (high-triglyceride, VLDL) in overweight postmenopausal women [473], and may be consistent with the key role of insulin observed in their lipid metabolism [474]. Carbohydrate intake has been shown to correlate positively to triglyceride and apo C-III concentrations, and negatively to LDL diameter. An associations between carbohydrate intake and either risk factors for or actual progression of coronary atherosclerosis has been observed in postmenopausal women [458].

N-3 PUFA: Women have significantly greater capacity for transformation from ALA to EPA and DHA than do men during the reproductive years, probably related to estrogen activity [475]. Thus, a decrease in this capacity parallel to estrogen loss, combined with the general age-related decline in delta-6-desaturase [291], may be relevant to postmenopausal acceleration of CVD processes. Association between higher plasma DHA and reduced progression of atherosclerosis in postmenopausal women with existing CAD has been described, though a relationship with EPA was not observed [476].

Soy: Increased consumption of soy foods has been associated with decrease in LDL-C, according to clinical and observational studies [477]. When low-fat diet was given to men and postmenopausal women with hypercholesterolemia, examining additional lipid-lowering benefits of soy, the diet reduced LDL-C, HDL-C and TG levels, independent of soy intake. Concurrent HRT treatment by the postmenopausal women changed the diet responsiveness: the lower at the entry LDL-C levels remained unchanged, but the higher at the entry TG levels improved, without lowering HDL-C [478]. In the Women's Healthy Lifestyle Project, no significant interaction between dietary intervention and use of hormone replacement therapy on changes in LDL or other

CHD risk factors was observed in postmenopausal women [472]. The effects of nutrients on sex hormone metabolism, particularly soy isoflavones as a means to mimic estrogenic activity, have been the subject of numerous studies: diet-based isoflavones have yielded inconsistent results. Consumption of soy has been associated with improvement of features of the metabolic syndrome in postmenopausal women, including better glycemic contol, lipid profiles [479, 480] and inflammatory markers [481], more than the DASH diet, used as a control diet [481]. Combining soy with a carbohydrate-control diet (low glycemic index), showed advantage in this population over that of the AHA Step 1 diet [480]. In contrast, modest reductions in blood lipids and oxidized LDL observed with use of soyfoods instead of animal products, were found to be independent of isoflavone content and related to reduced intake of high-SFA originating in animal foods. No gender differences were noted [482].

Soluble fiber: The lowering actions of dietary soluble fiber on lipids appear to differ with gender and hormonal status, as was shown with a psyllium-based supplement in guinea pigs, with overectomized females showing lower response compared to males and control females, pointing to the detrimental effect of estrogen deprivation on the lipid profile [483]. In other animal research flaxseed, a source of fiber and of n-3 PUFA, reduced plasma cholesterol and atherogenic plaque formation induced by ovarian hormone deficiency [484]. Rapid and significant lipid-lowering effect has been demonstrated in postmenopausal women, with daily consumption of two servings of oats associated with beneficial lipid alterations (lower TC and LDL-C) unresponsive to concomitant soy intake [485].

Compliance: Underutilization of lipid lowering therapy has been reported, particularly among women [486]. Non-adherence may play role: age <50 and female sex are predictors of treatment discontinuation [487]. Non-adherence to medication is influenced by patient educational and marital status and mental health [488].

Conclusion

The current chapter gives a short overview of CVD and CVD risk factors, with a focus on gender-related aspects, emphasizing the role of nutrition. The evidence for gender-based differences in the effect of nutrition and nutrition constituents on CVD risk and risk factors has been reviewed.

The importance of the gender-nutrition- CVD risk interrelation cannot be overstressed. The advancement of gender-specific nutritional interventions is critical for further improvement of the CVD risk management. The idea of gender-specific lifestyle intervention should be further investigated and promoted. The field of gender-specific nutritional health intervention is a critical area for further investigation.

References

[1]   Rosamond, W; Flegal, K; Friday, G; Furie, K; Go, A; Greenlund, K; Haase, N; Ho, M; Howard, W; Kissela, B; Kittner, S; Lloyd-Jones, D; McDermott, M; Meigs, J; Moy, C; Nichol, G; O'Donnell, CJ; Roger, V; Rumsfeld, J; Sorlie, P; Steinberger, J; Thom, T; Wasserthiel-Smoller, C; Hong, Y; American Heart Association Statistics Committee and Stroke Statistics Subcommittee. Heart disease and stroke statistics – 2007 update: a

report from the American Heart Association Statistics American Heart Association Statistics Committee and Stroke Statistics Subcommittee. Committee and Stroke Statistics Subcommittee. *Circulation*, 2007, 115, e69-e171.

[2]   Fox, CS; Evans, JC; Larson, MG; Kannel, WB; Levy, D. Temporal trends in coronary heart disease mortality and sudden cardiac death from 1950-1999: the Framingham Heart Study. *Circulation*, 2004, 110, 522-527.

[3]   Dawber, TR; Meadors, GF; Moore, FE. Epidemiological approaches to heart disease: the Framingham Study. *Am J Public Health*, 1951, 41, 279-281.

[4]   Kannel, WB; Feinleib, M; McNamara, PM; Garrison, RJ; Castelli, WP. An investigation of coronary heart disease in families. The Framingham offspring study. *Am J Epidemiol*, 1979, 110, 281-290.

[5]   Plan and operation of the Third National Health and Nutrition Examination Survey, 1988-1994. *Vital Health Stat 1*, 1994, 32, 1-407.

[6]   The Atherosclerosis Risk in Communities (ARIC) Study: design and objectives. The ARIC investigators. *Am. J. Epidemiol*, 1989, 129, 687-702.

[7]   Rosamond, WD; Folsom, AR; Chambless, LE; Wang, CH; ARIC Investigators. Atherosclerosis risk in communities. Coronary heart disease trends in four United States communities. The Atherosclerosis Risk in Communities (ARIC) study 1987-1996. *Int J Epidemiol*, 2001, 30 Suppl, S17-S22.

[8]   Fried, LP; Borhani, NO; Enright, P; Furberg, CD; Gardin, JM; Kronmal, RA; Kuller, LH; Manolio, TA; Mittelmark, MB; Newman A; et al. The Cardiovascular Health Study: design and rationale. *Ann Epidemiol*, 1991, 1, 263-276.

[9]   Powell-Griner, E; Anderson, JE; Murphy, W. State- and sex-specific prevalence of selected characteristics – Behavioral Risk Surveillance System, 1994 and 1995. *MMWR CDC Surveill Summ*, 1997, 46, 1-31.

[10]   Bonow, RO; Smaha, LA; Smith, SC; Jr, Mensah; GA, Lenfant C. World Heart Day 2002: the international burden of cardiovascular disease: responding to the global emerging epidemic. *Circulation*, 2002, 106, 1602-1605.

[11]   Yusuf, S; Reddy, S; Ounpuu, S; Anand, S. Global burden of cardiovascular diseases: Part I: General considerations, the epidemiological transition, risk factors, and impact of urbanization. Circulation, 2001, 104, 2746-2753.

[12]   Tobin, JN; Wassertheil -Smoller, S; Wexler, JP; et al. Sex bias in considering coronary bypass surgery. *Ann Intern Med*, 1987, 107, 19-25.

[13]   Lerner, DJ; Kannel, WB. Patterns of coronary heart disease morbidity and mortality in the sexes: a 26-year follow-up of the Framingham population. *Am Heart J,* 1986, 111, 383-390.

[14]   Vaccarino, Y; Parsons, L; Every, NR; Barron, HV; Krumholz, HM. Sex-based differences in early mortality after myocardial infarction: National Registry of Myocardial Infarction 2 participants. *N Engl J Med*, 1999, 341, 217-225.

[15]   Milcent, C; Dormont, B; Durand-Zaleski, I; Steg, PB. Gender differences in hospital mortality and use of percutaneous coronary intervention in acute myocardial infarction: microsimulation analysis of the 1999 nationwide French hospitals database. *Circulation*, 2007, 115, 823-826.

[16]   Ford, ES; Giles, WH. Changes in prevalence of nonfatal coronary heart disease in the United States from 1971-1994. *Ethn Dis* 2003, 13, 85-93.

[17] Redberg, RF. Gender differences in acute coronary syndrome: invasive versus conservative approach. *Cardiol Rev*, 2006, 14, 299-302.

[18] Reina, A; Colmenero, M; Aguayo de Hoyos, E; Aros, F; Marti, H; Claramonte, R; Cunat, J; PRIAMHO II Investigators. Gender differences in management and outcome of patients with acute myocardial infarction. *Int J Cardiol*, 2007, 116, 389-395.

[19] Gottlieb, S; Harpaz, D; Shotan, A; Boyko, V; Cohen, M; Mandelzveig, L; Mazouz, B; Stern, S; Behar, S. Sex differences in management and outcome after acute myocardial infarction in the 1990s: A prospective observational community-based study. Israeli Thrombolytic Survey Group. *Circulation*, 2000, 102, 2484-2490.

[20] Moriel, M; Behar, S; Tzivoni, D; Hod, H; Boyko, V; Gottlieb, S. Management and outcomes of elderly women and men with acute coronary syndromes in 2000 and 2002. *Arch Intern Med*, 2005, 165, 1521-1526.

[21] Narins, CR; Ling, FS; Fischi, M; Peterson, DR; Bausch, J; Zareba, W. In-hospital mortality among women undergoing contemporary elective percutaneous coronary intervention: a reexamination of the gender gap. *Clin Cardiol*, 2006, 29, 254-258.

[22] Alfredsson, J; Stenestrand, U; Wallentin, L; Swahn, E. Gender differences in management and outcome in Non-ST-elevation acute coronary syndrome. *Heart,* 2006, 10, 1-14.

[23] Levy, D; Garrison, RJ; Savage, DD; Kannel, WB; Castelli, WP. Prognostic implications of echocardiographically determined left ventricular mass in the Framingham Heart Study. *New Engl J Med*, 1990, 322, 1561-1566.

[24] Anversa, P; Leri, A; Kajstura, J; Nadal-Ginard, B. Myocyte growth and cardiac repair. *J Mol Cell Cardiol*, 2002, 34, 91-105.

[25] Guerra, S; Leri, A; Wang, X; Finato, N; Loreto, C; Beltrami, CA; Kajstura, J; Anversa, P. Myocyte death in the failing human heart is gender dependent. *Circ Res*, 1999, 85, 856-866.

[26] Luchner, A; Brockel, U; Muscholl, M; Hense, HW; Doring, A; Riegger, GA; Schunkert, H. Gender-specific differences of cardiac remodeling in subjects with left ventricular dysfunction: A population based study. *Cardiovasc Res*, 2002, 53, 720-727.

[27] Larsen, JA; Kadish, AH. Effects of gender on cardiac arrhytmias. *J Cardiovasc Electrophysiol*, 1998, 9, 655-664.

[28] Madden, K; Savard, GK. Effects of mental state on heart rate and blood pressure variability in men and women. *Clin Physiol*, 1995, 15, 557-569.

[29] Mallat, Z; Fornes, P; Costagliola, R; Esposito, B; Belmin, J; Lecomte, D; Tedgui, A. Age and gender effects on cardiomyocyte apoptosis in the normal human heart. *J Gerontol A Biol Sci Med Sci*, 2001, 56, M719-M723.

[30] Olivetti, G; Giordano, G; Corradi, D. Gender differences in aging: Effects on the human heart. *J Am Coll Cardiol*, 1995, 26, 1068-1079.

[31] Quyyumi, AA. Women and ischemic heart disease: pathophysiologic implications from the Women's Ischemia Syndrome Evaluation (WISE) Study and future research steps. *J Am Coll Cardiol*, 2006, 47(3 Suppl), 66-71.

[32] Merz, CNB; Shaw, LJ; Reis, SE; Bittner, V; Kelsey, SF; Olson, M; Johnson, D; Pepine, CJ; Mankad, S; Sharaf, BL; Rogers, WJ; Pohost, GM; Lerman, A; Quyymi, AA; Sopko, G; for the WISE investigators. Insights from the NHLBI-Sponsored Women's Ischemia Syndrome Evaluation (WISE) Study. Part II: Gender Differences in Presentation, Diagnosis, and Outcome With Regards to Gender-Based Pathophysiology

of Atherosclerosis and Microvascular Coronary Disease. *J Am Coll Cardiol*, 2006, 47, 21S-29S.

[33] Greenland, P; Knoll, MD; Stamler, J; Neaton, JD; Dyer, AR; Garside, DB; Wilson, PW. Major risk factors as antecedents of fatal and nonfatal coronary heart disease events. *JAMA*, 2003, 290, 891-897.

[34] Kannel, WB; McGee, D; Gordon, T. A general cardiovascular risk profile: the Framingham study. *Am J Cardiol*, 1976, 38, 46-51.

[35] Yusuf, S; Hawken, S; Ounpuu, S; Dans, T; Avezum, A; Lanas, F; McQueen, M; Budaj, A; Pais, P; Varigos, J; Lisheng, L; INTERHEART Study Investigators. Effect of potentially modifiable risk factors associated with myocardial infarction in 52 countries (the INTERHEART study): case-control study. *Lancet*, 2004, 364, 937-952.

[36] Ford, ES; Giles, WH; Mokdad, AH. The distribution of 10-year risk for coronary heart disease among US adults: findings from the National Health and Nutrition Survey III. *J Am Coll Cardiol*, 2004, 43, 1791-1796.

[37] Ajani, UA; Ford, ES; McGuire, LC. Distribution of lifestyle and emerging risk factors by 10-year risk for coronary heart disease. *Eur J Cardiovasc Prev Rehabil*, 2006, 13, 745-752.

[38] Hayes, DK; Greenlund, KJ; Denny, CH; Croft, JB; Keenan, NL. Racial/ethnic and socioeconomic disparities in multiple risk factors for heart disease and stroke – United States, 2003. *JAMA*, 2005, 293, 1441-1443.

[39] Vasan, RS; Sullivan, LM; Wilson, PW; Sempos, CT; Sundstrom, J; Kannel, WB; Levy, D; D'Agostino, RB. Relative importance of borderline and elevated levels of coronary risk factors. *Ann Intern Med*, 2005, 142, 393-402.

[40] Lloyd-Jones, DM; Leip, EP; Larson, MG; D'Agostino, RB; Beiser, A; Wilson, PW; Wolf, PA; Levy, D. Prediction of lifetime risk for cardiovascular disease by risk factor burden at 50 years of age. *Circulation*, 2006, 113, 791-798.

[41] Barret-Connor, E; Suarez, L; Khaw, K; Criqui, MH; Wingard, DL. Ischemic heart disease risk factors after age 50. *J Chronic Dis*, 1984, 37, 903-908.

[42] Asia Pacific Study Collaboration. Does sex matter in the associations between classic risk factors and fatal coronary heart disease in populations from the Asia-Pacific region? *J Womens' Health*, 2005, 14, 820-828.

[43] Mosca, L; Grundy, SM, MD; Judelson, D; King, K; Limacher, M; Oparil, S; Pasternak, R; Pearson, TA; Redberg, RF; Smith, CS; Winston, M; Zinberg. Guide to Preventive Cardiology for Women. AHA/ACC Scientific Statement Consensus panel statement. *Circulation*, 1999, 99, 2480-2484.

[44] Rowland, M; Roberts, J. Blood pressure levels and hypertension in persons aged 6-74 years: United States 1976-1980. *National Health and Nutrition Examination Survey* II. Hyattsville, Maryland. US Department of Health and Human Services, 1982 (Advanced data from vital and health statistics of the Centers for Disease Control and Prevention, National Center for Health Statistics, No. 84).

[45] Jousilahti, P; Vartiainen, E; Toumilehto, J; Puska, P. Sex, age, cardiovascular risk factors, and coronary heart disease. A prospective follow-up study of 14 786 middle-aged men and women in Finland. *Circulation*, 1999, 99, 1165-1172.

[46] Fowkes, FGR; Pell, JP; Donnan, PT; Housley, E; Low, GDO; Riemersma, RA; Prescott, RJ. Sex differences in susceptibility to etiologic factors for peripheral

atherosclerosis: importance of plasma fibrinogen and blood viscosity. *Arterioscler Thromb*, 1994, 14, 862-868.

[47] Tunstall, PH; Kuulasmss, P et al. Myocardial infarction and coronary deaths in the World Health Organization MONICA Project. Registration procedures, event rates, and case fatality rates in 38 populations from 21 countries in four continents. *Circulation*, 1994, 90, 583-612.

[48] Chrysohoou, C; Panagiotakos, DB; Pitsavos, C; Kokkinos, P; Marinakis, N; Stefanidis, C; Toutouzas, PK. Gender differences on the risk evaluation of acute coronary syndromes: the CARDIO2000 study. *Prev Cardiol*, 2003, 6, 71-77.

[49] Isles, CG; Hole, DJ; Hawthorne, VM; Lever, AF. Relation between coronary risk and coronary mortality in women of the Renfrew and Paisley survey: comparison with men. *Lancet*, 1992, 339, 702-706.

[50] Grundy, SM; Balady, GJ; Criqui, MH; Fletcher, G; Greenland, P; Hiratzka, LF; Houston-Miller, N; Kris-Etherton, P; Krumholz, HM; LaRosa, J; Ockene, IS; Pearson, TA; Reed, J; Washington, R; Smith, SC Jr. Guide to primary prevention of cardiovascular diseases: a statement for healthcare professionals from the Task Force on Risk Reduction. *Circulation*, 1997, 95, 2329-2331.

[51] Manolio, TA; Pearson, TA; Wenger, NK; Barrett-Connor, E; Payne, GH; Harlan, WR. Cholesterol and heart disease in older persons and women: review of an NHLBI workshop. *Ann Epidemiol*, 1992, 2, 161-176.

[52] Califf, RM; Armstrong, PW; Carver, JR; D'Agostino, RB; Strauss, WE (Task Force 5). 27th Bethesda Conference: matching the intensity of risk factor management with the hazard for coronary disease events: stratification of patients into high, medium and low risk subgroups for purposes of risk factor management. *J Am Coll Cardiol*, 1996, 27, 1007-19.

[53] Clinical guidelines on the identification, evaluation, and treatment of overweight and obesity in adults – the evidence report. National Institutes of Health. *Obes Res*, 1998, 2 (suppl 6), 51S-209S.

[54] Willet, WC; Dietz, WH; Colditz, GA. Guidelines for healthy weight. *N Engl J Med*, 1999, 341, 427-434.

[55] Willet, WC; Manson, JE; Stampfer, MJ; Colditz, GA; Rosner, B; Speizer, FE; Hennekens, CH. Weight, weight change, and coronary heart disease in women. Risk within the 'normal' weight range. *JAMA*.1995, 273, 461-465.

[56] Hubert, HB; Feinleib, M; McNamara, PM; Castelli, WP. Obesity as an independent risk factor for cardiovascular disease: A 26 year follow-up of participants in the Framingham Heart Study. *Circulation*, 1983, 67, 968-977.

[57] Flegal, KM; Carroll, MD; Ogden, CL; Johnson, CL. Prevalence and trends in obesity among US adults, 1999-2000. *JAMA*, 2002, 288, 1723-1727.

[58] Despres, JP; Lemieux, I. Abdominal obesity and metabolic syndrome. *Nature*, 2006, 444, 881-887.

[59] Carey, DG. Abdominal obesity. *Curr Opin Lipidol, 199*8, 9, 35-40.

[60] Kaplan, NM. The deadly quartet. Upper-body obesity, glucose intolerance, hypertriglyceridemia, and hypertension. *Arch Intern Med*, 1989, 149, 1514-1520.

[61] Sharma, AM. Adipose tissue: a mediator of cardiovascular risk *Int J Obes Relat Metab Disord*, 2002, 26(Suppl 4), S5-S7.

[62] Li, C; Ford, S; McGuire, LC; Mokdad, AH. Increasing trends in waist circumference and abdominal obesity among US adults. *Obesity (Silver Spring)*, 2007, 15, 216-224.

[63] Lakka, TA; Lakka, J; Tuomilehto, JT; Salonen, HM. Abdominal obesity is an independent risk factor for coronary heart disease in middle-aged men and even more important than overall obesity (Abdominal obesity is associated with increased risk of acute coronary events in men. *Eur Heart J*, 2002, 23, 706-713.

[64] Snijder, MB; Dam, RM; Visser, M; Seidell, JC. What aspects of body fat are particularly hazardous and how do we measure them? *Int J Epidemiol*, 2006, 35, 83-92.

[65] de Koning, L; Merchant, T; Pogue, J; Anand, SS. Waist circumference and waist-to-hip ratio as predictors of cardiovascular events: meta-regression analysis of prospective studies. *Eur Heart J*, 2007, 28, 850-856.

[66] Hu, FB. Obesity and mortality. Watch your waist, not just your weight. *Arch Intern Med*, 2007, 167, 875-876.

[67] Okosun, IS; Liao, Y; Rotimi, CN; Prewitt, TE; Cooper, RS. Abdominal adiposity and clustering of multiple metabolic syndrome in White, Black and Hispanic Americans. *Ann Epidemiol*, 2000, 105, 263-270.

[68] Visscher, TL; Seidell, JC; Molarius, A; van der Kuip, D; Hofman, A; Witteman, JC. A comparison of body mass index, waist-hip ratio and waist circumference as predictors of all-cause mortality among the elderly: the Rotterdam study *Int J Obes Relat Metab Disord*, 2001, 25, 1730-1735.

[69] Yusuf, S; Hawken, S; Oupuu, S; Bautista, L; Franzosi, MG; Commerford, P; Lang, CC; Rumboldt, Z; Onen, CL; Lisheng, L; Tanomsup, S; Wangai, P Jr; Razak, F; Sharma, AM; Anand, SS; INTERHEART Study Investigators. Obesity and the risk of myocardial infarction in 27,000 participants from 52 countries: a case controlled study. *Lancet*, 2005, 368, 1640-1649.

[70] Zhang, X; Shu, XO; Yang, G; Li, H; Cai, H; Gao, YT; Zheng, W. Abdominal adiposity and mortality in Chinese women. *Arch Intern Med*, 2007, 167, 886-892.

[71] Janssen, I; Katzmarzyk, PT; Ross, R. Body Mass Index, Waist Circumference, and Health Risk. Evidence in Support of National Institutes of Health Guidelines. *Arch Intern Med*, 2002, 162, 2074-2079.

[72] Alberti, KG; Zimmet, P; Shaw, J. Metabolic syndrome – a new world-wide definition. A consensus statement from the International Diabetes Federation. *Diabet Med*, 2006, 23, 469-480.

[73] Marinos, A. Obesity in the elderly. *Obes Res*, 2001, 9, S244-S248.

[74] Bose, K. Age trends in adiposity and central body fat distribution among adult white men resident in Peterborough, East Anglia, England. *Coll Antropol*, 2002, 26, 179-186.

[75] Shimokata, H; Tobin, JD; Muller, DC; Elahi, D; Coon, PJ; Andres, R. Studies in the distribution of body fat: I. Effects of age, sex, and obesity. *J Gerontol*, 1989, 44, M66-M73

[76] Okosun, IS; Chandra, KM; Boev, A; Boltri, JM; Choi, ST; Parish, DC; Dever, GE. Abdominal adiposity in U.S. adults: prevalence and trends, 1960-2000. *Prev Med*, 2004, 39, 197-206.

[77] Ford, ES; Mokdad, AH; Giles, WH. Trends in waist circumference among U.S. adults. *Obes Res*, 2003, 11, 1223-1231.

[78] Teh, BH; Pan, WH; Chen, CJ. The reallocation of body fat toward the abdomen persists to very old age, while body mass index declines after middle age in Chinese. *Int J Obes Relat Metab Disord,* 1996, 20, 683-687.

[79] DeNino, DF; Tchernof, A; Dionne, IJ; Toth, MJ; Ades PA, Sites CK, Poehlman FT. Contribution of abdominal adiposity to age-related differences in insulin sensitivity and plasma lipids in healthy nonobese women. *Diabetes Care,* 2001, 24, 925-932.

[80] Price, GM; Uauy, R; Breeze, E; Bulpitt, CJ; Fletcher, AE. Weight, shape, and mortality risk in older persons: elevated waist-hip ratio, not high body mass index, is associated with a greater risk of death. *Am J Clin Nutr,* 2006, 84, 449-460.

[81] Blaak, E. Gender differences in fat metabolism. *Curr Opin Clin Nutr Metab Care,* 2001, 4, 499-502.

[82] Krauss, RM; Winston, M; Fletcher, BJ; Grundy SM. Obesity: impact on cardiovascular disease. *Circulation,* 1998, 98, 1472-1476.

[83] Williams, CM. Lipid metabolism in women. *Proc Nutr Soc,* 2004, 63, 153-160.

[84] Rexrode, KM; Carey, VJ; Hennekens, CH; Walters, EE; Colditz, GA; Stampfer, M; Willett, WC; Manson, JE. Abdominal adiposity and coronary heart disease in women. *JAMA,* 1998, 280, 1843-1848.

[85] Rexrode, KM; Buring, JE; Manson, JE. Abdominal and total adiposity and risk of coronary heart disease in men. *Int J Obes Relat Metab Disord,* 2001, 25, 1047-1056.

[86] Mayes, JS; Watson, GH. Direct effects of sex steroid hormones on adipose tissues and obesity. *Obes Rev,* 2004, 5, 197-216.

[87] Zamboni, M; Zoico, E; Scartezzini, T; Mazzali, G; Tosoni, P; Zivelonghi, A; Gallagher, D; De Pergola, G; Di Francesco, V; Bosello, O. Body composition changes in stable-weight elderly subjects: the effect of sex. *Aging Clin Exp Res,* 2003, 15, 321-327.

[88] Hughes, VA; Roubenoff, R; Wood, M; Frontera, WR; Evans, WJ; Fiatarone Singh, MA. Anthropometric assessment of a 10-y changes in body composition in the elderly. *Am J Clin Nutr,* 2004, 80, 475-482.

[89] Li, C; Engstrom, G; Hedblad, B; Calling, S; Berglund, G; Janzon, L. Sex differences in the relationship between BMI, WHR and incidence of cardiovascular disease: a population-based cohort study. *Int J Obes,* 2006, 30, 1775-1781.

[90] Van Pelt, RE; Jankowski, CM; Gozansky, WS; Schwartz, RS; Kohrt, WM. Lower-body adiposity and metabolic protection in postmenopausal women. *J Clin Endocrinol Metab,* 2005, 90, 4573-4578.

[91] Horber, FF; Gruber, B; Thomi, F; Jensen, EX; Jaeger, P. Effect of sex and age on bone mass, body composition and fuel metabolism in humans. *Nutrition,* 1997, 13, 524-534.

[92] Westerterp, KR; Goran, MI. Relationship between physical activity related energy expenditure and body composition: a gender difference. *J Obes Relat Metab Disor,* 1997, 21, 184-188.

[93] Paul, DR; Novotny, JA; Rumpler,WV. Effects of the interaction of sex and food intake on the relation between energy expenditure and body composition. *Am J Clin Nutr,* 2004, 79, 385-389.

[94] Roca, P; Proenza, AM; Palou, A. Sex differences in the effect of obesity on human plasma tryptophan/large neutral amino acid ratio. *Ann Nutr Metab,* 1999, 43, 145-151.

[95] Hellstrom, L; Wahrenberg, H; Hruska, K; Reynisdottir, S; Arner, P. Mechanisms behind gender differences in circulating leptin levels. *J Intern Med,* 2000, 247, 457-462.

[96]. Bennett, FI; McFarlane-Anderson, N; Wilks, R; Luke, A; Cooper, RS; Forrester, TE. Leptin concentration in women is influenced by regional distribution of adipose tissue. *Am J Clin Nutr*, 1997, 66, 1340-1344.

[97] Ahmed, ML; Ong, KK; Morrell, DJ; Cox, L; Drayer, N; Perry, L; Preece, MA; Dunger, DB. Longitudinal study of leptin concentrations during puberty: sex differences and relationship to changes in body composition. *J Clin Endocrinol Metab*, 1999, 84, 899-905.

[98] Clegg, DJ; Brown, LM; Woods, SC; Benoit SC. Gonadal hormones determine sensitivity to central leptin and insulin. *Diabetes*, 2006, 55, 978-987.

[99] Clegg, DJ; Riedy, CA; Smith, KA; Benoit, SC; Woods, SC. Differential sensitivity to central leptin and insulin in male and female rats. *Diabetes*, 2003, 52, 682-687.

[100] Eckel, RH; Grundy, SM; Zimmet, PZ. The metabolic syndrome. *Lancet*, 2005, 365, 1415-1428.

[101] Haffner, SM; Valdez, RA; Hazuda, HP; Mitchell, BD; Morales, PA; Stern, MP. Prospective analysis of the insulin-resistance syndrome (syndrome X). *Diabetes*, 1992, 41, 715-722.

[102] Rader, DJ. Effect of insulin resistance, dyslipidemia, and intra-abdominal adiposity on the development of cardiovascular disease and diabetes mellitus. *Am J Med*, 2007, 120 (suppl), S12-S18.

[103] Weyer, C; Bogardus, C; Mott, DM; Pratley, RE. The natural history of insulin secretory dysfunction and insulin resistance in the pathogenesis of type 2 diabetes mellitus. *Clin Invest*, 1999, 104, 787-794.

[104] Wilson, PW; McGee, DL; and Kannel, WB. Obesity, very low density lipoproteins, and glucose intolerance over 14 years. The Framingham study. *Am J Epidemiol*, 1981, 114, 697-704.

[105] Meigs, JB. Epidemiology of the insulin resistance syndrome. *Curr Diab Rep*, 2003, 3, 73-79.

[106] Alberti, KG; Zimmet, PZ. Definition, diagnosis and classification of diabetes mellitus and it's complications. Part 1: diagnosis and classification of diabetes mellitus provisional report of a WHO consultation. *Diabet Med*, 1998, 15, 539-553.

[107] Grundy, SM; Brewer, HB; Cleeman, JI; Sidney, CS Jr; Lenfant, C for the Conference Participants. Definition of metabolic syndrome: report of the National Heart; Lung; and Blood Institute/American Heart Association conference on scientific issues related to definition. *Circulation, 2004*, 109, 433-438.

[108] Expert panel on detection, evaluation, and treatment of high blood cholesterol in Adults. Executive summary of the third report of the National Cholesterol Education Program (NCEP) expert panel on detection, evaluation, and treatment of high blood cholesterol in adults (Adult Treatment Panel III). *JAMA*, 2003, 285, 2486-2497.

[109] Balkau, B; Charles, MA; Drivsholm, T; Borch-Johnsen, K; Wareham, N; Yudkin, JS; Morris, R; Zavaroni, I; van Dam, R; Feskins, E; Gabriel, R; Diet, M; Nilsson, P; Hedblad, B; European Group for the Study of Insulin Resistance (EGIR). Frequency of the WHO metabolic syndrome in European cohorts; and an alternative definition of an insulin resistance syndrome. *Diabetes Metab, 2002*, 28, 364-376.

[110] Einhorn, D; Reaven, GM; Cobin, RH. American College of Endocrinology position statement on the insulin resistance syndrome. *Endocr Pract*, 2002, 9, 236-252.

[111] Daskalopoulou, SS; Athyros, VG; Kolovou, GD; Anagnostopoulou, KK; Mikhailidis, DP. Definitions of metabolic syndrome: Where are we now? *Curr Vasc Pharmacol*, 2006, 4, 185-197.

[112] Day, C. Metabolic syndrome; or what you will: definitions and epidemiology. *Diab Vasc Dis Res*, 2007, 4, 32-38.

[113] Ford, ES; Giles, WH; Dietz, WH. Prevalence of the metabolic syndrome among US adults: findings from the third National Health and Nutritional Examination Survey. *JAMA*, 2002, 287, 356-359.

[114] de Simone, G; Devereux, RB; Chinali, M; Best, LG; Lee, ET; Galloway, JM; Resnick, HE. Prognostic impact of metabolic syndrome by different definitions in a population with high prevalence of obesity and diabetes: the Strong Heart Study. *Diabetes Care*, 2007, 30, 1851-1856.

[115] Qiao, Q; Gao, W; Zhang, L; Nvamdori, R; Tuomilehto, J. Metabolic syndrome and cardiovascular disease. *Ann Clin Biochem*, 2007, 44, 232-263.

[116] Wilson, PW; D'Agostino, RB; Parise, H; Sullivan, L; Meigs, JB. Metabolic syndrome as a precursor of cardiovascular disease and type 2 diabetes mellitus. *Circulation*, 2005, 112, 3066-3072.

[117] Cankurtaran, M; Hail, M; Yavuz, BB; Dagli, N; Oyan, B; Ariogul, S. Prevalence and correlates of metabolic syndrome (MS) in older adults. *Arch Gerontol Geriatrics*, 2006, 42, 35-45.

[118] Lorenzo, C; Okoloise, M; Williams, K; Stern, MP; Haffner, SM; the San Antonio heart study. The metabolic syndrome as predictor of type 2 diabetes: the San Antonio heart study. *Diabetes Care*, 2003, 26, 3153-3159.

[119] Lorenzo, C; Williams, K; Hunt, KJ; Haffner, SM. The National Cholesterol Education Program – Adult Treatment Panel III; International Diabetes Federation; and World Health Organization definitions of the metabolic syndrome as predictors of incident cardiovascular disease and diabetes. *Diabetes Care*, 2007, 30, 8-13.

[120] Meigs, JB; Rutter, MK; Sullivan, LM; Fox, CS; D'Agostino, RB Sr; Wilson, PW. Impact of insulin resistance on risk of type 2 diabetes and cardiovascular disease in people with metabolic syndrome. *Diabetes Care*, 2007, 30, 1219-1225.

[121] Liu, J; Grundy, SM; Wang, W; Smith, SC Jr; Vega, GL; Wu, Z; Zeng, Z; Wang, W; Zhao, D. Ten-year risk of cardiovascular incidence related to diabetes; prediabetes; and the metabolic syndrome. *Am Heart J*, 2007, 153, 552-558.

[122] Malik, S; Wong, ND; Franklin, SS; Kamath, TV; L'Italien, GJ; Pio, JR; Williams, JR. Impact of the metabolic syndrome on mortality from coronary heart disease, cardiovascular disease, and all causes in United States adults. *Circulation*, 2004, 110, 1245-1250.

[123] Isomaa, B; Almgren, P; Tuomi, T; Forsen, B; Lahti, K; Nis, M; Taskinen, MR; Groop L. Cardiovascular morbidity and mortality associated with the metabolic syndrome. *Diabetes Care*, 2001, 24, 683-689.

[124] Girman, CJ; Rhodes, T; Mercuri, M; Pyorala, K; Kjeskhus, J; Pedersen, TR; Beere, PA; Gotto, AM; Clarfield, M. 4S Group and the AFCAPS/TexCAPS Research Group. The metabolic syndrome and risk of major coronary events in the Scandinavian Simvastatin Survival Study (4S) and the Air Force/Texas Coronary Atherosclerosis Prevention Study (AFCAPS/TexCAPS). *Am J Cardiol*, 2004, 93, 136-141.

[125] Simons, LA; Simons, J; Friedlander, Y; McCallum, J. Does a diagnosis of the metabolic syndrome provide additional prediction of cardiovascular disease and total mortality in the elderly? The Dubbo Study. *Med J Aust*, 2007, 186, 400-403.

[126] Lanz, JR; Pereira, AC; Martinez, E; Krieger, JE. Metabolic syndrome and coronary artery disease: is there a gender specific effect? *Int J Cardiol*, 2006, 107, 317-321.

[127] Han, TS; Sattar, N; Williams, K; Gonzales-Villalpando, C; Lean, ME; Haffner, SM. Prospective study of C-reactive protein in relation to the development of diabetes and metabolic syndrome in the Mexico City Diabetes Study. *Diabetes Care*, 2002, 25, 2016-2021.

[128] Lakka, HM; Laaksonen, DE; Lakka, TA; Niskanen, LK; Kumpusalo, E; Toumilehto, J; Salonen, JT. The metabolic syndrome and total and cardiovascular disease mortality in middle-aged men. *JAMA*, 2002, 288, 2709-2716.

[129] Fan, AZ; Dwyer, JH. Sex differences in the relation of HDL cholesterol to progression of carotid intima-media thickness: The Los Angeles Atherosclerosis Study. *Atherosclerosis*, 2007, 195, e191-196.

[130] Sundstrom, J; Riserus, U; Byberg, L; Zethelius, B; Lithell, H; Lind, L. Clinical value of the metabolic syndrome for long term prediction of total and cardiovascular mortality: prospective; population based cohort study. *Br Med J*, 2006, 2, 878-882.

[131] McNeill, AM; Katz, R; Girman, CJ; Rosamond, WD; Wagenknecht, LE; Barzilay, JL; Tracy, RP; Savage, PJ; Jackson, SA. Metabolic syndrome and cardiovascular disease in older people: The cardiovascular health study. *J Am Geriatr Soc*, 2006, 54, 1317-1324.

[132] Steinbaum, SR. The metabolic syndrome: an emerging health epidemic in women. *Prog Cardiovasc Dis*, 2004, 46, 321-336.

[133] Onat, A; Ceyhan, K; Basar, O; Erer, B; Sansoy, V. Metabolic syndrome: major impact on coronary risk in a population with low cholesterol levels – a prospective and cross-sectional evaluation. *Atherosclerosis*, 2002, 165, 285-292.

[134] Williams, JW; Zimmet, PZ; Shaw, JE; de Courten, MP; Cameron, AJ; Chitson, P; Tuomilehto, J; Alberti, KG. Gender differences in the prevalence of impaired fasting glycaemia and impaired glucose tolerance in Mauritius. Does sex matter? *Diabet Med*, 2003, 20, 915-920.

[135] Dallongeville J; Cottel D; Arveiler D; Tauber JP; Bingham A; Wagner A; Fauvel J; Ferrieres J; Ducimetiere P; Amouyel P. The association of metabolic disorders with the metabolic syndrome is different in men and women. *Ann Nutr Metab*, 2004;48(1): 43-50.

[136] Wajchenberg, BL. Subcutaneous and visceral adipose tissue: their relation to the metabolic syndrome. *Endocr Rev*, 2000, 21, 697-738.

[137] Rathmann, W; Haastert, B; Icks, A; Lowel, H; Meisinger, C; Holle, R; Giani G. High prevalence of undiagnosed diabetes mellitus in Southern Germany: target populations for efficient screening. The KORA survey 2000. *Diabetologia*, 2003, 46, 182-189.

[138] Zhu, S; St-Onge, MP; Heshka, S; Heymsfield, SB. Lifestyle behaviors associated with lower risk of having the metabolic syndrome. *Metabolism*, 2004, 53, 1503-1511.

[139] Loucks, EB; Rehkopf, DH; Thurston, RC; Kawachi, I. Socioeconomic disparities in metabolic syndrome differ by gender: evidence from NHANES III. *Ann Epidemiol*, 2007, 17, 19-26.

[140] Regitz-Zagrosek, V; Lehmkuhl, E; Weickert, MO. Gender differences in the metabolic syndrome and their role for cardiovascular disease. *Clin Res Cardiol*, 2006, 95, 136-147.

[141] Tong, W; Lai, H; Yang, C; Ren, S; Dai, S; Lai, S. Age; gender and metabolic syndrome-related coronary heart disease in U.S. adults. *Int J Cardiol*, 2005, 104, 288-291.

[142] Hong, Y; Jin, X; Mo, J; Lin, HM; Duan, Y; Pu M; Welbrette DL; Liao D. Metabolic syndrome, its preeminent clusters, incident coronary heart disease and all-cause mortality – results of prospective analysis for the Atherosclerosis Risk in Communities study. *J Intern Med*, 2007, 262, 113-122.

[143] The DECODE Study Group. Glucose tolerance and mortality: comparison of WHO and American Diabetes Association diagnostic criteria. *Lancet*, 1999, 354, 617-621.

[144] The DECODE Study Group. Comparison of different definitions of the metabolic syndrome in relation to cardiovascular mortality in European men and women. *Diabetologia*, 2006, 49, 2837-2846.

[145] Jacobs, DR Jr; Mebane, IL; Bangdiwala, SI; Criqui, MH; Tyroler, HA. High density lipoprotein cholesterol as a predictor of cardiovascular disease mortality in men and women: the follow-up study of the Lipid Research Clinics Prevalence Study. *Am J Epidemiol*, 1990, 131, 32-47.

[146] Austin, MA; Hokanson, JE; Edwards KL. Hypertriglyceridemia as a cardiovascular risk factor. *Am J Cardiol*, 1998, 81, 7B-12B.

[147] Gregg, EW; Qiuping, G; Cheng, YJ; Narayan, KMV; Cowie, CC. Mortality trends in men and women with diabetes, 1971-2000. *Ann Intern Med*, 2007, 147, 149-155.

[148] Williams, K; Hazuda, HP; Stern, MP; Haffner, SM. The metabolic syndrome and the impact of diabetes on coronary heart disease mortality in women and men: The San Antonio Study. *Ann Epidemiol*, 2007, 17, 870-877.

[149] Barrett-Connor, E; Cohn, BA; Wingard, DL; Edelstein, SL. Why is diabetes mellitus a stronger risk factor for fatal ischemic heart disease in women than in men? The Rancho Bernardo Study. *JAMA,* 1991, 265, 627-631.

[150] McNamara, JR; Campos, H; Ordovas, JM; Peterson, J; Wilson, PW; Schaefer, EJ. Effect of gender, age, and lipid status on low density lipoprotein subfraction distribution: results from the Framingham Offspring Study. *Arteriosclerosis,* 1987, 7, 483-490.

[151] Nikkila, M; Pitkajarvi, T; Koivula, T; Solakivi, T; Lehtimaki, T; Laippala, P; Jokela, H; Lehtomaki, E; Seppa, K; Sillanaukee, P. Women have a larger and less atherogenic low density lipoprotein particle size than men. *Atherosclerosis,* 1996, 119, 181-190.

[152] Kwiterovich, PO. Clinical relevance of the biochemical; metabolic; and genetic factors that influence low-density lipoprotein heterogeneity. *Am J Cardiol*, 2002, 90, 30i-47i.

[153] Ferrara, A; Barrett-Connor, E; Wingard, DL; Edelstein, SL. Sex differences in insulin levels in older adults and the effect of body size; estrogen replacement therapy; and glucose tolerance status: the Rancho Bernardo Study; 1984-1987. *Diabetes Care,* 1995, 18, 220-225.

[154] Welborn, TA; Knuiman, MW; Ward, N; Whittall, DE. Serum insulin is a risk marker for coronary heart disease mortality in men but not in women. *Diabetes Res Clin Pract,* 1994, 26, 51-59.

[155] Ferrara, A; Barrett-Connor, E; Edelstein, SL. Hyperinsulinemia does not increase the risk of fatal cardiovascular disease in elderly men or women without diabetes: the Rancho Bernardo Study, 1984-1991. *Am J Epidemiol,* 1994, 140, 857-869.

[156] Onat, A; Hergenc, G; Keles, I; Dogan, Y; Turkmen, S; Sansoy, V. Sex difference in development of diabetes and cardiovascular disease on the way from obesity and metabolic syndrome. *Metabolism,* 2005, 54, 800-808.

[157] Kawamoto, R; Tomita, H; Inoue, A; Ohtsuka, N; Kamitani, A. Metabolic syndrome may be a risk factor for early carotid atherosclerosis in women but not in men. *J Atheroscler Thromb,* 2007, 14, 36-43.

[158] Iglseder, B; Cip, P; Malaimare, L; Ladurner, G; Paulweber, B. The metabolic syndrome is a stronger risk factor for early carotid atherosclerosis in women than in men. *Stroke,* 2005, 36, 1212-1217.

[159] Skilton, MR; Moulin, P; Serusclat, A; Nony, P; Bonnet, F. A comparison of the NCEP-ATPIII; IDF and AHA/NHLBI metabolic syndrome definitions with relation to early carotid atherosclerosis in subjects with hypercholesterolemia or at risk of CVD: evidence for sex-specific differences. *Atherosclerosis,* 2007, 190, 416-422.

[160] Dokras, A; Bochner, M; Hollinrake, E; Markham, S; Vanvoorhis, B; Jagasia, DH. Screening women with polycystic ovary syndrome for metabolic syndrome. *Obstet Gynecol,* 2005, 106, 131-137.

[161] Ehrmann, DA; Liljenquist, DR; Kasza, K; Azziz, R ; Legro, RS ; Ghazzi, MN; PCOS/Troglitazone Study Group. Prevalence and predictors of the metabolic syndrome in women with polycystic ovary syndrome. *J Clin Endocrinol Metab,* 2006, 91, 48-53.

[162] Coviello, AD; Legro, RS; Dunaif, A. Adolescent girls with polycystic ovary syndrome have an increased risk of the metabolic syndrome associated with increasing androgen levels independent of obesity and insulin resistance. *J Endocrinol Metab,* 2006, 91, 492-497.

[163] Reaven, GM. Banting lecture 1988. Role of insulin resistance in human disease. *Diabetes,* 1988, 37, 1595-1607.

[164] Harris, ML. Epidemiology of diabetes mellitus among the elderly in the United States. *Clin Geriatr Med,* 1990, 6, 703-719.

[165] Field, AE; Cakley, EH; Must, A; Spadano, JL; Laird, N; Dietz, WH; Rimm, E; Colditz, GA. Impact of overweight on the risk of developing common chronic diseases during a 10-year period. *Arch Intern Med,* 2001, 161, 1581-1586.

[166] Must, A; Spadano, J; Coakley, EH; Field, AE; Colditz, G; Dietz, WH. The disease burden associated with overweight and obesity. *JAMA,* 1999, 282, 1523-1529.

[167] Folsom, AR; Kushi, LH; Hong, CP. Physical activity and incident diabetes mellitus in postmenopausal women. *Am J Public Health,* 2000, 90, 134-138.

[168] Knowler, WC; Barrett-Connor, E; Fowler, SE; Hamman, RF; Lachin, JM; Walker, EA; Nathan, DM; Diabetes Prevention Program Research Group. Reduction in the incidence of type 2 diabetes with lifestyle intervention or metformin. *N Engl J Med,* 2002, 346, 393-403.

[169] Haffner, SM. Epidemiology of type 2 diabetes: risk factors. *Diabetes Care,* 1998; Suppl 3:C3-6.

[170] Riserus, U; Arnlov, J; Berglund, L. Long-term predictors of insulin resistance: role of lifestyle and metabolic factors in middle-aged men. *Diabetes Care,* 2007, 30(11), 2928-2933.

[171] Haffner, SM. Management of dyslipidemia in adults with diabetes (technical review). *Diabetes Care*, 1998, 21, 160-178.

[172] Yamasa, T; Ikeda, S; Koga, S; Kawahara, E; Muroya, T; Shinboku, H; Kohno, S. Evaluation of glucose tolerance, post-prandial hyperglycemia and hyperinsulinemia influencing the incidence of coronary heart disease. *Intern Med*, 2007, 46, 543-546.

[173] Rader, DJ. Effect of insulin resistance; dyslipidemia; and intra-abdominal adiposity on the development of cardiovascular disease and diabetes mellitus. *Am J Med*, 2007, 120(Suppl 1), S12-8.

[174] Jørgen Jeppesen, J; Hansen, TW; Rasmussen, S; Ibsen, H; Torp-Pedersen, C; Madsbad, S. Insulin resistance; the metabolic sSyndrome, and risk of incident cardiovascular disease. *J Am Coll Cardiol*, 2007, 49, 2112-2119.

[175] Beckman, JA; Creager, MA; Libby, P. Diabetes and atherosclerosis: epidemiology; pathophysiology; and management. *JAMA*, 2002, 287, 2570-2581.

[176] Kannel, WB; McGee, DL: Diabetes and cardiovascular disease: the Framingham Study. *JAMA*, 1979, 241, 2035-2038.

[177] Fox, CS; Sullivan, L; D'Agostino, RB Sr; Wilson, PW. The significant effect of diabetes duration on coronary heart disease mortality: the Framingham Heart Study. *Diabetes Care* 2004, 27, 704-708.

[178] Almdal, T; Scharling H; Jensen, JS; Vestergaard, H. The independent effect of type 2 diabetes mellitus on ischemic heart disease, stroke, and death: a population-based study of 13,000 men and women with 20 years of follow-up. *Arch Intern Med*, 2004, 164, 1422-1426.

[179] Vaccaro, O; Eberly, LE; Neaton, JD; Yang, L; Riccardi, G; Stamler, J; Multiple Risk Factor Intervention Trial Research Group. Impact of diabetes and previous myocardial infarction on long-term survival: 25-year mortality follow-up of primary screenees of the Multiple Risk Factor Intervention Trial. *Arch Intern Med*, 2004, 164, 1438-1443.

[180] Held, C; Gerstein, HC; Yusuf, S; Zhao, F; Hilbrich, L; Anderson, C; Sleight, P; Teo, K; for the ONTARGET/TRANSCEND Investigators. Glucose Levels Predict Hospitalization for Congestive Heart Failure in Patients at High Cardiovascular Risk. *Circulation*, 2007, 115, 1371-1375.

[181] Tierney, EF; Geiss, LS; Engelgau, MM; Thompson, TJ; Schaubert, D; Shireley, LA; Vukelic, PJ; McDonough SL. Population-based estimates of mortality associated with diabetes: use of a death certificate check box in North Dakota. *Am J Public Health*, 2001, 91, 84-92.

[182] Lee, WL; Cheung, AM; Cape, D; Zinman, B. Impact of diabetes on coronary artery disease in women and men: a meta-analysis of prospective studies. *Diabetes Care*, 2000, 23, 962-968.

[183] Goldschmid, MG; Barrett-Connor, E; Edelstein, SL; Wingard, DL; Cohn, BA; Herman, WH. Dyslipidemia and ischemic heart disease mortality among men and women with diabetes. *Circulation*, 1994, 89, 991-997.

[184] Seeman, T; Mendes de Leon, C; Berkman, L; Ostfeld, A. Risk factors for coronary heart disease among older men and women: a prospective study of community-dwelling elderly. *Am J Epidemiol*, 1993, 138, 1037-1049.

[185] Barrett-Connor, EL; Cohn, BA; Wingard, DL; Edelstein, SL. Why is diabetes mellitus a stronger risk factor for fatal ischemic heart disease in women than in men? The Rancho Bernardo Study. *J Am Med Assoc*, 1992, 265, 627-631.

[186] Haffner, SM; Valdez, RA; Morales, PA; Hazuda, HP; Stern, MP. Decreased sex hormone-binding globulin predicts non-insulin dependent diabetes mellitus in women but not in men. *J Clin Endocrinol Metab*, 1993, 77, 56-60.

[187] Howard, BV; Cowan, LD; Go, O; Welty, TK; Robbins, DC; Lee, ET; the Strong Heart Investigators. Adverse effects of diabetes on multiple cardiovascular disease risk factors in women. *Diabetes Care*, 1998, 21, 1258-1265.

[188] Juutilainen, A; Kortelainen, S; Lehto, S. Gender difference in the impact of type 2 diabetes on coronary heart disease risk. *Diabetes Care*, 2004, 27, 2898-2904.

[189] Avogaro, A; Giorda, C; Maggini, M; Mannucci E; Raschetti, R; Lombardo, F; Spila-Alegiani, S; Turco, S; Velussi, M; Ferrannini, E; Diabetes and Informatics Study Group, Association of Clinical Diabetologists, Istituto Superiore di Sanita. Incidence of coronary heart disease in type 2 diabetic men and women: impact of microvscular complications, treatment, and geographic location. *Diabetes Care*, 2007, 30, 1241-1247.

[190] Kannel, WB; McGee, DL. Update on some epidemiologic features of intermittent claudication: the Framingham Study. *J Am Geriatr Soc*, 1985, 33, 13-18.

[191] Kuusisto, J; Mykkanen, L; Pyorala, K; Laakso, M. Non-insulin-dependent diabetes and its metabolic control are important predictors of stroke in elderly subjects. *Stroke*, 1994, 25, 1157-1164.

[192] Sowers, JR. Diabetes mellitus and cardiovascular disease in women. *Arch Intern Med*, 1998, 158, 617-621.

[193] Huxley, R; Barzi, F; Woodward, M. Excess risk of fatal coronary heart disease associated with diabetes in men and women: meta-analysis of 37 prospective cohort studies. *BMJ*, 2006, 332, 73-78.

[194] Hu, FB; Stampfer, MJ; Solomon, CG; Liu, S; Willett, WC; Speizer, FE; Nathan, DM; Manson, JE. The impact of diabetes mellitus on mortality from all causes and coronary heart disease in women. *Arch Intern Med*, 2001, 161, 1717-1723.

[195] Natarajan, S; Liao, Y; Cao, G; Lipsitz, SR; McGee, DL. Sex differences in risk for coronary heart disease mortality associated with diabetes and established coronary heart disease. *Arch Intern Med*, 2003, 163, 1735-1740.

[196] Gu, K; Cowie, CC; Harris, MI. Diabetes and decline in heart disease mortality in US adults. *JAMA*, 1999, 281, 1291-1297.

[197] Wenger, NK. Heightened cardiovascular risk in diabetic women: Can the tide be turned? *Ann Int Med*, 2007, 147, 208-210.

[198] Chou, AF; Scholle, SH; Weisman, CS; Bierman, AS; Correa-de-Araujo, R; Mosca, L. Gender disparities in the quality of cardiovascular disease care in private managed care plans. *Womens Health Issues*, 2007, 17, 120-130.

[199] Chou, AF; Wong, L; Weisman, CS; Chan, S; Bierman, AS; Correa-de-Araujo R; Scholle SH. Gender disparities in cardiovascular disease care among commercial and medicare managed care plans. *Womens Health Issues*, 2007, 17, 139-149.

[200] Kanaya, AM; Grady, D; Barrett-Connor, E. Explaining the sex difference in coronary heart disease mortality among patients with type 2 diabetes mellitus: a meta-analysis. *Arch Intern Med*, 2002, 162, 1737-1745.

[201] Hong, SC; Yoo, SW; Cho, GJ; Kim, T; Hur, JY; Park, YK; Lee, KW; Kim, SH. Correlation between estrogens and serum adipocytokines in premenopausal and postmenopausal women. *Menopause*, 2007, 14, 1-6.

[202] Borissova, AM; Tankova;,T; Kamenova, P; Dakovska, L; Kovacheva, R; Kirilov, G; Genov, N; Milcheva, B; Koev, D. Effect of hormone replacement therapy on insulin secretion and insulin sensitivity in postmenopausal diabetic women. *Gynecol Endocrinol*, 2002, 16, 67-74.

[203] Holmang, A; Larsson, BM; Brzezinska, Z; Bjorntorp, P. The effects of short term testosterone exposure on insulin sensitivity in female rats. *Am J Physiol*, 1992, 262, E851-E855.

[204] Perello, M; Castrogiovanni, D; Giovambattista, A; Gaillard, RC; Spinedi, E. Impairment in insulin sensitivity after early androgenization in the post-pubertal female rat. *Life Sci*, 2007, 80, 1792-1798.

[205] Choi, BG; McLaughlin, MA. Why men's heart break: cardiovascular effects of sex steroids. *Endocrinol Metab Clin North Am*, 2007, 36, 365-377.

[206] Oh, JY; Barrett-Connor, E; Wedick, NM; Wingard, DL; Rancho Bernardo Study. Endogenous sex hormones and the development of type 2 diabetes in older men and women: the Rancho Bernardo study. *Diabetes Care*, 2002, 25, 55-60.

[206a] Nishizawa, H; Shimomura, I; Kishida, K; Maeda, N; Kuriyama, H; Nagaretani H; Matsuda, M; Kondo, H; Furuyama, N; Kihara, S; Nakamura, T; Tochino, Y; Funahashi, T; Matsuzawa, Y. Androgens decrease plasma adiponectin, an insulin-sensitizing adipocyte-derived protein. *Diabetes*, 2002, 51, 2734-2741.

[207] Gau, GT; Wright, RS. The role of inflammation in atherosclerosis. *Curr Prob Cardiol*, 2006, 31, 445-486.

[208] Glass, CK; Witztum, JL. Atherosclerosis: The road ahead. *Cell*, 2001, 104, 503-516.

[209] Martin, MJ; Browner, WS; Hulley, SB; Kuller, LH; Wentworth, D. Serum cholesterol, blood pressure and mortality: implications from a cohort of 361,662 men. *Lancet*, 1986, 2, 933-936.

[210] Stamler J; Wentworth D; Neaton JD. Is relationship between serum cholesterol and risk of premature death from coronary heart disease continuous and graded? Findings in 356,222 primary screenees of the Multiple Risk Factor Intervention Trial (MRFIT). *JAMA*, 1986, 256, 2823-2828.

[211] Law, MR; Wald, MJ; Thompson, SG. By how much and how quickly does reduction in serum cholesterol concentration lower risk of ischemic heart disease. *BMJ*, 1994, 308, 367-373.

[212] Holme, I. An analysis of randomized trials evaluating the effect of cholesterol reduction on total mortality and coronary heart disease incidence. *Circulation*, 1990, 82, 1916-1924.

[213] LaRosa, JC; Vupputuri, S. Effect of statins on risk of coronary disease: a meta-analysis of randomized controlled studies. *JAMA*, 1999, 282, 2340-6.

[214] Wilt, TJ; Bloomfield, HE; MacDonald, R; Nelson, D; Rutks, I; Ho, M; Larsen, G; McCall, A; Pineros, S; Sales, A Effectiveness of statin therapy in adults with coronary heart disease. *Arch Intern Med*, 2004, 164, 1427-1436.

[215] Grundy SM, Cleeman JI, Merz CN, Brewer HB Jr, Clark LT, Hunninghake DB, Pasternak RC, Smith SC Jr, Stone NJ; Coordinating Committee of the National Cholesterol Education Program. Implications of recent clinical trials for the National

Cholesterol Education Program Adult Treatment Panel III guidelines. *Arterioscler Thromb Vasc Biol*, 2004, 24, e149-e161.

[216] Sarwar, N; Danesh, J; Eiriksdottir, G; Sigurdsson, G; Wareham, N; Bingham, S; Boekholdt, SM; Khaw, KT; Gudnason, V. Triglycerides and the risk of coronary heart disease. *Circulation*, 2007, 115, 450-458.

[217] Cullen, P. Evidence that triglycerides are an independent coronary heart disease risk factor. *Am J Cardiol*, 2000, 86, 943-949.

[218] Bansal, S; Buring, JE; Rifai, N; Mora, S; Sacks, FM; Ridker, PM. Fasting compared with nonfasting triglycerides and risk of cardiovascular events in women. *JAMA*, 2007, 297, 309-316.

[219] Nordestgaard, BG; Benn, M; Schnohr, P; Tybjærg-Hansen, A. Nonfasting triglycerides and risk of myocardial infarction, ischemic heart disease, and death in men and women. *JAMA*, 2007, 297, 299-308.

[220] Grundy, SM. Hypertriglyceridemia, atherogenic dyslipidemia, and the metabolic syndrome. *Am J Cardiol*, 1998, 81, 18B-25B.

[221] Austin, MA. Plasma triglyceride and coronary heart disease. *Arterioscler Thromb*, 1991, 11, 2-14.

[222] Otvos, JD; Jeyarajah, EJ; Cromwell, WC. Measurement issues related to lipoprotein heterogeneity. *Am J Cardiol*, 2002, 90, 22i-29i.

[223] Howard, BV; Ruotolo, G; Robbins, DC. Obesity and dyslipidemia. *Endocrinol Metab Clin North Am,*, 2003, 32, 855-867.

[224] Marcovina, SM; Koschinsky, ML. A critical evaluation of the role of Lp(a) in cardiovascular disease: can Lp(a) be useful in risk assessment? *Semin Vasc Med*, 2002, 2, 335-344.

[225] Loscalzo, J; Weinfeld, M; Fless, GM; Scanu, AM. Lipoprotein (a), fibrin binding, and plasminogen activation. *Arteriosclerosis*, 1990, 10, 240-245.

[226] Cambillau M; Simon A; Amar J; Giral, P; Atger, V; Segond, P; Levenson, J; Merli, I; Megnien, JL; Plainfosse, MC; et al. Serum Lp(a) as a discriminant marker of early atherosclerotic plaque at three extracoronary sites in hypercholesterolemic men. *Arterioscler Thromb*, 1992, 12, 1346-1352.

[227] Stubbs, P; Seed, M; Lane, D; Collinson, P; Kendall, F; Noble, M. Lipoprotein(a) as a risk predictor for cardiac mortality in patients with acute coronary syndromes. *Eur Heart J* 1998, 19, 1355-1364.

[228] Bostom AG; Cupples LA; Jenner JL; Ordovas, JM; Seman, LJ; Wilson, PW; Schaefer, EJ; Castelli, WP. Elevated plasma lipoprotein(a) and coronary heart disease in men aged 55 years and younger: a prospective study. *JAMA*, 1996, 276, 544-548.

[229] Ridker, PM; Hennekens, CH; Stampfer, MJ. A prospective study of lipoprotein(a) and the risk of myocardial infarction. *JAMA*, 1993, 270, 2195-2199.

[230] Ridker, PM. Novel risk factors and markers for coronary disease. *Adv Intern Med*, 2000, 45, 391-418.

[231] Bittner, V. State of the art paper: perspectives on dyslipidemia and coronary heart disease in women. *J Am Coll Cardiol*, 2005, 46, 1628-1635.

[232] Bittner, V. Perspectives on dyslipidemia and coronary heart disease in women: an update. *Curr Opinion Cardiol*, 2006, 21, 602-607.

[233] Carroll, MD; Lacher, DA; Sorlie, PD; Cleeman, JI; Gordon, DJ; Wolz, M; Grundy, SM; Johnson CL. Trends in serum lipids and lipoproteins of adults, 1960-2002. *JAMA*, 2000, 294, 1773-1781.

[234] Brown SA; Hutchinson R; Morrisett J; Boerwinkle, E; Davis, CE; Gotto, AM Jr; Patsch W. Plasma lipid, lipoprotein cholesterol, and apoprotein distributions in selected US communities. The Atherosclerosis Risk in Communities (ARIC) Study. *Arterioscler Thromb*, 1993, 13, 1139-1158.

[235] Laurier, D; Chau, NP and Segond, P. Cholesterol and other cardiovascular risk factors in a working population in Ile-de-France (France): first results of the PCV-METRA study. *Eur J Epidemiol*, 1992, 8, 693-701.

[236] Mittendorfer, B; Horowitz, JF; Klein, S. Gender differences in lipid and glucose kinetics during short-term fasting. *Am J Physiol Endocrinol Metab*, 2001, 281, E1333-E1339.

[237] Mittendorfer, B. Sexual dimorphism in human lipid metabolism. *J Nutr*, 2005, 135, 681-686.

[238] Mittendorfer, B; Patterson, BW; Klein, S. Effect of sex and obesity on basal VLDL-triacylglycerol kinetics. *Am J Clin Nutr*, 2003, 77, 573-579.

[239] Magkos, F; Patterson, BW; Mohammed, BS; Klein, S; Mittendorfer, B. Women produce fewer but triglyceride-richer very low-density lipoproteins than men. *J Clin Endocrinol Metab*, 2007, 92, 1311-1318.

[240] Kuhn, FE; Rackley, CE. Coronary artery disease in women. Risk factors; evaluation; treatment; and prevention. *Arch Intern Med*, 1993, 153, 2626-2636.

[241] Abbey, M; Owen, A; Suzakawa, M; Roach, P; Nestel, PJ. Effects of menopause and hormone replacement therapy on plasma lipids; lipoproteins and LDL-receptor activity. *Maturitas*, 1999, 33, 259-269.

[242] Downs, JR; Clearfield, M; Weis, S; Whitney, E; Shapiro, DR; Beere, PA; Langendorfer, A; Stein, EA; Kruyer, W; Gotto, AM Jr. Primary prevention of acute coronary events with lovastatin in men and women with average cholesterol levels: results of AFCAPS/TexCAPS. Air Force/Texas Coronary Atherosclerosis Prevention Study. *JAMA*, 1998, 279, 1615-1622.

[243] Miettinen, TA; Pyorala K; Olsson AG; Musliner, TA; Cook, TJ; Faergeman, O; Berg, K; Pedersen T, Kjekshus J. Cholesterol-lowering therapy in women and elderly patients with myocardial infarction or angina pectoris: findings from the Scandinavian Simvastatin Survival Study (4S). *Circulation* 1997, 96, 4211-4218.

[244] Randomised trial of cholesterol lowering in 4444 patients with coronary heart disease: the Scandinavian Simvastatin Survival Study (4S). *Lancet, 1994*, 19, 1383-1389.

[245] Jensen, J; Nilas, L; Christiansen, C. Influence of menopause on serum lipids and lipoproteins. *Maturitas*, 1990, 12, 321-331.

[246] Matthews KA; Meilahn E; Kuller LH; Kelsey, SF; Caggiula, AW; Wing RR. Menopause and risk factors for coronary heart disease. *New Engl J Med*, 1989, 321, 641-646.

[247] LaRosa, JC. Lipids and cardiovascular disease: do the findings and therapy apply equally to men and women? *Womens Health Issues*, 1992, 2, 102-111.

[248] Manolio, TA; Pearson, TA; Wenger, NK; Barrett-Connor, E; Payne, GH; Harlan, WR. Cholesterol and heart disease in older persons and women: review of an NHLBI workshop. *Ann Epidemiol, 199*2, 161-176.

[249] Austin, MA; Hokanson, JE; Edwards, KL. Hypertriglyceridemia as a cardiovascular risk factor. *Am J Cardiol*, 1998, 81, 7B-12B.

[250] Stensvold, I; Tverdal, A; Urdal, P; Graff-Iversen, S. Non-fasting serum triglyceride concentration and mortality from coronary heart disease and any cause in middle aged Norwegian women. *BMJ*, 1993, 307, 1318-1322

[251] Ikenoue, N; Wakatsuki, A; Okatami, Y. Small low-density lipoprotein particles in women with natural or surgically induced menopause. *Obstet Gynecol*, 1999, 93, 566-570.

[252] Nabeno, Y; Fukuchi, Y; Matsutani, Y; Naito, M. Influence of aging and menopause on postprandial lipoprotein responses in healthy adult women. *J Atheroscler Thromb*, 2007, 14, 142-150.

[253] Scanu, AM; Lawn, RM; Berg, K. Lipoprotein(a) and atherosclerosis. *Ann Intern Med*, 1991, 115, 209-218.

[254] Sunayama S; Daida H; Mokuno H; Miyano, H; Yokoi, H; Lee, YJ; Sakurai, H; Yamaguchi, H. Lack of increased coronary atherosclerotic risk due to elevated lipoprotein(a) in women ≥55 years of age. *Circulation*, 1996, 94, 1263-1268.

[255] Brown, SA; Morrisett, JD; Boerwinkle, E; Hutchinson, R; Patsch, W. The relation of lipoprotein(a) concentrations and apolipoprotein(a) phenotypes with asymptomatic atherosclerosis in subjects of the Atherosclerosis Risk in Communities (ARIC) Study. *Arterioscler Thromb*, 1993, 13, 1558-1566.

[256] Wild, SH; Fortmann, SP; Marcovina, SM. A prospective case-control study of lipoprotein(a) levels and apo(a) size and risk of coronary heart disease in Stanford Five-City Project participants. *Arterioscler Thromb Vasc Biol*, 1997, 17, 239-245.

[257] Seman LJ; de Luca C; Ordovas JM; Wilson, PWF; Cupples, LA; Schaefer, EJ. Lipoprotein(a)-cholesterol compared with sinking prebeta lipoprotein and associated relative risk of heart disease in the Framingham Heart Study. *Circulation, 1996*, 96(Suppl), I-304.

[258] Ariyo, AA; Thach, C; Tracy, R. Lp(a) Lipoprotein, vascular disease, and mortality in the elderly. *New Engl J Med*, 2003, 349, 2108-2115.

[259] Ross, R. Atherosclerosis – an inflammatory disease. *N Engl J Med*, 1999, 340, 115-126.

[260] Libby, P; Ridker, PM; Maseri, A. Inflammation and atherosclerosis. *Circulation.*, 2002, 105, 1135-1143.

[261] Libby, P. Inflammation in atherosclerosis. *Nature*, 2002, 321, 199-204.

[262] Fan, J; Watanabe, T. Inflammatory reactions in the pathogenesis of atherosclerosis. *J Atheroscler Thromb*, 2003, 10, 63-71.

[263] Nakajima, K; Nakano, T; Tanaka, A. The oxidative modification hypothesis of atherosclerosis: the comparison of atherogenic effects on oxidized LDL and remnant lipoproteins in plasma. *Clin Chim Acta*, 2006, 367, 36-47.

[264] Jacobs, M; Plane, F; Bruckdorfer, KR. Native and oxidized low-density lipoproteins have different inhibitory effects on endothelium-derived relaxing factor in the rabbit aorta. *Br J Pharmacol*, 1990, 100, 21-26.

[265] Schönbeck, U; Libby, P. The CD40/CD154 receptor/ligand dyad. *Cell Mol Life Sci*, 2001, 58, 4-43.

[266] Cai, H; Harrison, DG. Endothelial dysfunction in cardiovascular diseases: the role of oxidant stress. *Circ Res,* 2000, 87, 840-844.

[267] Esposito, K; Ciotola, M; Giugliano, D. Meditarranean diet, endothelial function and vascular inflammatory markers. *Public Health Nutr*, 2006, 9, 1073-1076.

[268] Poredos, S. Endothelial dysfunction and cardiovascular disease. *Pathophysiol Haemost Thromb*, 2002, 32, 274-277.

[269] Sattar, N; Gaw, A; Scherbakova, O; Ford, I; O'Reilly, DS; Haffner, SM; Isles, C; Macfarlane, PW; Packard, CJ; Cobbe, SM; Shepherd, J. Metabolic syndrome with and without C-reactive protein as a predictor of coronary heart disease and diabetes in the West of Scotland Coronary Prevention Study. *Circulation*, 2003, 108, 414-419.

[270] Ridker, PM; Buring, JE; Cook, NR; Rifai, N. C-reactive protein, the metabolic syndrome, and risk of incident cardiovascular events: An 8-year follow-up of 14,719 initially healthy American women. *Circulation*, 2003, 107, 391-397.

[271] Rutter, MK; Meigs, JB; Sullivan, LM; D'Agostino, RB Sr; Wilson, PW. C-reactive protein; the metabolic syndrome; and prediction of cardiovascular events in the Framingham Offspring Study. *Circulation*, 2004, 110, 380-385.

[272] Ridker PM; Hennekens CH; Buring JE; Rifai, N. C-reactive protein and other markers of inflammation in the prediction of cardiovascular disease in women. *N Engl J Med*, 2000, 342, 836-843.

[273] Ridker, PM; Buring, JE; Rifai, N. Soluble P-selectin and the risk of future cardiovascular events. *Circulation*, 2001, 103, 491-495.

[274] Ridker, PM; Stampfer, MJ; Rifai, N. Novel risk factors for systemic atherosclerosis: a comparison of C-reactive protein, fibrinogen, homocysteine, lipoprotein(a), and standard cholesterol screening as predictors of peripheral arterial disease. *JAMA*, 2001, 285, 2481-2485.

[275] Pearson ,TA; Mensah, GA; Alexander, RW; Anderson, J; Cannon, RO 3rd; Criqui, M; Fadl, YY; Fortmann, SP; Hong, Y; Myers, GL; Rifai, N; Smith, SC Jr; Taubert, K; Tracy, RP; Vinicor, F; Centers for Disease Control and Prevention; American Heart Association. Centers for Disease Control and Prevention. American Heart Association. Markers of inflammation and cardiovascular disease: application to clinical and public health practice: A statement for healthcare professionals from the Centers for Disease Control and Prevention and the American Heart Association. *Circulation*, 2003, 107, 499-511.

[276] Mayer, L; Jacobsen, DW; Robinson, K. Homocysteine and coronary atherosclerosis. *J Am Coll Cardiol*, 1996, 27, 517-27.

[277] Graham, IM; Daly, LE; Refsum, HM; Robinson, K; Brattström, LE; Ueland, PM; Palma-Reis, RJ; Boers, GH; Sheahan, RG; Israelsson, B; Uiterwaal, CS; Meleady, R; McMaster, D; Verhoef, P; Witteman, J; Rubba, P; Bellet, H; Wautrecht, JC; de Valk, HW; Sales Lúis, AC; Parrot-Rouland, FM; Tan, KS; Higgins, I; Garcon, D; Andria, G; et al. Plasma homocysteine as a risk factor for vascular disease: The European Concerted Action Project. *JAMA*, 1997, 277, 2743-2748.

[278] Loscalzo, J. The oxidant stress of hyperhomocyst(e)inemia. *J Clin Invest*, 1996, 98, 5-7.

[279] Jin, L; Caldwell, RB; Li-Masters, T; Caldwell, RW. Homocysteine induces endothelial dysfunction via inhibition of arginine transport. *J Physiol Pharmacol*, 2007, 58, 191-206.

[280] Pulvirenti D; Signorelli S; Sciacchitano S; Di Pino, L; Tsami, A; Ignaccolo, L; Neri, S.U.O. di Medicina Interna. Hyperhomocysteinemia; oxidative stress; endothelial dysfunction in postmenopausal women. *Clin Ter*, 2007, 158, 231-237.

[281] Powers, RW; Majors, AK; Lykins, DL; Sims, CJ; Lain, KY; Roberts, JM. Plasma homocysteine and malondialdehyde are correlated in an age- and gender- specific manner. *Metabolism*, 2002, 51, 1433-1438.

[282] Clarke, R; Armitage, J. Vitamin supplements and cardiovascular risk: review of the randomized trials of homocysteie-lowering vitamin supplements. *Semin Thromb Hemostat*, 2000, 26, 341-348.

[283] Ridker, PM; Cushman, M; Stampfer, MJ; Tracy, RP ; Hennekens, CH. Inflammation; aspirin, and the risk of cardiovascular disease in apparently healthy men. *New Engl J Med*, 1997, 336, 973-979.

[284] Ridker, PM; Glynn, RJ; Hennekens, CH. C-reactive protein adds to the predictive value of total and HDL cholesterol in determining risk of first myocardial infarction. *Circulation*, 1998, 97, 2007-2011.

[285] Ridker, PM; Buring, JE; Shih, J; Matias, M; Hennekens, CH. Prospective study of C-reactive protein and the risk of future cardiovascular events among apparently healthy women. *Circulation,* 1998, 98, 731-733.

[286]   Tracy, RP; Lemaitre, RN; Psaty, BM; Ives, DG; Evans, RW; Cushman, M; Meilahn, EN; Kuller, LH. Relationship of C-reactive protein to risk of cardiovascular disease in the elderly. Results from the Cardiovascular Health Study and the Rural Health Promotion Project. *Arterioscler Thromb Vasc Biol*, 1997, 17, 1121-1127.

[287] Nakanishi, N; Shiraishi, T; Wada, M. C-reactive protein concentration is more strongly related to metabolic syndrome in women than in men: the Minoh Study. *Circ J*, 2005, 69, 386-391.

[288]   Han, TS; Sattar, N; Williams, K; Gonzales-Villapando, C; Lean, ME; Haffner, SM. Prospective study of C-reactive protein in relation to the development of diabetes and metabolic syndrome in the Mexico City Diabetes Study. *Diabetes Care*, 2002, 25, 2016-2021.

[289] Fernandez-Real, JM; Broch, M; Vendrell, J; Ricart, W. Insulin resistance, inflammation, and serum fatty acid composition. *Diabetes Care*, 2003, 26,, 1362-1368.

[290] Burdge, GC; Calder, PC. Conversion of alpha-linoleic acid to longer-chain polyunsaturated fatty acids in human adults. *Reprod Nutr Dev*, 2005, 45, 581-597.

[291] Horrobin DF. Loss of delta-6-desaturase activity as a key factor in aging. *Med Hypotheses*, 1981, 7, 1211-1220.

[292] De Leo, V; la Marca, A; Morgante, G; Musacchio, MC; Luisi, S; Petraglia, F. Menopause, the cardiovascular risk factor homocysteine, and the effets of treatment. *Treat Endocrinol*, 2004, 3, 393-400.

[293] Rossi, GP; Maiolino, G; Seccia, TM; Burlina, A; Zavattiero, S; Cesari, M; Sticchi, D; Pedon, L; Zanchetta, M; Pessina, AC. Hyperhomocysteinemia predicts total and cardiovascular mortality in high-risk women. *J Hypertension,* 2006, 24, 851-859.

[294] Mueck, AO; Seeger, H. Biochemical markers surrogating on vascular effects of sex steroid hormones. *Gynecol Endocrinol,* 2006, 22, 163-173.

[295] Keys, A; Anderson, JT; Grande, F. Essential fatty acids, degree of unsaturation, and effect of corn oil on the serum cholesterol level in men. *Lancet*, 1957, 1, 66-68.

[296] Nicolosi, RJ. Dietary fat saturation effects on low-density-lipoprotein concentrations and metabolism in animal models. *Am J Clin Nutr*, 1997, 65, 1617S-1627S.

[297] Mensink, RP; Katan, MB. Effect of dietary fatty acids on serum lipids and lipoproteins: A meta-analysis of 27 trials. *Arterioscler Thromb*, 1992, 12, 911-919.

[298] Dayton, S; Pearce, ML; Hashimoto, S; Dixon, WJ; Tomiyasu, U. A controlled clinical diet of a diet high in unsaturated fat in preventing complications of atherosclerosis. *Circulation*, 1969, 40 (suppl II), 11-63.

[299] The Lipid Research Clinics Program. The Lipid Research Coronary Primary Prevention Trial.1. Reduction in incidence of coronary heart disease. *JAMA*, 1984, 251, 351-364.

[300] Manninen V; Elo O; Frick MH; Haapa, K; Heinonen, OP; Heinsalmi, P; Helo, P; Huttunen, JK; Kaitaniemi, P; Koskinen, P; et al. Lipid alterations and decline in the incidence of coronary heart disease in the Helsinki Heart Study. *JAMA*, 1988, 260, 641-651.

[301] Keys, A; Anderson, JT; Grande F. Prediction of serum cholesterol responses of man to changes in fats in the diet. *Lancet*, 1957, 2, 959-966.

[302] Hegsted, DM; McGandy, RB; Myers, ML; Stare FJ. Quantitative effects of dietary fat on serum cholesterol in man. *Am J Clin Nutr,* 1965, 17, 281-295.

[303] Keys, A; Anderson, JT; Grande, F. Serum cholesterol response to changes in the diet. *Metabolism*, 1965, 14, 747-758.

[304] Hegsted, DM. Serum-cholesterol response to dietary cholesterol: a re-evaluation. *Am J Clin Nutr,* 1986, 44, 299-305.

[305] Stamler, J; Shekelle, R. Dietary cholesterol and human coronary heart disease. The epidemiologic evidence. *Arch Pathol Lab Med*, 1988, 112, 1032-1040.

[306] Clarke, R; Frost, C; Collins, R; Appleby, P; Peto, R. Dietary lipids and blood cholesterol: quantitative meta-analysis of metabolic ward studies. *BMJ,* 1997, 314, 112-117.

[307] Hu, FB; Stampfer, MJ; Manson, JE; Rimm, E; Colditz, GA; Rosner, BA; Hennekens, CH; Willett, WC. Dietary fat intake and the risk of coronary heart disease in women. *N Engl J Med*, 1997, 337, 1491-1499.

[308] Ascherio, A; Rimm, EB; Giovannucci, EL; Spiegelman, D; Stampfer, M; Willett, WC. Dietary fat and risk of coronary heart disease in men: Cohort follow up study in the United States. *BMJ*, 1996, 313, 84-90.

[309] Esrey, KL; Joseph, L; Grover, SA. Relationship between dietary intake and coronary heart disease mortality: Lipid research clinics prevalence follow-up study. *J Clin Epidemiol*, 1996, 49, 211-216.

[310] Pietinen, P; Ascherio, A; Korhonen, P; Hartman, AM; Willett, WC; Albanes, D; Virtamo, J. Intake of fatty acids and risk of coronary heart disease in a cohort of Finnish men. The alpha-tocopherol, beta-carotene cancer prevention study. *Am J Epidemiol*, 1997, 145, 876-887.

[311] Millen, BE; Franz, MM; Quatromoni, PA; Gagnon, DR; Sonnenberg, LM; Ordovas, JM; Wilson, PW; Schaefer, EJ; Cupples, LA. Diet and plasma lipids in women. Macronutrients and plasma total and low-density lipoprotein cholesterol in women: The Framingham nutrition studies. *J Clin Epidemiol*, 1996, 49, 657-663.

[312] Sonnenberg LM; Quatromoni PA; Gagnon DR; Cupples, LA; Franz, MM; Ordovas JM ; Wilson, PW; Schaefer, EJ; Millen, BE. Diet and plasma lipid in women. II. Macronutrients and plasma triglycerides, HDL and total to HDL cholesterol ratio in women. The Framingham Nutrition Studies. *Am J Epidemiol*, 1996, 49, 657-663.

[313] Dawber, TR; Nickerson, RJ; Brand, FN; Pool J. Eggs, serum cholesterol, and coronary heart disease. *Am J Clin Nutr*, 1982, 36, 617-625.

[314] Gramenzi, A; Gentile, A; Fasoli, M; Negri, E; Parazzini, F; La Vecchia, C. Association between certain foods and risk of acute myocardial infarction in women. *BMJ*, 1990, 300, 771-773.

[315] Fraser, GE. Diet and coronary heart disease: beyond dietary fats and low-density-lipoprotein cholesterol. *Am J Clin Nutr*, 1994, 59, 1117S-1123S.

[316] Hu, FB; Stampfer, MJ; Rimm, EB; Manson, JE; Ascherio, A; Colditz, GC; Rosner, BA; Spiegelman, D; Speizer, FE; Sacks, FM; Hennekens, CH; Willett, WC. A prospective study of egg consumption and risk of cardiovascular disease in men and women. *JAMA*, 1999, 281, 1387-1394.

[317] Weggemans, RM; Zock, PL; Katan, MB. Dietary cholesterol from eggs increases the ratio of total cholesterol to high-density lipoprotein cholesterol in humans: a meta-analysis. *Am J Clin Nutr*, 2001, 73, 885-891.

[318] Katan, MB; Beynen, AC. Characteristics of human hypo- and hyperresponders to dietary cholesterol. *Am J Epidemiol*, 1987, 125, 1032-1040.

[319] Ginsberg, HN; Karmally, W; Siddiqui, M; Holleran, S; Tall, AR; Blaner, WS; Ramakrishnan, R. Increases in dietary cholesterol are associated with modest increases in both LDL and HDL cholesterol in healthy young women. *Arterioscler Thromb Vasc Biol, 1995*, 15, 169-178.

[320] Ginsberg, HN; Karmally, W; Siddiqui, M; Holleran, S; Tall, AR; Rumsey, SC; Deckelbaum, RJ; Blaner, WS; Ramakrishnan, R. A dose-response study of the effects of dietary cholesterol on fasting and postprandial lipid and lipoprotein metabolism in healthy young men. *Arterioscler Thromb, 1994*, 14, 576-586.

[321] Esposito, K; Giugliano, D. Diet and inflammation: a link to metabolic and cardiovascular diseases. *Eur Heart J*, 2006, 27, 15-20.

[322] Esposito, K; Giugliano, D; Nappo, F; Marfella, R for the Campanian Postprandial Hyperglycaemia Study Group. Regression of carotid atherosclerosis by control of post-prandial hyperglycaemia in type 2 diabetes mellitus. *Circulation*, 2004, 110, 214-219.

[323] Ebenbichler, CF; Kirchmair, R; Egger, JR; Patsch, JR. Postprandial state and atherosclerosis. *Curr Opin Lipidol*, 1995, 6, 286-290.

[324] Nappo, F; Esposito, K; Cioffi, M; Giugliano, G; Molinari, AM; Paolisso, G; Marfella, R; Giugliano, D. Postprandial endothelial activation in healthy subjects and in type 2 diabetic patients: role of fat and carbohydrate meals. *J Am Coll Cardiol*, 2002, 39, 1145-1450.

[325] Pankow, JS; Duncam, BB; Schmidt, MI; Ballantyne, CM; Couper, DJ; Hoogeveen, RC; Golden, SH. Atherosclerotic Risk in Community Study. Fasting plasma free fatty acids and risk of type 2 diabetes: the atherosclerotic risk in community study. *Diabetes Care*, 2004, 27, 77-82.

[326] Meigs, JB; Hu, FB; Rifai, N; Manson, JE. Biomarkers of endothelial dysfunction and risk of type 2 diabetes mellitus. *JAMA*, 2004, 91, 1978-1986.

[327] Kromhout, D. Serum cholesterol in cross-cultural perspective. The Seven Countries Study. *Acta Cardiol*, 1999, 54, 155-158.

[328] Kromhout D; Menotti A; Bloemberg B; Aravanis, C; Blackburn, H; Buzina, R; Dontas, AS; Fidanza, F; Giampaoli, S; Jansen, A; et al. Dietary saturated and *trans* fatty acids and cholesterol and 25-year mortality from coronary heart disease: the Seven Countries Study. *Prev Med*, 1995, 24, 308-315.

[329] McGee, DL; Reed, DM; Yano, K; Kagan, A; Tillotson, J. Ten-year incidence of coronary heart disease in the Honolulu Heart Program: relationship to nutrient intake. *Am J Epidemiol*, 1984, 119, 667-676.

[330] Kushi, LH; Lew, RA; Stare, FJ; Ellison, CR; el Lozy, M; Bourke, G; Daly, L; Graham, I; Hickey, N; Mulcahy, R; et al. Diet and 20-year mortality from coronary heart disease: the Ireland-Boston Diet-Heart Study. *N Engl J Med,* 1985, 312, 811-818.

[331] Lichtenstein, AH; Ausman, LM; Jalbert, SM; Schaefer, EJ. Effects of different forms of dietary hydrogenated fats on serum lipoprotein cholesterol levels [published correction appears in *N Engl J Med*, 1999;341:856]. *N Engl J Med,* 1999; 340: 1933-1940.

[332] Lapointe, A; Couillard, C; Lemieux, S. Effects of dietary factors on oxidation of low-density lipoprotein particles. *J Biochem*, 2006, 17, 645-658.

[333] Matthan, NR; Welty, FK; Barrett, PH; Harausz, C; Dolnikowski, GG; Parks, JS; Eckel, RH; Schaefer, EJ; Lichtenstein, AH. Dietary hydrogenated fat increases high-density lipoprotein apoA-I catabolism and decreases low-density apoB-100 catabolism in hypercholesterolemic women. *Artrioscler Thromb Vasc Biol*, 2004, 24, 1092-1097.

[334] Dattilo, AM; Kris-Etherton, PM. Effects of weight reduction on blood lipids and lipoproteins: a meta-analysis. *Am J Clin Nutr*, 1992, 56, 320-328.

[335] Howard, BV; Ruotolo, G; Robbins, DC. Obesity and dyslipidemia. *Endocrinol Metab Clin North* Am, 2003, 32, 855-867.

[336] Millen, BE; Franz, Q; Quatromoni, PA; Gagnon, DR; Sonnenberg, LM; Ordovas, JM; Wilson, PW; Schaefer, EJ; Cupples, LA. Diet and plasma lipid in women. I. Macronutrients and plasma total and LDL cholesterol in women. The Framingham Nutrition Studies. *Am J Epidemiol*.1996, 49, 657-663.

[337] Sonnenberg, LM; Quatromoni, PA; Gagnon, DR; Cupples, LA; Franz, MM; Ordovas, JM; Wilson, PW; Schaefer, EJ; Millen, BE. Diet and plasma lipids in women. II. Macronutrients and plasma triglycerides; high-density lipoprotein; and the ratio of total to high-density lipoprotein cholesterol in women: the Framingham nutrition studies. *J Clin Epidemiol*, 1996, 49, 665-672.

[338] West, SG. Effect of diet on vascular reactivity: an emerging marker for vascular risk. *Curr Atheroscler Rep*, 2001, 3, 446-455.

[339] Goode, GK; Garcia, S; Heagerty, AM. Dietary supplementation with marine fish oil improves in vitro small artery endothelial function in hypercholesterolemic patients: a double-blind placebo-controlled study. *Circulation*, 1997, 96, 2802-2807.

[340] De Caterina, R. Endothelial dysfunctions: common denominators in vascular disease. *Curr Opin Clin Nutr Metab Care*, 2000, 3, 453-467.

[341] Browning, LM; Krebs, JD; Moore, CS; Mishra, JD; O'Connell, MA; Jebb, SA. The impact of long chain n-3 polyunsaturated fatty acid supplementation on inflammation; risk in a group of overweight women with an inflammatory phenotype. *Diabetes Obes Metab*, 2007, 9, 70-80.

[342] Lopez-Garcia, E; Schulze, MB; Manson, JE; Meigs, JB; Albert, CM; Rifai, N; Willett, WC. Consumption of (n-3) fatty acids is related to plasma biomarkers of inflammation and endothelial activation in women. *J Nutr*, 2004, 134, 1806-1811.

[343] Ciubotaru, I; Lee, YS; Wander, RC. Dietary fish oil decreases C-reactive protein; interleukin-6; and triacylglycerol to HDL-cholesterol ratio in postmenopausal women on HRT. *J Nutr Biochem*, 2003, 14, 513-21.

[344] Leren, P. The Oslo Diet-Heart Study: eleven-year report. *Circulation, 1970, 42,* 935-942.

[345] Frantz, ID Jr; Dawson, EA; Ashman, PL; Gatewood, LC; Bartsch, GE; Kuba, K; Brewer ER. Test of effect of lipid lowering by diet on cardiovascular risk: the Minnesota Coronary Survey. *Arteriosclerosis,* 1989;9:129-135.

[346] Burr, ML; Fehily, AM; Gilbert, JF; Rogers, S; Holliday, RM; Sweetnam, PM; Elwood PC; Deadman, NM. Effects of changes in fat, fish, and fibre intakes on death and myocardial reinfarction: Diet and Reinfarction Trial (DART). *Lancet,* 1989, 2, 757-761.

[347] Katan, MB; Zock, PL; Mensink RP. *Trans* fatty acids and their effects on lipoproteins in humans. *Annu Rev Nutr,* 1995, 15, 473-493.

[348] Alice H. Lichtenstein. Thematic review series: Patient-Oriented Research. Dietary fat; carbohydrate; and protein: effects on plasma lipoprotein patterns. *J Lipid Res,* 2006, 47, 1661-1667.

[349] Hu, FB; Willett, WC. Optimal diets for prevention of coronary heart disease. *JAMA,* 2002, 288, 2569-2578.

[350] Brenna, J T. Efficiency of conversion of alpha-linolenic acid to long chain n-3 fatty acids in man. *Curr Opin Clin Nutr Metab Care, 2002,* 5, 127-132.

[351] Albert, CM; Campos, H; Stampfer, MJ; Ridker, PM; Manson, JE; Willett, WC; Ma, J. Blood levels of long-chain n-3 fatty acids and the risk of sudden death. *N Engl J Med,* 2002, 346, 1113-1118.

[352] Erkkila, AT; Lichtenstein, AH; Mozaffarian, D; Herrington, DM. Fish intake is associated with a reduced progression of coronary artery atherosclerosis in postmenopausal women with coronary artery disease. *Am J Clin Nutr,* 2004, 80, 626-632.

[353] Mozaffarian, D; Gottdiener, JS; Siscovick, DS. Intake of tuna or other broiled or baked fish versus fried fish and cardiac structure; function; and hemodynamics. *Am J Cardiol,* 2006, 97, 216-222.

[354] GISSI, 1999. Dietary supplementation with n-3 polyunsaturated fatty acids and vitamin E after myocardial infarction: results of the GISSI-Prevenzione trial. Gruppo Italiano per lo Studio della Sopravvivenza nell'Infarto miocardico. *Lancet,* 1999, 354, 447-455.

[355] Kris-Etherton, PM; Harris, WS; Appel, LJ; Nutrition Committee. Fish consumption, fish oil, omega-3 fatty acids, and cardiovascular disease. *Circulation, 2002,* 106, 2747-2757.

[356] Wang; C; Chung, M; Balk, E; Kupelnick, B; Jordan, H; Harris W; Lichtenstein, A; Lau, J. N-3 Fatty acids from fish or fish-oil supplements; but not α-linolenic acid; benefit cardiovascular disease outcomes in primary- and secondary-prevention studies: a systematic review. *Am J Clin Nutr,* 2006, 83, 5-17.

[357] Balk, EM; Lichtenstein, AH; Chung, M; Kupelnick, B; Chew, P; Lau, J. Effects of omega-3 fatty acids on coronary restenosis; intima-media thickness; and exercise tolerance: a systematic review. *Atherosclerosis,* 2006, 184, 237-246.

[358] Hooper, L; Thompson, RL; Harrison, RA; Summerbell, CD; Ness, AR; Moore, HJ; Worthington, HV; Durrington, PN; Higgins, JP; Capps, NE; Riemersma RA, Ebrahim SB, Davey Smith G. Risks and benefits of omega 3 fats for mortality; cardiovascular disease; and cancer: systematic review. *BMJ,* 2006, 332, 752-760.

[359] Kang, JX; Leaf, A. Antiarrhythmic effects of polyunsaturated fatty acids: recent studies. *Circulation,* 1996, 94, 1774-1780.

[360] Connor, SL; Connor ,WE. Are fish oils beneficial in the prevention and treatment of coronary artery disease? *Am J Clin Nutr,* 1997, 66(4 suppl), 1020S-1031S.

[361] Simopoulos, AP. Evolutionary aspects of diet, essential fatty acids and cardiovascular disease. *Europ Heart J,* 2001, 3 (suppl D), D8-D21.

[362] Mita ,T; Watada, H; Ogihara, T; Nomiyama ,T; Ogawa, O; Kinoshita, J; Shimizu, T; Hirose, T; Tanaka, Y; Hirose, T. Eicosapentaenoic acid reduces the progression of carotid intima-media thickness in patients with type 2 diabetes. *Atherosclerosis,* 2007, 191, 162-167.

[363] Mensink, RP; Katan, MB. Effect of dietary trans fatty acids on high-density and low-density lipoprotein cholesterol levels in healthy subjects. *N Engl J Med,* 1990, 323, 439-445.

[364] Mensink, RP; Zock, PL; Kester, ADM; Katan, MB. Effects of dietary fatty acids and carbohydrates on the ratio of serum total to HDL cholesterol and on serum lipids and apolipoproteins: a meta-analysis of 60 controlled trials. *Am J Clin Nutr,* 2003, 77, 1146-1155.

[365] Joshipura, KJ; Hu, FB; Manson, JE. The effect of fruit and vegetable intake on risk for coronary heart disease. *Ann Intern Med,* 2001, 134, 1106 -1114.

[366] Dauchet, L; Amouyel, P; Hercberg, S; Dallongeville, J. Fruit and vegetable consumption and risk of coronary heart disease: a meta-analysis of cohort studies. *J Nutr,* 2006, 136, 2588-93.

[367] Jenkins, DJ; Popovich, DG; Kendall, CW. Effect of a diet high in vegetables; fruit; and nuts on serum lipids. *Metabolism,* 1997, 46, 530-537.

[368] Appel, LJ; Moore, TJ; Obarzanek, E; Vollmer, WM; Svetkey, LP; Sacks, FM; Bray, GA; Vogt, TM; Cutler, JA; Windhauser, MM; Lin, PH; Karanja, N. A clinical trial of the effects of dietary patterns on blood pressure. DASH Collaborative Research Group *N Engl J Med,* 1997, 336, 1117-1124.

[369] Rimm, EB; Willett, WC; Hu, FB; Sampson, L; Colditz, GA; Manson, JE; Hennekens, C; Stampfer, MJ. Folate and vitamin B_6 from diet and supplements in relation to risk of coronary heart disease among women. *JAMA,* 1998, 279, 359-364.

[370] Rimm, EB; Stampfer, MJ; Ascherio, A; Giovannucci, E; Colditz, GA; Willett, WC. Vitamin E consumption and the risk of coronary heart disease in men. *N Engl J Med,* 1993, 328, 1450-1456.

[371] Stampfer, MJ; Hennekens, CH; Manson, JE; Colditz, GA; Rosner, B; Willett, WC. Vitamin E consumption and the risk of coronary disease in women. *N Engl J Med,* 1993, 328, 1444-1449.

[372] Kushi, LH; Folsom, AR; Prineas, RJ; Mink, PJ; Wu, Y; Bostick, RM. Dietary antioxidant vitamins and death from coronary heart disease in postmenopausal women. *N Engl J Med,* 1996, 334, 1156-1162.

[373] Khaw, KT; Barrett-Connor, E. Dietary fiber and reduced ischemic heart disease mortality rates in men and women: a 12-year prospective study. *Am J Epidemiol,* 1987, 126, 1093-1102.

[374] Miller, ER; Appel, LJ; Risby, TH. Effect of dietary patterns on measures of lipid peroxidation: results from a randomized clinical trial. *Circulation,* 1998, 98, 2390-2395.

[375] Cassidy, A; Hooper, L. Phytoestrogens and cardiovascular disease. *J Br Menopause Soc,* 2006, 12, 49-56.

[376] Rimm, EB; Ascherio, A; Giovannucci, E; Spiegelman, D; Stampfer, MJ; Willett, WC. Vegetable, fruit, and cereal fiber intake and risk of coronary heart disease among men. *JAMA, 1996,* 275, 447-451.

[377] Wolk, A; Manson, JE; Stampfer, MJ; Colditz, GA; Hu, FB; Speizer, FE; Hennekens, CH; Willett, WC. Long-term intake of dietary fiber and decreased risk of coronary heart disease among women. *JAMA,* 1999, 281, 1998-2004.

[378] Mozaffarian, D; Kumanyika, SK; Lemaitre, RN; Olson, JL; Burke, GL; Siscovick, DS. Cereal, fruit, and vegetable fiber intake and the risk of cardiovascular disease in elderly individual. *JAMA, 2003,* 289, 1659-1666.

[379] Pereira, MA; O'Reilly, E; Augustsson, K; Fraser, GE; Goldbourt, U; Heitmann, BL; Hallmans, G; Knekt, P; Liu, S; Pietinen, P; Spiegelman, D; Stevens, J; Virtamo, J; Willett, WC; Ascherio, A. Dietary fiber and risk of coronary heart disease: a pooled analysis of cohort studies. *Arch Intern Med,* 2004, 164, 370-376.

[380] Anderson, JW. Dietary fiber prevents carbohydrate-induced hypertriglyceridemia. *Curr Atheroscler Rep,* 2000, 2, 536-541.

[381] Galisteo, M; Duarte, J; Zarzuelo, A. Effects of dietary fibers on disturbances clustered in the metabolic syndrome. *J Nutr Biochem,* 2007 Jul 5 [Epub ahead of print].

[382] Burke, V; Hodgson, JM; Beilin, LJ; Giangiulioi, N; Rogers, P; Puddey, IB. Dietary protein and soluble fiber reduce ambulatory blood pressure in treated hypertensives. *Hypertension,* 2001, 38, 821-826.

[383] Glore, SR; Van Treeck, D; Knehans, AW; Guild, M. Soluble fiber and serum lipids: a literature review. *J Am Diet Assoc,* 1994, 94, 425-436.

[384] Jacobs, DR Jr; Myer, MA; Kushi, LH; Folsom, AR. Whole grain intake may reduce risk of coronary heart disease death in postmenopausal women: the Iowa Women's Health Study. *Am J Clin Nutr,* 1998, 68, 248-357.

[385] Jacobs, DR; Pereira, MA; Meyer, KA; Kushi, LH. Fiber from whole grain; but not refined grains; is inversely associated with all-cause mortality in older women: The Iowa Women's Health Study. *J Am Coll Nutr,* 2000, 19(3 Suppl), 326S-330S.

[386] Liu S; Stampfer, MJ; Hu, FB; Giovannucci, E; Rimm, E; Manson, JE; Hennekens, CH; Willett, WC. Whole-grain consumption and risk of coronary heart disease: results from the Nurses' Health Study. *Am J Clin Nutr,* 1999, 70, 412-419.

[387] McKeown, NM; Meigs, JB; Liu, S; Wilson, PWF; Jacques, PF. Whole-grain intake is favorably associated with metabolic risk factors for type 2 diabetes and cardiovascular disease in the Framingham Offspring Study. Am J Clin Nutr, *2002,* 76, 390-398.

[388] Krauss, RM; Eckel, RH; Howard, B; Appel, LJ; Daniels, SR; Deckelbaum, RJ; Erdman, JW Jr; Kris-Etherton, P; Goldberg, IJ; Kotchen, TA; Lichtenstein, AH; Mitch, WE; Mullis, R; Robinson, K; Wylie-Rosett, J; St Jeor, S; Suttie, J; Tribble, DL; Bazzarre, TL. Revision 2000: A statement for health professionals from the Nutrition Committee of the American Heart Association. *J Nutr,* 2001, 131, 132-146.

[389] Hu, FB; Stampfer, MJ; Manson, JE; Rimm, EB; Colditz, GA; Rosner, BA; Speizer, FE; Hennekens, CH; Willett, WC. Frequent nut consumption and risk of coronary heart disease in women: prospective cohort study. *BMJ,* 1998, 317, 1341-1345.

[390] Albert, CM; Gaziano, JM. Willett, WC; Manson, JE. Nut consumption and decreased risk of sudden cardiac death in the Physicians' Health Study. *Arch Intern Med,* 2002, 162, 1382-1387.

[391] Mukuddem-Petersen, J; Oosthuizen, W; Jerling, JC. A systematic review of the effects of nuts on blood lipid profiles in humans. *Nutr*, 2005, 135, 2082-2089.

[392] Hu, BF; Stampfer, MJ. Nut consumption and risk of coronary heart disease: a review of epidemiologic evidence. *Curr Atheroscler Rep*, 1999, 1, 204-209.

[393] Sabate, J; Fraser, GE; Burke, K; Knutsen, SF; Bennett H; Lindsted, KD. Effects of walnuts on serum lipid levels and blood pressure in normal men. *N Engl J Med*, 1993, 328, 603-607.

[394] Zambon, D; Sabate, J; Munoz, S; Campero, B; Casals, E; Merlos, M; Laguna, JC; Ros, E. Substituting walnuts for monounsaturated fat improves the serum lipid profile of hypercholesterolemic men and women. *Ann Intern Med*, 2000, 132, 538-546.

[395] Ros, E; Nunez, I; Perez-Heras, A; Serra, M; Gilabert, R; Casals, E; Deulofeu, R. A walnut diet improves endothelial function in hypercholesterolemic subjects: a randomized crossover trial. *Circulation*, 2004, 109, 1609-1614.

[396] Bazzano, LA; He, J; Ogden, LG; Loria, C; Vupputuri, S; Myers, L; Whelton, PL. Legume consumption and risk of coronary heart disease in U.S men and women. NHANES I Epidemiologic Follow-Up Study. *Arch Intern Med*, 2001, 161, 2573-2578.

[397] Anderson, JW; Johnstone, BM; Cook-Newell, M. Meta-analysis of the effects of soy protein intake on serum lipids. *N Engl J Med*, 1995, 333, 276-282.

[398] He, J; Ogden, LG; Vupputuri, S; Bazzano, LA; Loria, C; Whelton, PK. Dietary sodium intake and subsequent risk of cardiovascular disease in overweight adults. *JAMA*, 1999, 282, 2027-2034.

[399] Lichtenstein, AH. Soy protein, isoflavones and cardiovascular disease risk. *J Nutr*, 1998, 128, 1589-1592.

[400] Cassidy, A; Hooper, L. Phytoestrogens and cardiovascular disease. *J Br Menopause Soc*, 2006, 12, 49-56.

[401] Hallund J; Bugel S; Tholstrup T; Ferrari, M; Talbot, D; Hall, WL; Reimann, M; Williams, CM; Wiinberg, N. Soya isoflavone-enriched cereal bars affect markers of endothelial function in postmenopausal women. *Br J Nutr*, 2006, 95, 1120-1126.

[402] Cuevas, AM; Irribarra, VL; Castillo, OA; Yanez, MD; Germain, AM. Isolated soy protein improves endothelial function in postmenopausal hypercholesterolemic women. *Eur J Clin Nutr*, 2003, 57, 889-894.

[403] Colacurci, N; Chiantera, A; Fornaro, F; de Novellis, V; Manzella, D; Arciello, A; Chiàntera, V; Improta, L; Paolisso, G. Effects of soy isoflavones on endothelial function in healthy postmenopausal women. *Menopause*, 2005, 12, 299-307.

[404] Erdman, JW; Jr. Soy protein and cardiovascular disease. A statement for healthcare professionals from the nutrition committee of the AHA. *Circulation*, 2000, 102, 2555.

[405] Krauss, RM; Eckel, RH; Howard, B; Appel, LJ; Daniels, SR; Deckelbaum, RJ; Erdman, JW Jr; Kris-Etherton, P; Goldberg, IJ; Kotchen, TA; Lichtenstein, AH; Mitch, WE; Mullis, R; Robinson, K; Wylie-Rosett, J; St Jeor, S; Suttie, J; Tribble, DL; Bazzarre, TL. AHA dietary guidelines revision 2000: a statement for healthcare professionals from the Nutrition Committee of the American Heart Association. *Circulation*, 2000, 102, 2284-2299.

[406] Jenkins, DJ; Kendall, CW; Augustin, LS; Franceschi, S; Hamidi, M; Marchie, A; Jenkins, AL; Axelsen, M. Glycemic index: overview of implications in health and disease. *Am J Clin Nutr*, 2002, 76, 266S-273S.

[407] Salmeron, J; Ascherio, A; Rimm, EB; Colditz, GA; Spiegelman, D; Jenkins, DJ; Stampfer, MJ; Wing, AL; Willett, WC. Dietary fiber, glycemic load, and risk of NIDDM in men. *Diabetes Care,* 1997, 20, 545-550.

[408] Liu, S; Manson, JE; Stampfer, MJ; Holmes, MD; Hu, FB; Hankinson, SE; Willett, WC. Dietary glycemic load assessed by food frequency questionnaire in relation to plasma high-density lipoprotein cholesterol and fasting triglycerides in postmenopausal women. *Am J Clin Nutr,* 2001, 73, 560-566.

[409] Liu, S; Willett, WC; Stampfer, MJ; Hu, FB; Franz, M; Sampson, L; Hennekens CH; Manson, JE. A prospective study of dietary glycemic load and risk of myocardial infarction in women. *Am J Clin Nutr,* 2000, 71, 1455-1461.

[410] Jeppesen, J; Schaaf, P; Jones, C; Zhou, MY; Chen, YD; Reaven, GM. Effects of low-fat; high-carbohydrate diets on risk factors for ischemic heart disease in postmenopausal women. *Am J Clin Nutr,* 1997, 65, 1027-1033.

[411] Mann, GE; Rovvlands, DJ; Li, FY; de Winter, P; Siow, RC. Activation of endothelial nitric oxide synthase by dietary isoflavones: role of NO in Nrf2-mediated antioxidant gene expression. *Cardiovasc Res,* 2007, 75, 261-274.

[412] Meydani, M. Vitamin E modulation of cardiovascular disease. *Ann N Y Acad Sci,* 2004, 1031, 271-279.

[413] Buege, JA; Aust, SD. Microsomal lipid peroxidation. *Methods Enzymol,* 1978, 52, 302-310.

[414] Lowry, OH; Rosebrough, NJ; Farr, AL; Randall, RJ. Protein measurement with the Folin phenol reagent. *J Biol Chem,* 1951, 193, 265-275.

[415] Goulinet, S; Chapman, MJ. Plasma LDL and HDL subspecies are heterogenous in particle content of tocopherols and oxygenated and hydrocarbon carotenoids. Relevance to oxidative resistance and atherogenesis. *Arterioscler Thromb Vasc Biol,* 1997, 17, 786-796.

[416] Quatromoni, PA; Copenhafer, DL; Demissie, S; D'Agostino, RB; O'Horo Nam, BH; Millen, BE. The internal validity of a dietary pattern analysis. The Framingham Nutrition Studies. *J Epidemiol Community Health,* 2002, 56, 381-388.

[417] Sonnenberg, L; Pencina, M; Kimokoti, R; Quatromoni, P; Nam, BH; D'Agostino, R; Meigs, JB; Ordovas, J; Cobain, M; Millen, B. Dietary patterns and the metabolic syndrome in obese and non-obese Framingham women. *Obes Res,* 2005, 13, 153-162.

[418] Millen, BE; Pencina, MJ; Kimokoti, RQ; Zhu, L; Meigs, JB; Ordovas, JM; D'Agostino, RB. Nutritional risk and the metabolic syndrome in women: opportunities for preventive intervention from the Framingham Nutrition Study. *Am J Clin Nutr,* 2006, 84, 434-441.

[419] Esmaillzadeh, A; Kimiagar, M; Mehrabi, Y; Azadbakht, L; Hu, FB; Willet, WC. Dietary patterns; insulin resistance; and prevalence of the metabolic syndrome in women. *Am J Clin Nutr,* 2007, 85, 910-918.

[420] Fung, TT; Willett, WC; Stampfer, MJ; Manson, JE; Hu, FB. Dietary patterns and the risk of coronary heart disease in women. *Arch Intern Med,* 2001, 161, 1857-1862.

[421] Hu, FB; Rimm, EB; Stampfer, MJ; Ascherio, A; Spiegelman, D; Willett, WC. Prospective study of major dietary patterns and risk of coronary heart disease in men. *Am J Clin Nutr,* 2000, 72, 912-921.

[422] Willett, WC. Diet and health: what should we eat? *Science,* 1994, 264, 532-537.

[423] Trichopoulou, A; Costacou, T; Bamia, C; Trichopoulos, D. Adherence to a Mediterranean diet and survival in a Greek population. *N Engl J Med*, 2003, 348, 2599-2608.

[424] Knoops, KT; de Groot, L; Kromhout, D; Perrin, AE; Moreiras-Varela, O; Menotti, A; van Staveren, WA. Mediterranean diet, lifestyle factors, and 10-year mortality in elderly European men and women. *JAMA*, 2004, 292, 1433-1439.

[425] de Lorgeril, M; Salen, P; Martin, JL; Monjaud, I; Delaye, J; Mamelle, N. Mediterranean diet, traditional risk factors, and the rate of cardiovascular complications after myocardial infarction: final report of the Lyon Diet Heart Study. *Circulation*, 1999, 99, 779-785.

[426] Kris-Etherton, P; Eckel, RH; Howard, BV; St Jeor, S; Bazzarre, TL; Nutrition Committee Population Science Commettee and Clinical Science Committee of the American Heart Association.. AHA Science Advisory: Lyon Diet Heart Study. Benefits of a Mediterranean-style; National Cholesterol Education Program/American Heart Association Step I dietary pattern on cardiovascular disease. *Circulation*, 2001, 103, 1823-1825.

[427] de Lorgeril M; Salen P; Martin JL; Monjaud I; Delaye J; Mamelle N. Mediterranean diet; traditional risk factors and the rate of cardiovascular complications after myocardial infarction. Final report of the Lyon Diet Heart Study. *Circulation*, 1999, 99, 779-785.

[428] Salas-Salvado, J; Garcia-Arellano, A; Estruch, R; Marquez-Sandoval, F; Corella, D; Fiol, M; Gomez-Gracia, E; Vinoles, E; Aros, F; Herrera, C; Lahoz, C; Lapetra, J; Perona, JS; Munoz-Aguado, D; Martinez-Gonzalez, MA; Ros, E. Components of the Medirerranean-type food pattern and serum inflammatory markers among patients at high risk for cardiovascular disease. *Eur J Clin Nutr*, 2007 Apr 18 [Epub ahead of print].

[429] Jacobs, DR Jr; Andersen, LF; Blomhoff, R. Whole grain consumption is associated with a reduced risk of noncardiovascular; noncancer death attributed to inflammatory diseases in the Iowa Women's Health Study. *Am J Clin Nutr*, 2007, 85, 1606-1614.

[430] Salmeron, J; Manson, JE; Stampfer, MJ; Colditz, GA; Wing, AL; Willett, WC. Dietary fiber; glycemic load; and risk of non-insulin-dependent diabetes mellitus in women. *JAMA*, 1997, 277, 472-477.

[431] de Lorgeril, M; Salen, P. The Meditrranean-style diet for the prevention of cardiovascular diseases. *Public Health Nutr*, 2006, 9, 118-123

[432] American Heart Association. Dietary guidelines for healthy American adults: a statement for physicians and health professionals by the Nutrition Committee, American Heart Association. *Circulation*, 1988, 77, 721A-724A.

[433] Expert Panel on Detection, Evaluation, and Treatment of High Blood Cholesterol in Adults. Summary of the second report of the National Cholesterol Education Program (NCEP) Expert Panel on Detection; Evaluation; and Treatment of High Blood Cholesterol in Adults (Adult Treatment Panel II). *JAMA*, 1993, 269, 3015-3023.

[434] Yao, M; Roberts, SB. Dietary energy density and weight regulation. *Nutr Rev*, 2001, 59, 247-258.

[435] Howard, BV; Manson, JE; Stefanick, ML; Beresford, SA; Frank, G; Jones, B; Rodanbough, RJ; Snetselaar, L; Thomson, C; Tinker, L; Vitolins, M; Prentise, R. Low-

fat dietary pattern and weight change over 7 years. The Women's Health Initiative dietary modification trial. *JAMA*, 2006, 295, 39-49.

[436] Hays, NP; Starling, RD; Liu, X; Sullivan, DH; Trappe, TA; Fluckey, JD; Evans, WJ. Effects of ad libitum low-fat, high-carbohydrate diet on body weight, body composition, and fat distribution in older men and women. *Arch Intern Med*, 2004, 164, 210-217.

[437] Design of the Women's Health Initiative clinical trial and observational study. The Women's Health Initiative Study Group. *Control Clin Trials*, 1998, 19, 61-109.

[438] Ness, AR; Hughes, J; Elwood, PC; Whitley, E; Smith, GD; Burr, ML. Multiple Risk Factor Intervention Trial Research Group. Multiple risk factor intervention trial. Risk factor changes and mortality results. *JAMA*, 1982, 248, 1465-1477.

[439] Appel, LJ; Moore, TJ; Obarzanek, E; Vollmer, WM; Svetkey, LP; Sacks, FM; Bray, GA; Vogt, TM; Cutler, JA; Windhauser, MM; Lin, PH; Karanja, JA. Clinical trial of the effects of dietary patterns on blood pressure. DASH Collaborative Research Group. *N Engl J Med,* 1997, 336, 1117-1124.

[440] Atkins, R. *Dr Atkins' New Diet Revolution.* New York, NY: Harper Collins; 2002.

[441] Sears B; Lawren W. *Enter the Zone.* New York; NY: Harper Collins; 1995.

[442] Brownell KD. *The LEARN Manual for Weight Management.* Dallas, TX: American Health Publishing Co; 2000

[443] Gardner, CD; Kiazand, A; Alhassan, S; Kim, S; Stafford, RS; Balise, RR; Kraemer, HC; King, AC. Comparison of the Atkins, Zonem, Ornish, and LEARN Diets for change in weight and related risk factors among overweight premenopausal women. The A to Z weight loss study: a randomized trial. *JAMA,* 2007, 297, 969-977.

[444] Howard, BV; Van Horn, L; Hsia, J; Manson, JE; Stefanick, ML; Wassertheil-Smoller, S; Kuller, LH; LaCroix, AZ; Langer, RD; Lasser, NL; Lewis, CE; Limacher, MC; Margolis, KL; Mysiw, WJ; Ockene, JK; Parker, LM; Perri, MG; Phillips, L; Prentice, RL; Robbins, J; Rossouw, JE; Sarto, GE; Schatz, IJ; Snetselaar, LG; Stevens, VJ; Tinker, LF; Trevisan, M; Vitolins, MZ; Anderson, GL; Assaf, AR; Bassford, T; Beresford, SA; Black, HR; Brunner, RL; Brzyski, RG; Caan, B; Chlebowski, RT; Gass, M; Granek, I; Greenland, P; Hays, J; Heber, D; Heiss, G; Hendrix, SL; Hubbell, FA; Johnson, KC; Kotchen, JM. Low-fat dietary pattern and risk of cardiovascular disease. The Women's Health Initiative Randomized Controlled Dietary Modification Trial. *JAMA, 2006,* 295, 655-666.

[445] Nordmann AJ; Nordmann A; Briel M; Keller, U; Yancy, WS Jr; Brehm, BJ; Bucher, HC. Effects of low-carbohydrate vs low-fat diets on weight loss and cardiovascular risk factors: a meta-analysis of randomized controlled trials. *Arch Intern Med*, 2006, 166, 285-293.

[446] Cornier, MA; Donahoo, WT; Pereira, R; Gurevich, I; Westergren, R; Enerback, S; Eckel, PJ; Goalstone, ML; Hill, JO; Eckel, RH; Draznin, B. Insulin sensitivity determines the effectiveness of macronutrient composition on weight loss in obese women. *Obes Res*, 2005, 13, 703-709.

[447] Bravata, DM; Sanders, L; Huang, J; Krumholz, HM; Olkin, I; Gardner, CD; Bravata, DM. Efficacy and safety of low-carbohydrate diets: a systematic review. *JAMA,* 2003, 289, 1837-1850.

[448] Lichtenstein, AH; Van Horn, L. Very low fat diets. *Circulation*, 1998, 98, 935-939.

[449] Fletcher, B; Berra, K; Braun, LT; Burke, LE; Durstine, JL; Fair, JM; Fletcher, GF; Goff, D; Miller, H; Krauss, R; Kris-Etherton, P; Stone, N; Wilterdink, J; Winston, M. Managing Abnormal Blood Lipids. A Collaborative Approach. *Circulation*, 2005, 112, 3184-3209.

[450] Ervin, RB; Wright, JD; Wang, CY; Kennedy-Stephenson, J. Dietary intake of fats and fatty acids for the United States population: 1999-2000. *Adv Data*, 2004, 348, 1-6.

[451] Horrobin, DF. Loss of delta-6-desaturase activityas a key factor in aging. *Med Hypotheses*, 1981, 7, 1211-1220.

[452] Jenkins, DJ; Kendall, CW; Marchie, A; Faulkner, DA; Wong, JM; de Souza, R; Emam, A; Parker, TL; Vidgen, E; Lapsley, KG; Trautwein, EA; Josse, RG; Leiter, LA; Connelly, PW. Effects of a dietary portfolio of cholesterol-lowering foods vs lovastatin on serum lipids and C-reactive protein. *JAMA*, 2003, 290, 502-510.

[453] Hickey MS; Houmard JA; Considine RV; Tyndall, GL; Midgette, JB; Gavigan, KE; Weidner, ML; McCammon, MR; Israel, RG; Caro, JF. Gender-dependent effects of exercise training on serum leptin levels in humans. *Am J Physiol*, 1997, 272, E562-E566.

[453a] US Food and Drug Administration. FDA Announces Qualified Health Claims for Omega-3 Fatty Acids (September 8, 2004).

[454] Wirth, A; Steinmetz, B. Gender differences in changes in subcutaneous and intra-abdominal fat during weight reduction: an ultrasound study. *Obes Res*, 1998, 6, 393-399.

[455] Wing, RR; Jeffery, RW. Effect of modest weight loss on changes in cardiovascular risk factors: Are there differences between men and women or between weight loss and maintenance? *Int J Obes*, 1995, 19, 67-73.

[456] Rice, B; Jansen, I; Hudson, R; Ross, R. Effects of exercise and/or diet on insulin; glucose and abdominal adipose tissue in obese men. *Diabetes Care*, 1999, 22, 684-691.

[457] Jansen, I; Fortier, A; Hudson, R; Ross, R. Effects of an energy-restrictive diet with or without exercise on abdominal fat, intermuscular fat, and metabolic risk factors in obese women. *Diabetes Care*, 2002, 25, 431-438.

[458] Mozaffarian, D; Rimm, EB; Herrington, DM. Dietary fats, carbohydrate, and progression of coronary atherosclerosis in post menopausal women. *Am J Clin Nutr*, 2004, 80, 1175-1184.

[459] Parker, B; Moakes, M; Luscombe, N; Clifton, P. Effect of a high-protein; high-monounsaturated fat weight loss diet on glycemic control and lipid levels in type 2 diabetes. *Diabetes Care*, 2002, 25, 425-430.

[460] Manolio, TA; Pearson, TA; Wenger, NK; Barrett-Connor, E; Payne, GH; Harlan, WR. Cholesterol and heart disease in older persons and women: review of an NHLBI workshop. *Ann Epidemiol*, 1992, 2, 161-176.

[461] National Cholesterol Education Program Expert Panel. Second report of the National Cholesterol Education Program Expert Panel on Detection; Evaluation; and Treatment of High Blood Cholesterol in Adults (Adult Treatment Panel). *Circulation*, 1994, 89, 1333-1445.

[462] Gotto, AM Jr. Cholesterol management in theory and practice. *Circulation*, 1997, 96, 4424-4430.

[463] Pleiner, J; Schaller, G; Mittermayer, F; Marsik, C; Macallister, RJ; Kapiotis, S; Ziegler, S; Ferlitsch, A; Wolzt, M. Intra-arterial vitamin C prevents endothelial dysfunction caused by ischemia-reperfusion. *Atherosclerosis*, 2007 Jul 21 [Epub ahead of print]

[464] Naissides, M; Pal, S; Mamo, JC; James, AP; Dhaliwal, S. The effect of chronic consumption of red wine polyphenols on vascular function in postmenopausal women. *Eur J Clin Nutr*, 2006, 60, 740-745.

[465] Katz, DL; Evans, MA; Chan, W; Nawaz, H; Comerford, BP; Hoxley, ML; Njike, VY; Sarrel, PM. Oats, antioxidants and endothelial function in overweight; dyslipidemic adults. *J Am Coll Nutr*, 2004, 23, 397-403.

[466] Kelemen M; Vaidya D; Waters DD; Howard BV; Cobb F; Younes N; Tripputti M; Ouyang P. Hormone therapy and antioxidant vitamins do not improve endothelial vasodilator function in postmenopausal women with established coronary artery disease: a substudy of the Women's Angiographic Vitamin and Estrogen (WAVE) trial. *Atherosclerosis*, 2005, 179, 193-200.

[467] Arteaga, E; Rojas, A; Villaseca, P; Bianchi, M. The effect of 17beta-estradiol and alpha-tocopherol on the oxidation of LDL cholesterol from postmenopausal women and the minor effect of gamma-tocopherol and melatonin. *Menopause*, 2000, 7, 112-116.

[468] Guetta, V; Panza, JA; Waclawiw, MA; Cannon, RO 3rd. Effect of combined 17 beta-estradiol and vitamin E on low-density lipoprotein oxidation in postmenopausal women. *Am J Cardiol*, 1995, 75, 1274-1276.

[469] Li, Z; Otvos, JD; Lamon-Fava, S; Carrasco,WV; Lichtenstein, AH; McNamara, JR; Ordovas, JM; Schaefer, EJ. *J Nutr*, 2003, 133, 3428-3433.

[470] Liu, S; Manson, JE; Burin, JE; Stampfer, MJ; Willett, WC; Ridker, PM. Relation between a diet with high glycemic load and plasma concentrations of high-sensitivity C-reactive protein in middle-aged women. *Am J Clin Nutr*, 2002, 75, 492-498.

[471] Turley, ML; Skeaff, CM; Mann, JI; Cox, B. The effect of a low-fat, high-carbohydrate diet on serum high density lipoprotein cholesterol and triglyceride. *Eur J Clin Nutr*, 1998, 52, 728-732.

[472] Kuller, LH; Simkin-Silverman, LR; Wing, RR; Meilahn, EN; Ives, DG. Women's Healthy Lifestyle Project: A randomized clinical trial: results at 54 months. *Circulation*, 2001, 103, 32-37.

[473] Lofgren, IE; Herron, KL; West, KL. Zern, TL; Patalay, M; Koo, SI; Fernandez, ML. Carbohydrate intake is correlated with biomarkers for coronary heart disease in a population of overweight premenopausal women. *J Nutr Biochem*, 2005, 16, 245-250.

[474] Mittendorfer, B. Insulin resistance: sex matters. *Curr Opin Clin Nutr Metab Care*, 2005, 8, 367-372.

[475] Burdge, GC; Calder, PC. Conversion of alpha-linoleic acid to longer-chain polyunsaturated fatty acids in human adults. *Reprod Nutr Rev*, 2005, 45, 581-597.

[476] Erkkilä, AT; Matthan, NR; Herrington, DM; Lichtenstein, AH. Higher plasma docosahexaenoic acid is associated with reduced progression of coronary atherosclerosis in women with CAD. *J Lipid Res*, 2006, 47, 14-19.

[477] Cassidy, R; Hooper, L. Phytoestrogens and cardiovascular disease. *J Br Menopause Soc*, 2006, 12, 49-56.

[478] West, SG; Hilpert, KF; Juturu, V; Bordi, PL; Lampe, JW; Mousa, SA; Kris-Etherton, PM. Effects of including soy protein in a blood cholesterol-lowering diet on markers of

cardiac risk in men and in postmenopausal women with and without hormone replacement therapy. *J Womens Health*, 2005, 14, 253-262.

[479] Lukaczer, D; Liska, DJ; Lerman, RH; Darland, G; Schiltz, B; Tripp, M; Bland, JS. Effect of a low glycemic index diet with soy protein and phytosterols on CVD risk factors in postmenopausal women. *Nutrition*, 2006, 22, 104-113.

[480] Azadbakht, L; Kimiagar, M; Mehrabi, Y; Esmaillzadeh, A; Hu, FB; Willett, WC. Soy inclusion in the diet improves features of the metabolic syndrome: a randomized crossover study in postmenopausal women. *Am J Clin Nutr*, 2007, 85, 735-741.

[481] Azadbakht, L; Kimiagar, M; Mehrabi, Y; Esmaillzadeh, A; Hu, FB; Willett, WC. Soy consumption, markers of inflammation, and endothelial function: a cross-over study in postmenopausal women with the metabolic syndrome. *Diabetes Care*, 2007, 30, 967-973.

[482] Jenkins, DJ; Kendall, CW; Jackson, CJ; Connelly, PW; Parker, T; Faulkner, D; Vidgen, E; Cunnane, SC; Leiter, LA; Josse, RG. Effects of high- and low-isoflavone soyfoods on blood lipids, oxidized LDL, homocysteine, and blood pressure in hyperlipidemic men and women. *Am J Clin Nutr*, 2002, 76, 365-372.

[483] Roy, S; Vega-Lopez, S; Fernandez, ML. Gender and hormonal status affect the hypolipidemic mechanisms of dietary soluble fiber in guinea pigs. *J Nutr*, 2000, 130, 600-607.

[484] Lucas, EA; Lightfoot, SA; Hammond, LJ; Devareddy, L; Khalil, DA; Daggy, BP; Smith, BJ; Westcott, N; Mocanu, V; Soung, DY; Arjmandi, BH. Flaxseed reduces plasma cholesterol and atherosclerotic lesion formation in ovariectomized Golden Syrian hamsters. *Atherosclerosis*, 2004, 173, 223-229.

[485] Van Horn, L; Liu, K; Gerber, J; Garside, D; Schiffer, L; Gernhofer, N; Greenland, P. Oats and soy in lipid-lowering diets for women with hypercholesterolemia: is there synergy? *J Am Diet Assoc*, 2001, 101, 1319-1325.

[486] Miller, M; Byington, R; Hunninghake, D; Pitt, B; Furberg, CD. Sex bias and underutilization of lipid-lowering therapy in patients with coronary artery disease at academic medical centers in the United States and Canada. *Arch Intern Med*, 2000, 160, 343-347.

[487] Caspard, H; Chan, AK; Walker, AM. Compliance with a statin treatment in a usual-care setting: retrospective database analysis over 3 years after treatment initiation in health maintenance organization enrollees with dyslipidemia. *Clin Ther*, 2005, 27, 1639-1646.

[488] Kulkarni, SP; Alexander, KP; Lytle, B; Heiss, G; Peterson, ED. Long-term adherence with cardiovascular drug regimens. *Amer Heart J*, 2006, 151, 185S-191S.

In: Research Trends in Nutrition…
Editor: Johan P. Urster, pp. 129-149

ISBN: 978-1-60456-147-0
© 2008 Nova Science Publishers, Inc.

Chapter 3

Diet and Type 2 Diabetes in Older Population – Focus on Primary Prevention

Joanna Myszkowska-Ryciak, Danuta Gajewska and Anna Harton
Chair of Dietetics, Faculty of Human Nutrition and Consumer Sciences, Warsaw
University of Life Sciences, Poland

Abstract

Diabetes mellitus is a group of metabolic diseases characterized by hyperglycemia resulting from defects in insulin secretion, insulin action, or both. The chronic hyperglycemia is associated with long-term damage causing dysfunction and failure of various organs, especially the eyes, kidneys, nerves, heart, and blood vessels. The prevalence of type 2 diabetes is increasing dramatically across the globe and in some regions has reached almost epidemic proportions. An estimated 135 million people worldwide had diagnosed diabetes in 1995, and this number is expected to rise to at least 300 million by 2025. This increase in prevalence is primarily being driven by environmental factors: "western" type of diet and more sedentary lifestyle. In addition, the ageing of the world population, particularly the western population, will increase the number of type 2 diabetes over the next years, unless adequate preventative actions are undertaken. Indeed, there are strong evidences that diabetes may be preventable, even in high-risk groups. Therefore, this chapter is focused on dietary factors which are important in the type 2 diabetes prevention in the elderly. The paper has been written based on research and epidemiological data. Topics include epidemiology informations as well as nutrients and recommendation. Special attention is paid on energy, fats, carbohydrates supply in prevention of the disease. In this paper, each of these nutrients is discussed separately. The efficacy of selected vitamins and minerals as well as alcohol at preventing type 2 diabetes in elderly are also discussed.

Introduction

Diabetes mellitus is a group of metabolic diseases characterized by hyperglycemia resulting from defects in insulin secretion, insulin action, or both. The chronic hyperglycemia is associated with long-term damage causing dysfunction and failure of various organs, especially the eyes, kidneys, nerves, heart, and blood vessels [1].

Type 2 diabetes results from an interactions between genetic (non-modifiable risk factors) and environmental factors (modifiable risk factors) [2]. The risk of developing type 2 diabetes increases with age, obesity, lack of physical activity but is also related to hypertension, dyslipidemia and even depression [1],[3]. In all societies overweight and obesity, especially centrally distributed, are associated with higher risk of type 2 diabetes [2].

Economic costs of diabetes mellitus are increasing dramatically. In UK they reached 4-5% of total healthcare expenditure [4] , whereas in USA in 2002 was $132 billion [5]. As the prevention is believed to be more economic than treatment, there is an urgent need for strategies which could reduce the global epidemic of type 2 diabetes. Increasingly more attention is paid to modifiable risk factors: body weight, well-balanced diet and physical activity. Several intervention studies have strongly proved that type 2 diabetes may be prevented or delayed, mainly by lifestyle modification [6], [7], [8].

Hereunder is a short review about the role of selected nutrients, dietary pattern and scientific evidence-based nutritional recommendations for the primary prevention of type 2 diabetes.

Epidemiology

Worldwide, the number of cases of diabetes in 2003 was estimated to be around 150 million and predictable by year 2030 will reach 366 million [2], [9] . By this year the number of people with diabetes aged above 64 years will be more than 82 million in developing countries and 48 million in developed countries, respectively [10] . In England and Wales 50% of new cases of diabetes mellitus in 1998 were people aged 55-74 [11] . The most common is type 2 diabetes, which accounts for ~90-95% of those with diabetes [1] . Moreover, the incidence of type 2 diabetes has increased dramatically during the last decades, mainly as a consequence of ageing of the population and increasing obesity rates [12] . Data from National Health Interview Survey [13] show that the incidence of diabetes increased 65% in population aged 65 to 79 during recent 7 years. As type 2 diabetes is frequently not diagnosed until complications appear, presumably one-third cases of diabetes may be undiagnosed [7] .

Nutrients and Recommendation

Energy

Excessive energy supply associated with prevalence of overweight and obesity is observed in almost all Western European countries, Australia, the USA as well as in China [14] . An excessive weight gain is considered by far as the most important risk factor for type

2 diabetes. The association between overweight, obesity, especially abdominal adiposity and the increased risk of type 2 diabetes is almost certain as it was reported in many population-based studies [15],[16],[17],[18],[19] . Furthermore these studies clearly showed that type 2 diabetes can be prevent or delay by substantial weight loss. In Malmö feasibility study weight reduction of 2.3-3.7% was correlated to improvement in glucose tolerance and in more than 50% of subjects glucose tolerance was normalized [20] . In Japanese trial [21] dietary intervention including reduction of the amount of each food by 10%, not exceeding 50g of fat and 50g of alcohol per day as well as recommendation of consuming a larger amount of vegetables and increasing physical activity produced a decrease of ~2kg in body weight. In this group such intervention reduced the development of diabetes by 67%. Data from the Framingham Study on 618 overweight individuals showed that sustained weigh loss reduced risk of type 2 diabetes by 37%. This effect was even more pronounced for subject with BMI >29; thus people who lost more than 4.5kg had a 51% reduction in diabetes risk [22] .

In epidemiological investigations separation of different components of high energy diet might be difficult. Consumption of this type of diet may influence insulin resistance, even independently of central obesity. Population-based survey of U.S. adults showed that increased standardized dietary energy-density was independently associated with elevated fasting insulin [23] . Commonly, excessive intake of fats and refined carbohydrates has been linked with high energy-dense diet. According to Astrup [24] energy intake is often high when fat-dense foods are consumed in large amounts, however excessive consumption of carbohydrate-rich products (e.g. soft drinks) may also led to weight gain [25],[26] . In the Nurses' Health Study [27] the association between percentage of calories from animal, saturated, trans fat and weight gain among women aged 41-68 was reported. However, it should be emphasized that in case of body weight control, the total calories amount is rather more important than the proportions of protein, fats and carbohydrates in the diet. Thus, available research has not demonstrated a long-term weight loss benefit with diets extreme in their macronutrient content [28] .

Considering that in a majority of adults and elderly weight gain process is slow and elongated in time, usually a substantial reducing of energy intake can prevent it. According to Dietary Guidelines for Americans [29] for most adults a reduction of only 50 to 100 calories per day may prevent gradual weight gain, whereas a reduction of 500 calories or more per day is a common initial goal in weight-loss programs. The subjects for reduction the total energy intake are: sugars, fats, and alcohol, as they provide calories but few or no essential nutrients. *Ad libitum* consumption of diets low in fat and high in protein and complex carbohydrates, with a low glycemic index, contributes to the prevention of weight gain in normal weight subjects [24] .

In the light of present knowledge, individuals who losing weight should follow a diet that is within the Acceptable Macronutrient Distribution Ranges (AMDR) for fat, carbohydrates, and protein, which are 20 to 35 percent of total calories, 45 to 65 percent of total calories, and 10 to 35 percent of total calories, respectively [29] .

Fats, Saturated Fats, n-3 Fatty Acids and Trans Fatty Acids

Fats are the most energy-dense macronutrients, with calorie value of 9 kcal per gram. Thus, the association between fat intake and body weight gain has been examined for a long time [rev. in [30] . However, the role of fat in etiology and prevention of type 2 diabetes has been also considered. Almost 40 years ago, West and Kalbfleisch [31] reported that the total fat intake was positively associated with the risk of development of diabetes. In animal experiments high-fat diets (with the exception of n-3 fatty acids) have been shown to cause insulin resistance relative to high carbohydrate diets [32],[33],[34],[35],[36] . Additionally, a diets high in saturated fat decreased insulin sensitivity [36] . A fat-dense diets might result in deterioration of glucose tolerance by several mechanisms including decreased binding of insulin to its receptors, impaired glucose transport, reduced proportion of glycogen synthase and accumulation of stored triglycerides in skeletal muscle [37] . Moreover, dietary fat can influence insulin sensitivity independently of any change in body weight [38] . The fatty acid composition of the diet may affect tissue phospholipid composition, which may relate to insulin action by altering membrane fluidity and insulin signaling [32] . The results of human studies consistently show that the fatty acid composition of body tissues (serum lipids, phospholipid in erythrocyte membranes, triacylglycerol in adipose tissue, phospholipid in skeletal muscle membranes) reflects, at least in part, the fat composition of the habitual diet [39] . The strength of the relationships between the proportion of a specific fatty acid in the diet and in body tissues varies between different fatty acids and for different tissues [40] . Number of studies demonstrated that both the amount and quality of dietary fat may influence glucose tolerance and insulin sensitivity [32],[41],[42] .

The evidence that total amount of fat consumed is associated with the development of type 2 diabetes is inconsistent, however, the WHO experts [2] consider it as the possible risk factor for diabetes. In the San Luis Valley Diabetes Study [43] an increase in total fat intake (40g/d) was associated with a 6% greater risk of developing diabetes in 134 subjects with impaired glucose tolerance. Similarly, in the Finnish and the Dutch cohorts of the Seven Countries Study total fat consumption also contributed to the risk of disease incidence [44] . In the Health Professionals' Study [45] carried on 42 504 male subjects for 12 years, total fat intake was associated with a higher risk of type 2 diabetes, however the association disappeared after adjustments for BMI. On the contrary, in the Nurses' Health Study [46] included 84 204 women no association between total fat intake and risk of type 2 diabetes was observed. These observations were also reported by Lundgren *et al* [47] , Meyer *et al* [48] and Colditz *et al* [49] . Thus, the total fat intake does not seem to predict *per se* the development of type 2 diabetes, although when consumed in excessive amount it might indirectly influence the development of disease by promoting the body weight gain [50],[51] . This is in accordance with results from KANWU study [52] . This intervention study carried out on 162 healthy individuals strongly indicated that the total amount of fat can influence insulin sensitivity and possibly the risk of type 2 diabetes, but only when it exceeds a threshold level of 35–40% of total energy intake. According to Dietary Guidelines for Americans [29] energy from fat consumed should not exceed 30% of total energy intake.

In animal studies saturated fats have been reported to trigger insulin resistance when fed as high-fat diets [32],[33],[35],[36] . In human studies similar association has been observed. In the San Luis Valley Diabetes Study [43],[53] saturated fat was only marginally associated with an increased risk of diabetes. These data were confirmed both by the Finnish and the Dutch cohorts of the Seven Countries Study [44] carried out on 338 subjects and followed for 30 years as well as by the Health Professionals' Study [45] included 42 504 male subjects followed for 12 years. Additionally, Van Dam *et al.* [45] observed an increased risk of development of type 2 diabetes in men consuming processed meat at least five times per week compared with those who consumed processed meats less than once per month. In the Nurses'

Health Study Salmeròn *et al.* [46] reported a relationship between intake of animal fat and incidence of diabetes, however no statistically significant after correcting for vegetable fat consumption. Evidence on effects of single fatty acids on glucose and insulin metabolism are limited. Data from Schwab *et al* [54],[55] and Louheranta *et al* [56] showed no effect of single saturated fatty acids: lauric, palmitic and stearic on glucose and insulin metabolism when these saturated fatty acids were compared with an equivalent energy exchange with monounsaturated. The role of saturated fat as a risk factor for type 2 diabetes, inversely to the protective character of vegetable (unsaturated) fat, has been recently confirmed in a cross-sectional study on a European population [57] and is further supported by evidence from studies where dietary fat composition was assessed by objective markers of fat intake [58], [59],[60] . However, evidence from controlled intervention studies are contradictory. Whereas detrimental effect of saturated fat versus polyunsaturated fat on insulin sensitivity was observed by Summers *et al* [61] , data from Lovejoy *et al.* [62] did not confirm previous findings. As animal (saturated) fat is generally consider to be a risk factor for type 2 diabetes, thus vegetable (unsaturated) fat is rather thought to have a beneficial effect on the risk of disease development. Data from Iowa study [48] on 35 988 elderly women followed for 11 years indicated that vegetable fat consumption was inversely related to incidence of type 2 diabetes. WHO [2] recognized saturated fats as probable risk factor of developing type 2 diabetes and recommended that saturated fat intake should not exceed 10% of total energy in general population and 7% of total energy in high-risk groups. The main sources of saturated fats in Western diet are: whole milk, cream, ice cream, whole-milk cheeses, butter, lard and meats and certain plant oils (palm, coconut oils), cocoa butter.

In the prevention of type 2 diabetes long-chain *n-3* fatty acids seem to be important. The rich sources of these fatty acids, mainly EPA and docosahexaenoic acid, are fish and fish oil [63] . Number of studies examined the effects of long-chain *n-3* fatty acids on the risk of diabetes [44],[46],[48],[64] . In Feskens *et al* [64] study of 175 elderly subjects an inverse association between fish intake and incidence of impaired glucose tolerance or diabetes was noticed for individuals consuming any type of fish (mean 24.2g/day). Similarly, in the large Nurses' Health Study [46] increased fish consumption had a protective effect on the development of disease in women. On the contrary, in the Iowa Women's Study a higher *n-3* intake was even associated with an increased risk of type 2 diabetes [48] . Data from the intervention study [52] did not confirmed any benefits from the *n-3* fatty acid supplementation regarding prevention of developing of type 2 diabetes in healthy subjects. Modest amount of *n-3* fatty acids (1-2g/day) probably has no significant effect on glucose metabolism in patients with type 2 diabetes [65] . In the light of present knowledge there is no specific recommendation regarding the *n-3* fatty acids intake in the prevention of type 2 diabetes, however according to WHO [2] they might possible reduce the risk of disease. According to recommendation for a general population by WHO [2] the *n-3* fatty acids should provide 1-2% of total energy. The main sources of the *n-3* fatty acids are marine-fish. People should consume fish, especially oily fish, at least twice per week [66] .

Even though WHO experts [2] consider trans fatty acids as possible risk factor of developing type 2 diabetes, data on the effects of trans fatty acids on glucose metabolism are limited. Data from the Nurses Health Study [46] demonstrated a positive association between trans fatty acid intake and development of type 2 diabetes. On the contrary, consumption of diet with 5% of energy from trans fatty acids for 4 weeks had no significant influence on insulin sensitivity in healthy women compared to an oleic acid enriched diet [67] . The main sources of trans fatty acids in Western diet are: processed and fried food, hydrogenated fats, and spreads as well as shortened and cooked fats.

In the light of present knowledge regarding the relationship between type 2 diabetes and dietary fat, shifting from a diet rich with fat from animal sources to a diet based on vegetable fat might be beneficial in relation to the prevention of disease, however more experiments are needed to establish clear dietary recommendations.

Carbohydrates and Fiber

A lot of controversy in the literature exists considering the relations between the amount and types of dietary carbohydrate and the risk of type 2 diabetes. There are also ambiguity regarding to the definitions of dietary fiber and non-starch polysaccharides [2] . Carbohydrates are classified as sugars, oligosaccharides and polysaccharides on the basis of its chemical structure [68]. However, in respect of their influence on human health, classification based on their ability to be digested and absorbed in the human small intestine is used [38] . Carbohydrate-rich foods can also be classified on the basis of their effects on postprandial glycemia, which can be expressed as glycemic index (GI; defined as the glycemic response elicited by a 50g carbohydrate portion of a food expressed as a percentage of that elicited by a 50g portion of a reference food - glucose or white bread). Fibre-rich foods often have a low GI, although some foods with a low-fibre content may also have a low GI [69],[70],[71] . As the postprandial blood glucose response is influenced not only by the glycemic index value of the food but also by the amount of carbohydrate ingested in epidemiological studies, the concept of glycemic load has been introduced as representing both quantity and quality of consumed carbohydrates [2]. A high carbohydrate intake increases the requirement for endogenous insulin secretion in order to maintain glucose homeostasis [72] . Insulin secretion by beta-cells is glucose sensitive and a high intake of carbohydrate in relation to energy intake, produces higher postprandial insulin levels. It is hypothesis that repeated stimulation of a high insulin output by a high carbohydrate diet might speed up an age-related decline in insulin secretion and lead to an earlier onset of type 2 diabetes [73] . However, in epidemiological studies the intake of either total carbohydrate or sugars (sucrose) was not associated with the higher risk of diabetes [74] . Large cohort study carried on 39 345 women over age 45 (the Women's Health Study) reported by Janket *et al* [74] found no association between sugar intake and diabetes risk. So far no clear carbohydrate guideline regarding the prevention of type 2 diabetes has been formulated. American Dietary Guidelines [29] recommend intake of a variety of grain products (including whole grains) equating to six or more servings a day depending on energy level. According to the FAO/WHO [68] carbohydrates in the diet should comprise at least 55% of total energy intake in healthy individuals.

Conversely, there is strong evidence that a diet rich in carbohydrate and fibre and with low GI may contribute to the prevention of type 2 diabetes. According to WHO [2] non-starch polysaccharides have been reported as probable factor playing role in the prevention of type 2 diabetes, whereas low-glycemic index food possibly decreased risk of development of disease. Two large cohort studies: the Health Professionals Follow-up study [75],[76],[77] and the Nurses Health Study [75],[76],[78] , evaluated the effects of fibre and glycemic load on risk of developing diabetes. All obtained data clearly showed that a relatively low intake of dietary fibre significantly increased the risk of type 2 diabetes. The association was stronger for cereal fibre, a rich source of insoluble fibre, but much weaker for sources of soluble fibre [rev. in [37] . Also fruit and vegetable consumption was associated with a reduced risk of type 2 diabetes [79],[80],[81] . On the contrary, in the Iowa Women's Health Study [83] carried out on women aged 55–69 years no effect of GI on the risk of diabetes was observed. ADA [28] recommended 14g of fibre/1000kcal, whereas WHO [2] suggested 20g of non-starch polysaccharides (NSP) as a minimum in prevention of type 2 diabetes. In American Dietary Guidelines [29] as a good sources of fibre (>4g per portion) are proposed: navy beans, ready-to-eat cereals, kidney beans, split peas, lentils, variety of beans, green peas and blackberries.

Vitamins and Minerals

Majority of research focused on role of macronutrients in prevention of type 2 diabetes. However, there are a lot of studies reporting micronutrients and phytochemicals effects on risk of type 2 diabetes.

As chromium plays the important role in glucose metabolism, its possible effect on prevention of type 2 diabetes has been examined. Studies on animal and *in vitro* proved positive effect of chromium on insulin resistance [84],[85] . However, Gunton *et al* [86] did not observed any beneficial effect of supplementation with 800 µg of chromium picolinate in patients with impaired glucose tolerance on their glucose control after 3 months of treatment. Similarly, Usitupa *et al* [87] reported no improvement in glucose tolerance in elderly individuals with impaired glucose tolerance after 6 months of supplementation with 160 µg of chromium per day. On the contrary, Offenbacher and Pi-Sunyer [88] observed positive effect of 9 g chromium-rich brewers' yeast on glucose tolerance in elderly non-diabetes subjects. The authors assumed that elderly people may have a low level of chromium and that an effective source for chromium repletion, such as brewers' yeast, may improve their carbohydrate tolerance. Offenbacher *et al* [89] presumed that benefits of chromium supplementation may occurs in elderly with low intake of chromium but age *per se* was not a factor leading to this deficiency. Similarly, Anderson *et al* [90] reported an improvement in glucose tolerance after supplementation with 200 µg of chromium in individuals with low intake of this micronutrient. So far, there is no evidence that chromium supplementation can prevent from type 2 diabetes. According to WHO report [2] there is insufficient evidence to confirm or refute the suggestion that chromium might protect against the development of disease. However, considering that mineral bioavailability may change due to ageing and a number of surveys show chromium intakes by old persons to be lower than the corresponding reference nutrient intakes [91],[92] , recommendations to increase the consumption of chromium rich food might be reasonable. Even though chromium occurs naturally in a wide variety of foods, deficiency is possible, as food processing methods often remove the naturally occurring chromium. The good dietary sources of chromium are: romaine lettuce, onions, tomatoes, brewer's yeast, oysters, whole grains, bran cereals, and potatoes.

Magnesium is a essential cofactor for several enzymes that plays an important role in glucose metabolism [93] . In several studies on animals [94] a negative effect on the post-receptor signaling of insulin was observed in case of magnesium deficiency. Although WHO [2] stated that evidence to confirm or negate protective role of magnesium in type 2 diabetes is insufficient, some recently published studies might suggest rehearing this opinion. Van Dam *et al* [95] in 8-year prospective population study of black women in U.S. observed significant association between higher dietary magnesium intake and a lower risk of type 2 diabetes. Lopez-Ridaura *et al* [96] in large prospective studies on 85,060 women and 42,872 men reported a consistent inverse association between magnesium intake and risk of type 2 diabetes. This association was independent of other risk factors for type 2 diabetes, including several dietary factors. Earlier, large American cohort studies have demonstrated a strong negative association between intake of magnesium and risk of type 2 diabetes, both in men and women [rew. in [37] . In The Health Professionals Follow-up Study [76] independent inverse association between magnesium intake and risk of type 2 diabetes was reported in men of age 40-75. Similar results were obtained for women aged 40-65 in the Nurses Study [75] . As reported by Ford *et al* [82] , the most important sources of magnesium for U.S. population were: vegetables, bread and cold cereals, and milk.

As oxidative stress may contribute to the pathogenesis of type 2 diabetes by increasing insulin resistance or impairing insulin secretion [97] , thus vitamin E as an efficient chain-breaking antioxidant have been hypothesized to play a protective role for development of type 2 diabetes [98] . Studies on animals strongly suggest that sufficient dietary intake of vitamin E can prevent the development of diabetes [99],[100],[101] . The 5-year follow-up study on 895 individuals with either normal or impaired glucose tolerance showed a significantly protective effect of increasing concentration of plasma α-tocopherol with reduced risk of diabetes incidence; however, this effect was limited to subjects who did not take vitamin E supplements. Among these supplement nonusers, the statistically significant protective effect was independent of potentially confounding variables (e.g. total energy intake, total fat, fiber, vitamin C, and magnesium) [102] . Similarly, The Finnish Mobile Clinic Health Examination Survey including 10,054 people aged 40–69 reported a reduced risk of type 2 diabetes associated with the intakes of total vitamin E, α-tocopherol, γ-tocopherol, ß-tocotrienol, and ß-cryptoxanthin [103] . On the contrary, in recent double-blind, placebo-controlled, primary-prevention trial in 38,716 initially healthy women, vitamin E supplementation at a dose of 600 IU every other day for 10 years was not associated with a significant reduction in the risk of type 2 diabetes [104] . Thus, according to WHO report [2] the evidence of potentially preventing role of vitamin E in developing type 2 diabetes is insufficient. However, the effect of vitamin E supplementation in general or high-risk populations requires further research, ideally in randomized clinical trials. It may be most appropriate to emphasize the dietary recommendation to increase consumption of major food sources of vitamin E, such as fortified ready-to-eat cereals, sunflower seeds, almonds, vegetable oils, and nuts.

Alcohol

Number of studies have examined the relationship between alcohol consumption and the risk of development of type 2 diabetes [105],[106],[107],[108],[109] . Facchini *et al* [110] observed in healthy men and women association between light-to-moderate alcohol consumption and enhanced insulin-mediated glucose uptake, lower plasma glucose, and insulin concentrations in response to oral glucose.

Koppes *et al* [111] in meta-analysis of 15 studies reported a U-shaped relationship with a highly significant ~30% reduced risk of type 2 diabetes in alcohol consumers of 6-48g/day compared with heavier consumers or abstainers. Recently, similar association was observed in population of older women consuming alcohol, moreover beverage type did not influence this association [112] . In prospective study by Hodge *et al* [113] total alcohol intake was associated with reduced risk only in women, whereas alcohol from wine reduced risk of type

2 diabetes both in male and female. In a large Japanese cohort study [114] moderate alcohol consumption was associated with a reduced risk of type 2 diabetes only among men with a BMI≥22.1 kg/m², whereas among lean men (BMI≤22.0 kg/m²) heavy alcohol consumption was related to an increased risk of type 2 diabetes. Wannamethee *et al* [115] in prospective study of 5221 men aged 40-59 years noticed a non-linear relation between alcohol intake and age adjusted risk of type 2 diabetes, with risk lowest in light to moderate drinkers and highest in heavy drinkers. As alcohol has high energy value, excessive intake may trigger body weight gain, which is independent risk factor for diabetes development. The relationship between high alcohol consumption (≥30g/day) and excessive weight gain was demonstrated in older men, irrespective of the type of alcohol consumed [116] .

On the contrary, in large population-based study Harding *et al* [117] observed higher occurrence of diabetes incidents among people (mean age 58.9) drinking alcohol compared to those who did not consume alcohol. Additionally, Hodge *et al* [113] reported that a high daily intake of alcohol, even on only 1-3 days a week, may increase the risk of diabetes in men. Similarly, the results of the Atherosclerosis Risk in Communities Study [118] suggested that high alcohol intake (≥36g/day) predicts type 2 diabetes among middle-aged men, and the relationship is even more pronounced for spirits

The apparent inconsistencies in the results of performed studies and more the detrimental consequences of alcoholism on health preclude clear recommendations regarding alcohol as a prevention factor in type 2 diabetes. According to WHO report [2] there is still insufficient evidence to confirm or refute the suggestion that moderate alcohol consumption might protect against the type 2 diabetes.

Diet for the Elderly

Prospects for healthy ageing are affected by nutrition at every stage of life. As generally people eat less as they get older [119] , consequently special attention should be paid when making food choices. Foote *et al* [120] in study carried on 1740 elderly Americans reported that more than half of the population were at risk of inadequate vitamin E, folate and calcium intake. Thus, selection of fortified and whole grain foods, vegetables and fruits might have reduced not only possible deficiencies but also risk of age-related diseases.

Dietary patterns characterized by higher diary intake, especially low-fat dairy products, might contribute to prevention of the development of type 2 diabetes both in men aged 40-75 [121] and middle-aged and elderly women [122] .

Higher consumption of total red meat, especially various processed meat was positively associated with an increase risk of developing type 2 diabetes in women. Moreover total red meat and processed meat intake were correlated with total energy, fats and cholesterol intake and inversely associated with dietary carbohydrate, fiber, magnesium and glycemic load [123] . Similarly, in men frequent consumption of processed meats was related to higher risk of diabetes development [124] .

Consumption of whole grains and low-fat dairy products, but not high-fat dairy, were associated with a lower risk of development of type 2 diabetes [95] .

Nut and peanut butter consumption was associated with a lower risk of type 2 diabetes in women [125] . However nuts are energy- and fat-dense products, no relationship was observed between nuts consumption and body weight gain [125] . As nuts are a good source of fiber, vitamins, minerals and antioxidants, it would be reasonable to encourage individuals to consumed them *e.g.* as a snack.

Generally, the risk of development of type 2 diabetes is inversely related to the Alternate Healthy Eating Index (AHEI) score, which measures diet quality using nine dietary components [126] .

The potential benefit of coffee consumption on risk of type 2 diabetes is more likely for obese compared to non-obese individuals [127] . However, in a large study of Finish population, strong inverse relationship between coffee consumption and the risk of diabetes development [128] . was Moreover, some types of coffee might give additional health benefits. Consumption paper-filtered coffee instead of unfiltered may lower low-density lipoprotein cholesterol concentration [129] whereas decaffeinated besides reduction of risk of type 2 diabetes is deprived of detrimental effects of caffeine [127] .

As pointed Schulze *et al* [130] diet high in sugar-sweetened soft drinks, refined grains, diet soft drinks, and processed meat and low in wine, coffee, cruciferous vegetables, and yellow vegetables may contribute to development of type 2 diabetes in adults.

With regard to dietary interventions, it should be targeted to increase the consumption of fish, vegetables, whole-grained bread and cereals and fruit, and decrease the intake of foods containing animal and trans fatty acids as well as sugar. Furthermore, an increasing amount of physical activity should be strongly advised. In a view of presented findings, avoiding a Western dietary pattern might substantially reduce risk of developing type 2 diabetes [124] .

Although diet and nutrients are generally believed to play an important role in the development of type 2 diabetes (table 1), specific dietary recommendations have not been clearly establish till now.

Table 1. Summary of strength of evidence on dietary factors and risk of development of type 2 diabetes [adapted from [2]

Evidence	Decreased risk	Increased risk
Convicting	Voluntary weight loss in overweight and obese individuals (limited energy supply/lower energy-dense diet)	Overweight and obesity (excess of energy/high energy-dense diet)
Probable Possible	Non-starch polysaccharides (NSP) n-3 fatty acids Low glycemic index foods	Saturated fats Total fat intake Trans fatty acids
Insufficient	Chromium Magnesium Vitamin E Moderate alcohol consumption	Excess of alcohol

Dietary guidelines for individuals at high risk for developing type 2 diabetes including elderly according to the present knowledge are presented in table 2.

**Table 2. Summary of practical dietary recommendations
for individuals at high risk for developing type 2 diabetes**

Factor	Recommendations	Practical clue
Energy	For overweight/obese individuals: reduce energy (7% weight loss)[132]; For normal weigh individuals: 1.4–1.8 multiples of the basal metabolic rate (BMR) to maintain body weight at different levels of physical activity[131]	Reduce intake of added sugars, fats and alcohol Pay attention to serving size
Fats	<7% saturated fatty acids[2] Minimize trans-fatty acids[29]	Choose lean meat and low-fat dairy products Avoid processed vegetable fats, processed cookies, cakes, crackers, potatoes
NSP	14g fibre/1000kcal[132] or min. 20g/day[2] Introduce low-glycemic index foods[132]	Choose whole-grain products, vegetable, fruits, cereals
Chromium	50µg/day[131]	Choose romaine lettuce, onions, tomatoes, brewer's yeast, oysters, whole grains
Magnesium	225-280mg/day[131]	Choose whole-grain products, nuts, cereals, vegetables
Vitamin E	100-400 IU/day[131]	Choose cereals, sunflower seeds, almonds, vegetable oils, and nuts
Alcohol	If consumed, not more than 30g/day for men and 15g/day for women [29]	Not exceed 1 drink for women and 2 drink for men per day

Conclusion

Aging of population is related to an increasing risk of chronic diseases such as type 2 diabetes. Despite that type 2 diabetes has a genetic background, only the importance of lifestyle factors can explain the global epidemic of disease. In type 2 diabetes, both insulin secretion defect and insulin resistance are genetically determined, but the latest is highly modifiable by lifestyle [133] . On the basis of current research it should be emphasized that lifestyle modification remains the best way to prevent type 2 diabetes. Harding *et al* [117] suggested that primary prevention of the development of type 2 diabetes should be aimed to obese men and women aged over 55 years, irrespectively of their physical activity. As reported Colditz *et al* [134] body mass index (BMI) of 23.0 to 25.0 kg/m^2 was associated with fourfold increased risk for type 2 diabetes in female subjects compared to those with BMI lower than 22.0 kg/ m^2. Contrary, loosing more than 5 kg in middle life reduced this risk substantially. Data from The European Prospective Investigation into Cancer and Nutrition (EPIC) – Potsdam Study [19] showed that weight gain in early adulthood (25-40 y) strongly predicts the the risk of type 2 diabetes with a latency period of ~ 15-23 years. According to Astrup [135] maintenance of a healthy body weight in susceptible individuals requires 45-60 minutes physical activity daily, a fat-reduced diet with plenty of fruit, vegetables, whole grain, and lean meat and dairy products, and moderate consumption of calorie containing beverages. The replacement of starchy carbohydrates with protein from lean meat and lean dairy products enhances satiety, and facilitate weight control [135] . McAuley *et al* [136] observed insulin sensitivity improvement in adults who underwent the vigorous exercise program including training 5 times a week for at least 20 minutes per session at an intensity of 80-90% of age-predicted maximum heart rate.

Number of migration studies in different population groups point a significant association between adoption of a "Western lifestyle" and type 2 diabetes prevalence [63],[137],[138] . Shifting to a higher calorie intake, high protein diet, higher alcohol consumption, a greater weight gain and altered levels of physical activity in the migrants are most likely to contribute to this situation.

It should be emphasized that although diet and food components are generally believed to play an important role in the development of type 2 diabetes, specific dietary recommendations have not been clearly establish till now.

References

[1]   American Diabetes Association (ADA). Diagnosis and classification of diabetes mellitus. *Diabetes Care*, 30, 2007, 30(suppl. 1), 42-47.
[2]   WHO/FAO. Diet, nutritional and the prevention of chronic diseases. Report of Joint WHO/FAO Expert Consultation. World Health Organization: Geneva 2003.
[3]   Knol, MJ; Twisk, JW; Beekman, AT;, Heine, RJ; Snoek, FJ; Pouwer, F. Depression as a risk factor for the onset of type 2 diabetes mellitus. A meta-analysis. *Diabetologia*, 2006, 49, 837-845.
[4]   Dixon, S; Currie, CJ; Peters JR. The cost of diabetes: time for a different approach. *Diabet Med*, 2000, 17, 820-822.
[5]   Thom, T; Haase, N; Rosamond, W; Howard, VJ; Rumsfeld, J; Manolio, T; Zheng, Z-J; Flegal, K; O'Donnell, Ch; Kittner, S; Lloyd-Jones, D; Goff, DC; Hong, Y; Adams, R; Friday, G; Furie, K; Gorelick, P; Kissela, B; Marler, J; Meigs, J; Roger, V; Sidney, S; Sorlie, P; Steinberger, J; Wasserthiel-Smoller, S; Wilson, M; Wolf, P. Heart Disease and Stroke Statistics-2006 Update. A Report From the American Heart Association Statistics Committee and Stroke Statistics Subcommittee. *Circulation*, 2006, 113, 85-151.
[6]   Lindström, J; Ilanne-Parikka, P; Peltonen, M; Aunola, S; Eriksson, JG; Hemiö, K; Hämäläinen, H; Härkönen, P; Keinänen-Kiukaanniemi, S; Laakso, M; Louheranta, A; Mannelin, M; Paturi, M; Sundvall, J; Valle, TT; Uusitupa, M; Tuomilehto, J; Finnish Diabetes Prevention Study Group. Sustained reduction in the incidence of type 2 diabetes by lifestyle intervention: follow-up of the Finnish Diabetes Prevention Study. *Lancet*, 2006, 368,1673-1679.

[7]   American Diabetes Association (ADA). Standards of medical care in diabetes - 2007. *Diabetes Care*, 30, 2007, 30(suppl. 1), 4-41.

[8]   American Diabetes Association (ADA); National Institute of Diabetes and Digestive and Kidney Diseases. Prevention or Delay of Type 2 Diabetes. *Diabetes Care*, 2004, 27(suppl. 1), 47-54.

[9]   WHO. Prevalence of diabetes worldwide. Available from: URL: http://www.who.int/diabetes/facts/world_figures/en/index.html

[10]   Wild, S; Roglic, G; Green, A; Sicree, R; King, H. Global Prevalence of Diabetes, Estimates for the year 2000 and projections for 2030. *Diabetes Care*, 2004, 27, 1047-1053.

[11]   Ryan, R; Newnhamk, A; Khuntik, K; Majeedk, A. New cases of diabetes mellitus in England and Wales, 1994-1998: Database study. *Public Health*, 2005, 119, 892-899.

[12]   Lipscombe, LL; Hux, JE. Trends in diabetes prevalence, incidence, and mortality in Ontario, Canada 1995-2005: a population-based study. *Lancet*, 2007, 369, 750-756.

[13]   Geiss, LS; Pan, L; Cadwell, B; Gregg, EW; Benjamin, SM; Engelgau, WW. Changes in incidence of diabetes in U.S. adults, 1997-2003. *Am J Prev Med*, 2006, 30, 371-377.

[14]   Silventoinen, K; Sans, S; Tolonen, H; Monterde, D; Kuulasmaa, K; Kesteloot, H; Tuomilehto, J. Trends in obesity and energy supply in the WHO MONICA Project. *Int J Obes Relat Metab Disord*, 2004, 28, 710-718.

[15]   Meisinger, C; Doring, A; Thorand, B; Heier, M; Lowel, H. Body fat distribution and risk of type 2 diabetes in the general population: are there differences between men and women? The MONICA/KORA Augsburg cohort study. *Am J Clin Nutr*, 2006, 84, 483-489.

[16]   Harding, AH; Griffin, SJ; Wareham, NJ. Population impact of strategies for identifying groups at high risk of type 2 diabetes. *Preventive Medicine*, 2006, 42, 364-368.

[17]   Tuomilehto, J; Lindström, J; Eriksson, JG; Valle, TT; Hämäläinen, H; Ilanne-Parikka, P; Keinänen-Kiukaanniemi, S; Laakso, M; Louheranta, A; Rastas, M; Salminen, V; Uusitupa, M; Finnish Diabetes Prevention Study Group. Prevention of type 2 diabetes mellitus by changes in lifestyle among subjects with impaired glucose tolerance. *N Engl J Med*, 2001, 344, 1343-1350.

[18]   Knowler, WC; Barrett-Connor, E; Fowler, SE; Hamman, RF; Lachin, JM; Walker, EA; Nathan, DM; Diabetes Prevention Program Research Group. Reduction in the incidence of type 2 diabetes with lifestyle intervention or metformin. *N Engl J Med*, 2002, 346, 393-403.

[19]   Schienkiewitz, A; Schulze, MB; Hoffmann, K; Kroke, A; Boeing, H. Body mass index history and risk of type 2 diabetes: results from the European Prospective Investigation into Cancer and Nutrition (EPIC)-Potsdam Study. *Am J Clin Nutr*, 2006, 84, 427-433.

[20]   Eriksson, KF; Lindgärde, F. Prevention of type 2 (non-insulin-dependent) diabetes mellitus by diet and physical exercise. The 6-year Malmö feasibility study. *Diabetologia*, 1991, 34, 891-898.

[21]   Kosaka, K; Noda, M; Kuzuya T. Prevention of type 2 diabetes by lifestyle intervention: a Japanese trial in IGT males. *Diabetes Res Clin Pract*, 2005, 67, 152-62.

[22]   Moore, LL; Visioni, AJ; Wilson, PW; D'Agostino, RB; Finkle, WD; Ellison, RC. Can sustained weight loss in overweight individuals reduce the risk of diabetes mellitus? *Epidemiology*, 2000, 11, 269-273.

[23]   Mendoza, JA; Drewnowski, A; Christakis, DA. Dietary energy density is associated with obesity and the metabolic syndrome in U.S. adults. *Diabetes Care*, 2007, 30, 974-979.

[24]   Astrup, A. Healthy lifestyles in Europe: prevention of obesity and type II diabetes by diet and physical activity. *Public Health Nutr*, 2001, 4, 499-515.

[25]   Ludwig, DS; Peterson, KE; Gortmaker, SL. Relation between consumption of sugar-sweetened drinks and childhood obesity: a prospective, observational analysis. *Lancet*, 2001, 357, 505-508.

[26]   Schulze, MB; Manson, JE; Ludwig, DS; Colditz, GA; Stampfer, MJ; Willett, WC; Hu, FB. Sugar-sweetened beverages, weight gain, and incidence of type 2 diabetes in young and middle-aged women. *JAMA*, 2004, 292, 927-934.

[27]   Field, AE; Willett, WC; Lissner, L; Colditz, GA. Dietary fat and weight gain among women in the Nurses' Health Study. *Obesity*, 2007,15, 967-976.

[28]   American Diabetes Association (ADA). Nutrition recommendations and interventions for diabetes. A position statement of the American Diabetes Association. *Diabetes Care*, 2007, 30(suppl. 1), 48-65.

[29]   Dietary   Guidelines   for   Americans   2005.   Availabe   at: www.healthierus.gov/dietaryguidelines.

[30]   Bray, GA; Paeratakul, S; Popkin, BM. Dietary fat and obesity: a review of animal, clinical and epidemiological studies. *Physiology and Behavior*, 2004, 83, 549– 555.

[31]   West, KM; Kalbfleisch, JM. Influence of nutritional factors on prevalence of diabetes. *Diabetes*. 1971, 20, 99-108.

[32]   Storlien, LH; Baur, LA; Kriketos, AD; Pan, DA; Cooney, GJ; Jenkins, AB; Calvert, GD; Campbell, LV. Dietary fats and insulin action. *Diabetologia*, 1996, 39, 621-631.

[33]   Hedeskov, CJ; Capito, K; Islin, H; Hansen, SE; Thams, P.Long-term fat-feeding-induced insulin resistance in normal NMRI mice: postreceptor changes of liver, muscle and adipose tissue metabolism resembling those of type 2 diabetes. *Acta Diabetologica*, 1992, 29, 14-19.

[34]   Storlien, LH; Kraegen, EW; Chisholm, DJ; Ford, GL; Bruce, DG; Pascoe, WS. Fish oil prevents insulin resistance induced by high-fat feeding in rats. *Science*, 1987, 237, 885-888.

[35]   Storlien, LH; James, DE; Burleigh, KM; Chisholm, DJ; Kraegen, EW. Fat feeding causes widespread in vivo insulin resistance, decreased energy expenditure, and obesity in rats. *Am J Physiol*, 1986, 251,576-583.

[36]   Storlien, LH; Jenkins, AB; Chisholm, DJ; Pascoe, WS; Khouri, S; Kraegen, EW. Influence of dietary fat composition on development of insulin resistance in rats. Relationship to muscle triglyceride and omega-3 fatty acids in muscle phospholipid. *Diabetes*, 1991, 40, 280-289.

[37]   Steyn, NP; Mann, J; Bennett, PH; Temple, N; Zimmet, P; Tuomilehto, J; Lindstrom, J; Louheranta, A.   Diet, nutrition and the prevention of type 2 diabetes. *Public Health Nutr*, 2004, 7, 147-165.

[38]   Parillo, M; Riccardo, G. Diet composition and the risk of type 2 diabetes: epidemiological and clinical evidence. *Br J Nutr*, 2004, 92, 7-19.

[39]   Riccardi, G; Aggett, P; Brighenti, F; Delzenne, N; Frayn, K; Nieuwenhuizen, A; Pannemans, D; Theis, S; Tuijtelaars, S; Vessby, B. Body weight regulation, insulin sensitivity and diabetes risk. *Eur J Nutr*, 2004, 43, 7-46.

[40] Aro, A. Fatty acid composition of serum lipids: is this marker of fat intake still relevant for identifying metabolic and cardiovascular disorders? Nutr Metab Cardiovasc Dis, 2003, 13, 253-255.

[41] Lichtenstein, AH; Schwab, US. Relationship of dietary fat to glucose metabolism *Atherosclerosis*, 2000, 150, 227-243.

[42] Hu, FB; van Dam, RM; Liu, S. Diet and risk of type II diabetes: the role of types of fat and carbohydrate. Diabetologia, 2001, 44, 805-817.

[43] Marshall, JA; Hoag, S; Shetterly, S; Hamman, RF. Dietary fat predicts conversion from impaired glucose tolerance to NIDDM. The San Luis Valley Diabetes Study. *Diabetes Care*, 1994, 17, 50-56.

[44] Feskens, EJ; Virtanen, SM; Rasanen, L; Tuomilehto, J; Stengard, J; Pekkanen, J; Nissinen, A; Kromhout, D. Dietary factors determining diabetes and impaired glucose tolerance. A 20-year follow-up of the Finnish and Dutch cohorts of the Seven Countries Study. *Diabetes Care*, 1995, 18, 1104-1112.

[45] van Dam, RM; Willett, WC; Rimm, EB; Stampfer, MJ; Hu, FB. Dietary fat and meat intake in relation to risk of type 2 diabetes in men. *Diabetes Care*, 2002, 25, 417-424.

[46] Salmeron; J; Hu, FB; Manson, JE; Stampfer, MJ; Colditz, GA; Rimm, EB; Willett, WC. Dietary fat intake and risk of type 2 diabetes in women. *Am J Clin Nutr*, 2001, 73, 1019-1026.

[47] Lundgren, H; Bengtsson, C; Blohme, G; Isaksson, B; Lapidus, L; Lenner, RA; Saaek, A; Winther, E. Dietary habits and incidence on noninsulin-dependent diabetes mellitus in a population study of women in Gothenburg, Sweden. *Am J Clin Nutr*, 1989, 49, 708-712.

[48] Meyer, KA; Kushi, LH; Jacobs, DR; Folsom, AR. Dietary fat and incidence of type 2 diabetes in older Iowa women. *Diabetes Care*, 2001, 24, 1528-1535.

[49] Colditz, GA; Manson, JE; Stampfer, MJ; Rosner, B; Willett, WC; Speizer, FE. Diet and risk of clinical diabetes in women. *Am J Clin Nutr*, 1992, 55, 1018-1023.

[50] Mayer-Davis, EJ; Monaco, JH; Hoen, HM; Carmichael, S; Vitolins, MZ; Rewers, MJ; Haffner, SM; Ayad, MF; Bergman, RN; Karter, AJ.Dietary fat and insulin sensitivity in a triethnic population: the role of obesity. The Insulin Resistance Atherosclerosis Study (IRAS). *Am J Clin Nutr*, 1997, 65, 79-87.

[51] Marshall, JA; Bessensen, DH. Dietary fat and the development of type 2 diabetes. *Diabetes Care*, 2002, 25, 620-622.

[52] Vessby, B; Uusitupa, M; Hermansen, K. Substituting dietary saturated for monounsaturated fat impairs insulin sensitivity in healthy men and women: the KANWU study. *Diabetologia*, 2001, 44, 312-319.

[53] Marshall, JA; Bessesen, DH; Hamman, RF. High saturated fat and low starch and fibre are associated with hyperinsulinaemia in a non-diabetic population: the San Luis Diabetes Study *Diabetologia*, 1997, 40, 430-438.

[54] Schwab, US; Maliranta, HM; Sarkkinen, ES; Savolainen, MJ; Kesaniemi, YA; Uusitupa, MI. Different effects of palmitic and stearic acid-enriched diets on serum lipids and lipoproteins and plasma cholesteryl ester transfer protein activity in healthy young women. *Metabolism*, 1996, 45, 143-149.

[55] Schwab, US; Niskanen, LK; Maliranta, HM; Savolainen, MJ; Kesäniemi, YA; Uusitupa, MIJ Lauric and palmitic acid-enriched diets have minimal impact on serum

lipid and lipoprotein concentrations and glucose metabolism in healthy young women. *J Nutr*, 1995, 25, 466-473.

[56] Louheranta, AM; Turpeinen, AK; Schwab, US; Vidgren, HM; Parviainen, MT; Uusitupa, MIJ. A high-stearic acid diet does not impair glucose tolerance and insulin sensitivity in healthy women. *Metabolism*, 1998, 47, 529-534.

[57] Thanopoulou, AC; Karamanos, BG; Angelico, FV. Dietary fat intake as a risk factor for the development of diabetes. *Diabetes Care*, 2003, 26, 302-307.

[58] Vessby, B; Aro, A; Skarfors, E; Berglund, L; Saltinen, I; Lithell H. The risk to develop NIDDM is related to the fatty acid composition of the serum cholesterol esters. *Diabetes*, 1994, 43, 1353-1357.

[59] Laaksonen, DE; Lakka, TA; Lakka, HM; Nyyssonen, K; Rissanen, T; Niskanen, LK; Salonen, JT. Serum fatty acid composition predicts development of impaired fasting glycaemia and diabetes in middle-aged men. *Diabet Med*, 2002, 19, 456-464.

[60] Wang, L; Folsom, AR; Zheng, Z-J; Pankow, JS; Eckfeldt, JH; for the ARIC Study Investigators. Plasma fatty acid composition and incidence of diabetes in middle-aged adults: the Atherosclerosis Risk in Communities (ARIC) Study. *Am J Clin Nutr*, 2003, 78, 91-98.

[61] Summers, LKM; Fielding, BA; Bradshow, HA; Ilic, V; Beysen, C; Clark, ML; Moore, NR; Frayn, KN. Substituting dietary saturated fat with polyunsaturated fat changes abdominal fat distribution and improves insulin sensitivity. *Diabetologia*, 2002, 45, 369-377.

[62] Lovejoy, JC; Smith, SR; Champagne, CM; Most, MM; Lefevre, M; DeLany, JP; Denkind, YM; Rood, JC; Veldhuis, J; Bray, GA. Effects of diets enriched in saturated (palmitic), monounsaturated (oleic) or trans (elaidic) fatty acids on insulin sensitivity and substrate oxidation in healthy adults *Diabetes Care*, 2002, 25, 1283-1288.

[63] Feskens, EJ; van Dam, RM. Dietary fat and the etiology of type 2 diabetes: an epidemiological perspective. *Nutr Metab Cardiovasc Dis*, 1999, 9, 87-95.

[64] Feskens, EJ; Bowles, CH; Kromhout D. Inverse association between fish intake and risk of glucose intolerance in normoglycemic elderly men and women. *Diabetes Care*, 1991, 14, 935-941.

[65] Nettleton, JA; Katz, R. n-3 long-chain polyunsaturated fatty acids in type 2 diabetes: a review. *J Am Diet Assoc*, 2005, 105, 428-440.

[66] American Heart Association Nutrition Committee, Lichtenstein, AH; Appel, LJ; Brands, M; Carnethon, M; Daniels, S; Franch, HA; Franklin, B; Kris-Etherton, P; Harris, WS; Howard, B; Karanja, N; Lefevre, M; Rudel, L; Sacks, F; Van Horn, L; Winston, M; Wylie-Rosett, J. Diet and lifestyle recommendations revision 2006: a scientific statement from the American Heart Association Nutrition Committee. *Circulation*, 2006, 114, 82-96.

[67] Louheranta, AM; Turpeinen, AK; Vidgren, HM; Schwab, US; Uusitupa, MIJ. A high-trans fatty acid diet and insulin sensitivity in young healthy women. *Metabolism*, 1999, 8, 870-875.

[68] Food and Agriculture Organization/World Health Organization. Report of a Joint Expert Consultation: Carbohydrates in Human Nutrition. Rome FAO, 1989.

[69] Jenkins, DJA; Ghafari, H; Wolever, TMS; Taylor, RH; Jenkins, AL; Barker, HM; Fielden, H; Bowling, AC. Relationship between the rate of digestion of foods and post-prandial glycaemia. *Diabetologia*, 1982, 22, 450-455.

[70] Jenkins, DJA; Wolever, TMS; Jenkins, AL; Josse, RG; Wong, GS. The glycaemic response to carbohydrate foods. *Lancet*, 1984, 2, 388-391.

[71] Bjorck, I; Liljeberg, H; Ostman, E. Low glycaemic index foods. *Br J Nutr*, 2000, 83, 149-155.

[72] Reaven, GM. Pathophysiology of insulin resistance in human disease. *Physiol Rev*, 1995, 75, 473-486.

[73] Grundy, SM. Obesity, metabolic syndrome, and cardiovascular disease. *J Clin Endocrinol Metab*, 2004, 89, 2595-2600.

[74] Yang, EJ; Kerver, JM; Park, UK; Kayitsinga, J; Allison, DB; Song, WO. Carbohydrate intake and biomarkers of glycemic control among US adults: the third National Health and Nutrition Examination Survey (NHANES III). *Am J Clin Nutr*, 2003, 77, 1426-1433.

[75] Salmeron, J; Manson, JE; Stampfer, MJ; Colditz, GA; Wing, AL; Willett, WC. Dietary fiber, glycemic load, and risk of non-insulin-dependent diabetes mellitus in women. *JAMA*, 1997, 277, 472-477.

[76] Salmeron, J; Ascherio, A; Rimm, EB; Colditz, GA; Spiegelman, D; Jenkins, DJ; Stampfer, MJ; Wing, AL; Willett, WC. Dietary fiber, glycemic load, and risk of NIDDM in men. *Diabetes Care*, 1997, 20, 545-550.

[77] Fung, TT; Hu, FB; Pereira, MA; Liu, S; Stampfer, MJ; Colditz, GA; Willett, WC. Whole-grain intake and the risk of type 2 diabetes: a prospective study in men. *Am J Clin Nutr*, 2002, 76, 535-540.

[78] Liu, S; Manson, JE; Stampfer, MJ; Hu, FB; Giovannucci, E; Colditz, GA; Hennekens, CH; Willett, WC. A prospective study of whole-grain consumption and risk of type 2 diabetes mellitus in US women. *Am J Public Health,* 2000, 90, 1409-1415.

[79] Williams, DE; Wareham, NJ; Cox, BD; Byrne, CD; Hales, CN; Day, NE. Frequent salad vegetable consumption is associated with a reduction in the risk of diabetes mellitus. *J Clin Epidemiol*, 1999, 52, 329- 335.

[80] Ford, ES; Mokdad, AH. Fruit and vegetable consumption and diabetes mellitus incidence among U.S. adults. *Prev Med*, 2001, 32, 33-39.

[81] Sargeant, LA; Khaw, KT; Bingham, S; Day, NE; Luben, RN; Okaes, S; Welch, ; Wareham, NJ. Fruit and vegetable intake and population glycosylated haemoglobin levels: the EPIC-Norfolk Study. *Eur J Clin Nutr*, 2001, 55, 342-348.

[82] Ford, ES; Mokdad, AH: Dietary magnesium intake in a national sample of US adults. *J Nutr*, 2003, 133, 2879–2882.

[83] Meyer, KA; Kushi, LH; Jacobs, DR; Slavin, J; Sellers, TA; Folsom, AR. Carbohydrate, dietary fiber and the incident type 2 diabetes in older women. *Am J Clin Nutr*, 2000, 71, 921-930.

[84] Shindea, UA; Sharma, G; Xu, YJ; Dhalla, NS; Goyal, RK: Insulin sensitising action of chromium picolinate in various experimental models of diabetes mellitus. *J Trace Elem Med Bid*, 2004, 18, 23-32.

[85] Davis, CM; Vincent, JB: Chromium oligopeptide activates insulin receptor tyrosine kinase activity. *Biochemistry*, 1997, 36, 4382-4385.

[86] Gunton, JE; Cheung, NW; Hitchman, R; Hams, G; O'Sullivan, C; Foster-Powell, K; McElduff, A. Chromium supplementation does not improve glucose tolerance, insulin sensitivity, or lipid profile: a randomized, placebo-controlled, double-blind trial of

supplementation in subjects with impaired glucose tolerance. *Diabetes Care*, 2005, 28, 712-713.

[87]   Uusitupa, MI; Mykkänen, L; Siitonen, O; Laakso, M; Sarlund, H; Kolehmainen, P; Räsänen, T; Kumpulainen, J; Pyörälä, K. Chromium supplementation in impaired glucose tolerance of elderly: effects on blood glucose, plasma insulin, C-peptide and lipid levels. *Br J Nutr*, 1992, 68, 209-216.

[88]   Offenbacher, EG; Pi-Sunyer, FX: Beneficial effect of chromium-rich yeast on glucose tolerance and blood lipids in elderly subjects. *Diabetes*, 1980, 29, 919-925.

[89]   Offenbacher, EG; Rinko, CJ; Pi-Sunyer, FX: The effects of inorganic chromium and brewer's yeast on glucose tolerance, plasma lipids, and plasma chromium in elderly subjects. *Am J Clin Nutr*, 1985, 42, 454-461.

[90]   Anderson, RA; Polansky, MM; Bryden, NA; Canary, JJ. Supplemental-chromium effects on glucose, insulin, glucagon, and urinary chromium losses in subjects consuming controlled low-chromium diets. *Am J Clin Nutr,* 1991, 54, 909-916.

[91]   Vaquero, MP. Magnesium and trace elements in the elderly: intake, status and recommendations. *J Nutr Health Aging*, 2002, 6, 147-53.

[92]   Wood, RJ; Suter, PM; Russell, RM. Mineral requirements of elderly people. *Am J Clin Nutr*, 1995, 62, 493-505.

[93]   Paolisso, G; Scheen, A; D'Onofrio, F; Lefebvre, P. Magnesium and glucose homeostasis. *Diabetologia,* 1990, 33 511–514.

[94]   Dzurik R; Stefikova K; Spustova V; Fetkovska N. The role of magnesium deficiency in insulin resistance: an in vitro study. *J Hypertens*, 1991, 9, S312–S313.

[95]   van Dam, RM; Hu, FB; Rosenberg, L; Krishnan, S; Palme, JR. Dietary calcium and magnesium, major food sources, and risk of type 2 diabetes in U.S. black women. *Diabetes Care*, 2006, 29, 2238-2243.

[96]   Lopez-Ridaura R, Willett WC, Rimm EB, Liu S, Stampfer MJ, Manson JE, Hu FB. Magnesium intake and risk of type 2 diabetes in men and women. *Diabetes Care*, 2004, 27, 134-140.

[97]   Oberley, LW. Free radicals and diabetes. *Free Radic Biol Med*, 1988, 5, 113-124.

[98]   Halliwell, B; Gutteridge, JMC. Free radicals in biology and medicine. New York, Oxford Univewrsity Press, 1989.

[99]   Murthy, VK; Shipp, JC; Hanson, C; Shipp, DM. Delayed onset and decreased incidence of diabetes in BB rats fed free radical scavengers. *Diabetes Res Clin Pract*, 1992, 18, 11–16.

[100] Beales, PE, Williams, AJ, Albertini, MC, Pozzilli, P. Vitamin E delays diabetes onset in the non-obese diabetic mouse. *Horm Metab Res*, 1994, 26, 450–452.

[101] Slonim, AE, Surber, ML, Page, DL, Sharp, RA, Burr, IM. Modification of chemically induced diabetes in rats by vitamin E: supplementation minimizes and depletion enhances development of diabetes. *J Clin Invest*, 1983, 71, 1282–1288.

[102] Mayer-Davis, EJ; Costacou, T; King, I; Zaccaro, DJ; Bell, RA. The Insulin Resistance and Atherosclerosis Study (IRAS). Plasma and dietary vitamin E in relation to incidence of type 2 diabetes: The Insulin Resistance and Atherosclerosis Study (IRAS). *Diabetes Care*, 2002, 25, 2172-2177.

[103] Montonen, J, Knekt, P, Jarvinen, R, Reunanen, A. Dietary antioxidant intake and risk of type 2 diabetes. *Diabetes Care*, 2004, 27, 362-366.

[104] Liu, S; Lee, IM; Song, Y; Van, Denburgh M; Cook, NR; Manson, JE; Buring, JE. Vitamin E and risk of type 2 diabetes in the women's health study randomized controlled trial. *Diabetes*, 2006, 55, 2856-2862.

[105] Stampfer, MJ; Colditz, GA; Willett, WC; Manson, JE; Arky, RA; Hennekens, CH; Speizer, FE. A prospective study of moderate alcohol drinking and risk of diabetes in women. *Am J Epidemiol*, 1988, 28, 549-558.

[106] Ajani, UA; Hennekens, CH; Spelsberg, A; Manson, JE. Alcohol consumption and risk of type 2 diabetes mellitus among US male physicians. *Arch Intern Med*, 2000, 160, 1025-1030.

[107] Conigrave, KM; Hu, BF; Camargo, CA Jr; Stampfer, MJ; Willett, WC; Rimm, EB. A prospective study of drinking patterns in relation to risk of type 2 diabetes among men. *Diabetes*, 2001, 50, 2390-2395.

[108] Carlsson, S; Hammar, N; Grill, V; Kaprio, J. Alcohol consumption and the incidence of type 2 diabetes: a 20-year follow-up of the Finnish twin cohort study. *Diabetes Care*, 2003, 26, 2785-2790.

[109] Nakanishi, N; Suzuki, K; Tatara K. Alcohol consumption and risk for development of impaired fasting glucose or type 2 diabetes in middle-aged Japanese men. *Diabetes Care*, 2003, 26, 48-54.

[110] Facchini, F, Chen, YD; Reaven, GM. Light-to-moderate alcohol intake is associated with enhanced insulin sensitivity. *Diabetes Care*, 1994, 17, 115-119.

[111] Koppes, LL; Dekker, JM; Hendriks, HF; Bouter, LM; Heine, RJ. Moderate alcohol consumption lowers the risk of type 2 diabetes: a meta-analysis of prospective observational studies. *Diabetes Care*, 2005, 28, 719-725.

[112] Beulens, JW; Stolk, RP, van der Schouw, YT; Grobbee, DE; Hendriks, HF; Bots, ML. Alcohol consumption and risk of type 2 diabetes among older women. *Diabetes Care*, 2005, 28, 2933-2938.

[113] Hodge, AM; English, DR; O'Dea, K; Giles, GG. Alcohol intake, consumption pattern and beverage type, and the risk of Type 2 diabetes. *Diabet Med*, 2006, 23, 690-697.

[114] Tsumura, K; Hayashi, T; Suematsu, C; Endo, G; Fujii, S; Okada, K. Daily alcohol consumption and the risk of type 2 diabetes in Japanese men: the Osaka Health Survey. *Diabetes Care*, 1999, 22, 1432-1437.

[115] Wannamethee, SG; Shaper, AG; Perry, IJ; Alberti, KG. Alcohol consumption and the incidence of type II diabetes. *J Epidemiol Community Health*, 2002, 56, 542-548.

[116] Wannamethee, SG; Shaper AG. Alcohol, body weight, and weight gain in middle-aged men. *Am J Clin Nutr*, 2003, 77, 1312-1317.

[117] Harding, AH; Griffin, SJ; Wareham, NJ. Population impact of strategies for identifying groups at high risk of type 2 diabetes. *Prev Med*, 2006, 42, 364-368.

[118] Kao, WH; Puddey, IB; Boland, LL; Watson, RL; Brancati FL. Alcohol consumption and the risk of type 2 diabetes mellitus: atherosclerosis risk in communities study. *Am J Epidemiol*, 2001, 54, 748-757.

[119] Drewnowski, A; Shultz, JM. Impact of aging on eating behaviors, food choices, nutrition, and health status. *J Nutr Health Aging*, 2001, 5, 75-79.

[120] Foote, JA; Giuliano, AR; Harris, RB. Older adults need guidance to meet nutritional recommendations. *J Am Coll Nutr*, 2000, 19, 628-640.

[121] Choi, HK; Willett, WC; Stampfer, MJ; Rimm, E; Hu, FB. Dairy consumption and risk of type 2 diabetes mellitus in men: a prospective study. *Arch Intern Med*, 2005, 165, 997-1003.

[122] Liu, S; Choi, HK; Ford, E; Song, Y; Klevak, A; Buring, JE; Manson JE. A prospective study of dairy intake and the risk of type 2 diabetes in women. *Diabetes Care*, 2006, 29, 1579-1584.

[123] Song, Y; Manson, JE; Buring, JE; Liu, S. A prospective study of red meat consumption and type 2 diabetes in middle-aged and elderly women: the women's health study. *Diabetes Care*, 2004, 27, 2108-2115.

[124] van Dam, RM; Rimm, EB; Willett, WC; Stampfer, MJ; Hu, FB. Dietary patterns and risk for type 2 diabetes mellitus in U.S. men. *Ann Intern Med*, 2002, 136, 201-209.

[125] Jiang R, Manson JE, Stampfer MJ, Liu S, Willett WC, Hu FB. Nut and peanut butter consumption and risk of type 2 diabetes in women. *JAMA*, 2002, 288, 2554-2560.

[126] Fung TT, McCullough M, van Dam RM, Hu FB. A prospective study of overall diet quality and risk of type 2 diabetes in women. Diabetes Care, 2007, 30, 1753-1757.

[127] van Dam, RM. Coffee and type 2 diabetes: from beans to beta-cells. Nutr Metab Cardiovasc Dis, 2006, 16, 69-77.

[128] Tuomilehto, J; Hu, G; Bidel, S; Lindström, J; Jousilahti, P. Coffee consumption and risk of type 2 diabetes mellitus among middle-aged Finnish men and women. *JAMA*, 2004, 291, 1213-1219.

[129] Jee, SH; He J, Appel, LJ; Whelton, PK; Suh, I; Klag, MJ. Coffee consumption and serum lipids: a meta-analysis of randomized controlled clinical trials. *Am J Epidemiol*, 2001, 153, 353-362.

[130] Schulze, MB; Hoffmann, K; Manson, JE; Willett, WC; Meigs, JB; Weikert, C; Heidemann, C; Colditz, GA; Hu, FB. Dietary pattern, inflammation, and incidence of type 2 diabetes in women. *Am J Clin Nutr*, 2005, 82, 675-684.

[131] WHO. Keep fit for life. Meeting the nutritional needs of older persons. Geneva: World Health Organization; 2002.

[132] Wylie-Rosett, J; Albright, AA; Apovian, C; Clark, NG; Delahanty, L; Franz, MJ; Hoogwerf, B; Kulkarni, K; Lichtenstein, AH; Mayer-Davis, E; Mooradian, AD; Wheeler, M. 2006-2007 American Diabetes Association Nutrition Recommendations: issues for practice translation. *J Am Diet Assoc*, 2007, 107, 1296-304.

[133] Uusitupa, M. Gene-diet interaction in relation to the prevention of obesity and type 2 diabetes: evidence from the Finnish Diabetes Prevention Study. *Nutr Metab Cardiovasc Dis*, 2005, 15, 225-233.

[134] Colditz, GA; Willett, WC; Rotnitzky, A; Manson, JE. Weight gain as a risk factor for clinical diabetes mellitus in women. *Ann Intern Med*, 1995, 122, 481-486.

[135] Astrup, A. How to maintain a healthy body weight. *Int J Vitam Nutr Res*, 2006, 76, 208-215.

[136] McAuley, KA; Williams, SM; Mann, JI; Goulding, A; Chisholm, A; Wilson, N; Story, G; McLay, RT; Harper, MJ; Jones, IE. Intensive lifestyle changes are necessary to improve insulin sensitivity: a randomized controlled trial. *Diabetes Care*, 2002, 25, 445-452.

[137] Ostbye, T; Welby, TJ; Prior, IA; Salmond, CE; Stokes, YM. Type 2 (non-insulin-dependent) diabetes mellitus, migration and westernisation: the Tokelau Island Migrant Study. *Diabetologia*, 1989, 32, 585-590.

[138] Ferreira, SR; Lerario, DD; Gimeno, SG; Sanudo, A; Franco, LJ; Japanese-Brazilian Diabetes Study Group. Obesity and central adiposity in Japanese immigrants: role of the Western dietary pattern. *J Epidemiol*. 2002, 12, 431-438.

In: Research Trends in Nutrition…
Editor: Johan P. Urster, pp. 151-170

ISBN: 978-1-60456-147-0
© 2008 Nova Science Publishers, Inc.

Chapter 4

Diet and Cardiovascular Disease in Older Adults

Anna Harton, Joanna Myszkowska-Ryciak and Danuta Gajewska
Chair of Dietetics, Faculty of Human Nutrition and Consumer Sciences,
Warsaw University of Life Sciences, Poland

Abstract

Nutrition has been recognized as a major determinant of health for centuries. Many studies showed that both food overabundance and macronutrient deficiency in older people increase the risk of many metabolic diseases. The costs associated with hospitalization resulting from many chronic diseases are usually higher than the costs of their prevention. The role of nutrition in health promotion and prevention of non-communicable or diet related diseases has not been given proper consideration. Aging of population is related to an increasing risk of chronic diseases such as cardiovascular disease (CVD) because an age has been included in groups of independent heart disease risk factors. Therefore, the primary target of this chapter is focus on the CVD prevention in the elderly. The paper has been written based on research and epidemiological data. Topics include epidemiology as well as nutrients and recommendation. In this paper, each of important diet ingredients in the prevention of cardiovascular disease such as fats, saturated fatty acids, cholesterol, carbohydrates, fiber, protein and B-groups vitamins, antioxidants, minerals as well as flavonoids is discussed separately. In conclusion there is a diet for the elderly. This chapter gives practical dietary recommendation for older people. Nutritional education of people even above 60 years old might be effective and useful because it is never too late to change nutritional habits for healthy ageing.

Introduction

Epidemiology

Cardiovascular diseases (CVD) are the major contributor to the global burden of disease among the non-communicable diseases [1],[2] which tends to almost 50% of all deaths in the developing countries [3],[4] An age was included in groups of independent CVD risk factor [5] It was estimated that above 38% of all of CVD concerned the elderly (aged 65 and older) [AHA statistics]. The leading cause of CVD worldwide mortality is a coronary heart disease (CHD) and the mortality rates from CHD will double from 1990 to 2020 [6] The American data showed that an average age of heaving first heart attack is almost the age of 70 [1] Besides the age, there are other non modifiable and modifiable risk factors [5] In the primary prevention, factors having influence on it, should be taken into account. One of them is a healthy and well balanced diet. An association between a diet and heart diseases and an effectiveness of a diet therapy, in the primary prevention of CVD, were researched in many studies [7],[8] There is a briefly review about the role of important nutrients, a dietary pattern and a recently related recommendations to the primary prevention of CVD.

Nutrients and Recommendation

Fats, Saturated Fatty Acids and a Dietary Cholesterol

Several studies found that an intake of fats (especially high calories fats) and saturated fatty acids (SFAs), as well as dietary cholesterol, raise total cholesterol (TC) and low-density lipoprotein cholesterol (LDL-C) [9] The profitable changes of the lipids profile have been observed in lots of studies after fats and the level of SFAs consumption were decreased [10],[11] A high level of LDL-C is the most important risk factor of CHD [12] Grundy [13] showed that people with a low level of LDL had a lower frequency of CHD even if they smoked cigarettes, had hypertension and diabetes type 2.

Saturated fatty acids without hypercholesterolemic effect had moreover pro-clot [14] and pro-arrhythmic effects [15] SFAs tend to elevate LDL, but not to all of them [16],[17] Stearic acid has not been shown to increase the level of cholesterol (it is rapidly converted to oleic acid) but other SFAs such as lauric, myristic and palmitic acids raise the cholesterol level [18]

Kelly et al. [19] showed that this is probable because of the fact that stearic acid, compared to palmitic one, increases the risk of CHD because it had trombogenic and atherogenic effects (without an impact on the cholesterol level). A strong positive association between SFAs and the risk of CVD was observed in the Nursers` Health Study (NHS) and Health Professionals` Follow-up Study (HPFS) [20],[21] In the NHS it was estimated that 5% of the SFAs energy, compared to an equivalent energy from carbohydrates, was associated with a 17% greater risk of CHD. On the other hand, total fat was not significantly related to that risk. For that reason, replacing SFAs with mono- and polyunsaturated fats (MUFAs and PUFAs) is more effective from preventing CHD than reducing an overall fat intake. According to dietary guidelines for general public by Third Report of the National Cholesterol Education Program - Adult Treatment Panel Step I [12] as well as WHO [2] saturated fatty acids intake should be limited no more than 10% of total calories. The Diet and Lifestyle Recommendation for Cardiovascular Disease Risk Reduction made by American Heart Association (AHA) [22] for general population is more restricted. According to them, the same like for people at higher risk of CVD by Step II NCEP ATP III [12] men should limit SFAs <7% of total calories. The main sources of SFAs are red meat, butter, whole milk and dairy products.

Sjögren et al. [23] proved that SFAs, derived from dairy products (about 4-10 and 14-carbons), have a positive association with a lower atherogenic profile of LDL cholesterol because there is a possible increase of contribution of small, dense LDL-C. An inverse association between SFAs derived from dairy products such as lauric and myristic fatty acid and TC concentration was found by Samuelson et al. [24] The above results indicate that fatty milk consumption may not be as harmful for health as it is commonly reputed. There is no evidence that a high frequency intake of whole milk tends to cardiovascular or other cause of mortality [25] Moreover, Sjögren et al. [23] indicate that there is a possible diminishes of atherogenic LDL profile by the other ingredients; without SFAs. Elwood et al. [26] showed that people drinking high and moderate milk amount have a lower risk of a stroke and a cardiac incident.

Moreover, milk and dairy products supply conjugated linoleic acid (CLA). It is possible that CLA plays a cardioprotective role from an atherogenesis development [27],[28],[29] In the animals study a profitable influence CLA on lipids profile were also proved [30]

It is clear that a high level of blood cholesterol is a risk factor of CVD. Cholesterol is derived from two sources: endogenous synthesis and from a diet. But the role of dietary cholesterol is not clear nowadays. In many previous studies it was indicated that the association between dietary cholesterol and the risk of CHD is equally the same as well as deaths from it [31],[32] in the Nurses' Health Study [20] and Health Professionals Follow-up Study [21] that link was not confirmed. de Lorgeril et al. [33] showed that even though a decreasing cholesterol level during the diet therapy did not decrease mortality. Many studies indicate that cholesterol concentration is not regulated by dietary cholesterol but a number of genes; once people are responsive, while the others not. It was also suggested that about 70% of humans are hyporesponsive to an excess of the dietary cholesterol consumption [34]

In a casual diet the major source of cholesterol are eggs. Studies have found no association between eggs consumption and the risk of CHD [35],[36],[37] Thus, a widespread belief that eggs are a major cause of heart diseases is not true. According to Fernandez, [38] there is a lack of a justification recommending people a reducing an intake of eggs nowadays. Nutritional guidelines for healthy people suggest eating moderate eggs as a part of well balanced diet. According to AHA, [22] the same like WHO [2] people should reduce dietary cholesterol in to<300 mg per day. The main sources of cholesterol are butter, fatty meat and their products, giblets, whole milk and dairy products as well as eggs.

In the prevention of CVD, polyunsaturated fatty acids are more important. Monounsaturated fatty acids (MUFAs) lower TC and LDL cholesterol, without influence on HDL cholesterol. MUFAs lower serum concentration of triglyceride (TG), glucose and blood pressure of patients with type 2 diabetes reveal moreover platelet antiaggregation [39]

MUFAs are derived from olive oil, rape-oil, almonds and nuts. Several prospective cohort studies found an inverse association between nuts consumption and the risk of CHD [40] Other studies showed that regular, varied type nut consumption may improve lipids profiles (reduction of total and LDL cholesterol) in co-operation with moderate of hypercholesterolemia [41],[42]. According to the above authors, consumption of 50–100 g of nuts >5 times per week has a profitable influence. These findings are supported by results from other numerous studies [43],[44],[45] Moreover, Bes-Rastrollo et al. [46] it was evidenced that frequent nuts consumption, compared to traditional snacks, which are usually rich in calories and may promote an energy imbalance resulting in obesity, was associated with a risk of weight gaining.

Another type of unsaturated fatty acid is a polyunsaturated fatty acid (PUFAs), which includes long-chain fatty acids omega-6 (e.g. linoleic acid) and omega-3 (EPA+DHA). Studies have found convincing evidence which has adverse effects on CHD risk by PUFAs [47] Omega-6 fatty acid lowers TC level without any impact on TG, but a higher intake of omega-6 (> 10% of energy) may increase susceptibility to LDL oxidation and speed up atherogenesis development [48],[49]

Fatty acid omega-3 has antiaggregation [50] and antiarrhythmic effect [51],[52] as well as improving lipids profile. The largest prospective Randomized Controlled Trials study - the GISSI-Prevenzione [53] showed, that a daily intake by the patients with myocardial infarction (MI) of 1 g PUFA such as long-chain fatty acid omega-3 (EPA+DHA) tends to 15% reduction of the primary end point of death, nonfatal MI and stroke. There was a 20% reduction in all-cause mortality and a 45% reduction in sudden death compared to a controlled group. This finding is supported by results of Indian Study [54] Moreover, PUFAs are more useful with the patients with insulin resistance and with type 2 diabetes [55]

The Nurses' Health Study showed that a higher fish intake (above 5 serving per week) was associated with a lower risk of cardiac events and total mortality [56] The profitable results of fish consumption were presented by the others [57],[58]

According to recommendations for a general population by WHO [2003] all PUFAs should provide 6-10% of total energy (from this 1-2% derived from omega-3). The main sources of PUFAs omega-3 are marine-fish. People should consume fish, especially oily fish, at least twice per week [22]

From the prevention of CVD point of view, trans fatty acids should be reduced in the casual diet [22] Trans fat has more atherogenic effect on plasma lipids (raising LDL-C), TG and lipoprotein (a) level as well as decreasing concentration of HDL-C [18] High trans fat intake contributes to an increase of risk of CHD [20],[47],[59],[60] For that reason people should avoid consumption of products, which contain trans fat acids such as processed and fried food, hydrogenated fats, and spreads as well as shortened and cooked fats.

Carbohydrates, and Fiber

Low in fat (low in SFAs) but rich in carbohydrates diet, which are usually recommended, especially for people with obesity, has no profitable effect on profile lipids. This type of dietary pattern leads to decrease of LDL-C, HDL-C and apolipoproteina A1 (apo A1) level elevates TG concentration at the same time [27],[61] Similar results were found by Williams et al. [62] in study about twins. In this situation more profitable would be a replacement of saturated fatty acids by monounsaturated fatty acids [63] or by use of a complex carbohydrates diet plus suitable amount of soluble fiber [12] Quality and quantity of carbohydrates and fiber contain food related to glycemic index (GI) and glycemic load (GL). High GI and GL products compared to low GI and GL products quickly and more efficiently increase level of glucose and TG as well as decrease level of HDL-C. A Population-Based Follow-Up Study has found that risk of CHD increased by consumption of high dietary GI and GL food, is especially accompanied with overweight [64] Moreover, a chronic consumption of high GI food may lead to chronically high oxidative stress [65] According to Hu and Willett, [66] the GI and GL concepts are more useful in prediction of risk of CHD than a traditional division based on chemical structure carbohydrates (simple vs. complex). A new dietary pyramid by United States Department of Agriculture (USDA) [67] based on products with low GI. with references for this pyramid says, that every day people should intake whole-grain products, oatmeal, brown rice etc. Numerous prospective studies proved, that whole-grain food intake correlates with a lower risk of CVD, mortality from CHD and MI [68],[69],[70] as well as reduction of potential risk factors such as diabetes type 2 [71],[72] and hypertension [73]

Whole-grain foods supply fiber, as well as vegetables and fruit. Soluble fraction of dietary fiber, compared to insoluble fiber, reveals profitable effect on total and LDL cholesterol concentration [74],[75] Among the elderly, only fiber from cereals sources, in comparison to that derived from vegetables and fruit, is much more strongly linked with the risk of CVD incident [76] This finding is supported by a result from other studies [77],[78],[79] Moreyra et al. [80] that have found that supplementation of psyllium may lower pharmacology simvastatin dose. The meta-analysis by Anderson [81] showed, that people intaking a large amount of dietary fiber compared to a consumption of a small portion of them, have lower risk of CHD for about 29%. The inverse correlation between a dietary fiber intake and risk of total and ischemic stroke was found in the other studies [55],[82] According to AHA Diet and Lifestyle Recommendation [22] people for CVD risk reduction should choose whole-grain and high-fiber foods and minimize an intake of beverages as well as food with added sugars.

Protein and B-Group Vitamins

These studies, which have been done so far, have found no association between protein intake and heart disease or myocardial infarction mortality. Numerous researchers emphasize that the replacement of animals protein by protein derived from plants is more profitable in the prevention of CVD. Lawrence [83] said that higher plant proteins intake decreased blood pressure and risk of heart disease. Animal proteins may be substituted by soy protein, which tends to improve lipids profile through reduction of total and LDL cholesterol level [84] The above-mentioned meta-analysis showed that the reduction of blood cholesterol depends on the level of hypercholesterolemia. The US Food and Drug Administration [85] based on clinical studies, shows that intake of at least 25g of soy protein per day reduces total and LDL cholesterol. The next randomized trials proved that isolated soy protein with isoflavones rich diet, as an alternative of animal proteins, gives a benefit to improve lipids profile (a very small benefit related to a large amount of soy protein, averaging 50g). For that reason an intake of large dose of soy protein (in contrast soy products) is not recommended by AHA [86]

The animal proteins are rich in sulphuric amino acids such as methionine. Methionine in the metabolic pathway is converted to homocysteine. A high level of homocysteine is an independent risk factor leading to atherosclerosis development [87] A higher intake of animal proteins, as well as folate, B_6, B_{12} vitamins deficiency, elevates methionine concentration. Profitable results of supplementation of B-group vitamins are both noticeable among healthy people aged 50-70 [88] and patients after coronary intervention were proved [89] This finding is no supported by other results [90] Although supplementation of B-group vitamins is recognized of hyperhomocysteinemia treatment [91],[92] it is not recommended nowadays based on results of clinical randomized studies [93],[94],[95],[96] Taking into account that a high B-group vitamins intake is beneficial in preventing CVD and lowers the intake among the elderly [97],[98] these ingredients should be derived from a diet. The major sources of folate are green leafy vegetable; B_6 and B_{12} – meat, their products and some alternatives e.g. soy products or nuts.

Antioxidants, Minerals and Flavonoids

Antioxidants such as vitamins C, E as well as beta-carotene play more important preventive role in CVD. Vitamin C neutralizes free radicals and improves a vascular reactivity among people with hypercholesterolemia and CHD [99],[100] Vitamin E prevents the LDL cholesterol oxidation, inhibits platelet activation and monocyte adhesion [101]

An association between the intakes of antioxidants was affirmed in the Health Professionals Follow-up Study [102] These findings are consistent with several other studies [103],[104],[105] Another result was noted in large studies related to a primary prevention. The Randomized Controlled Trials such as Alpha-Tocopherol Beta-Carotene Cancer Prevention Study (ATBC) [106] Beta-Carotene and Retinol Efficacy Trial (CARET) [107] Chinese Cancer Prevention Trial [[108] and Physicians' Health Study [[109] showed significant, negative effects or had no influence of antioxidants on CHD.

In spite of a few above-mentioned facts related to link antioxidants and CVD risk, according to NCEP ATP III [12] there are no recommendations of antioxidants a diet supplementation. The Institute of Medicine [110] recommends a high intake of vitamin C for smokers.

In the prevention of CVD more important are minerals such as sodium and potassium. There is convincing evidence that an increase of sodium intake increases blood pressure [111] The International Study of Sodium, Potassium and Blood Pressure (INTERSALT) showed that the sodium intake above 100 mmol per day tends to elevate both diastolic and systolic pressure respectively (3-6 and 0-3 mmHg) [112] A high risk of a stroke in Japan and China compared to the population of the United Kingdom (UK) and US is associated to a high consumption of dietary sodium and low potassium in these populations [113] The benefits of reduction decrease of sodium intake in the Dietary Approaches to Stop Hypertension (DASH) were showed [114],[115] It was estimated that about 80% of salt intake by US and Europe populations was derived from take-away food usually consumed by people [116] Thus, more important is a population strategy of a progressively reduction of a salt level in products which salt is added during the technology process. If people want to reduce a salt intake, according to the AHA Diet and Lifestyle Recommendation [22] they should choose and prepare food with little or no salt amount or choose low-sodium and low-salty products. For the group of products with a little amount of sodium vegetables and fruit may be accepted, which likewise legumes, potatoes contain potassium. Suitable proportions of sodium and potassium in a diet are more important to reduce blood pressure [117]

In the prevention of heart diseases, the role of flavonoids should be considered. Flavonoids are widely distributed in vegetables, fruit and other products such as red wine, cocoa and tea. Cardioprotective property of flavonoids has been revealed in numerous studies [118],[119],[120] Flavonoids inhibit oxidative stress and platelet aggregation, reduce LDL cholesterol oxidation' atherosclerosis plaque development, and improve endothelial function. Many types of flavonoids have varied impact on CVD risk. Cocoa products contain greater antioxidant capacity than red wine and teas per serving [121],[122] Properties of products containing cocoa such as dark chocolate were proved in many studies [123] It was estimated that the intake of 50g dark chocolate per day may reduce risk of CVD by 10.5% [124]

Moreover, other studies showed that chocolate preference in an old age was associated with better health, optimism and better psychological well-being [122]

In the meta-analysis by Hyxley and Neil [125] all of the flavonoids have beneficial impact on CHD mortality. On the other hand, there are studies which do not confirm the correlation between flavonoids intake and CVD incidents [126],[127]

Diet for the Elderly

Nutritional habits have influence on nutrition statues and health statues, which guarantee longevity. Unhealthy nutritional habits (caloric, fat and cholesterol rich diet as well as low in fruit, vegetables and whole-grain products one) appear to have associations with risk of cardiovascular diseases what the above-mentioned was proved. Many studies showed do not promote nutrition guidelines for public of an intake of major nutritional ingredients and do not suggest the minimum Food Guide Pyramid in food group consumption by the elderly [128],[129][130] The greatest abnormalities have been noted in association with diet high in fat, refined grains, added sugar and salt as well as low in vegetables, fruit, whole grains and dairy products. The other disadvantage of that, with reference for nutritional habits of older people, is high prevalence of snaking [130]

That above-presented unhealthy, dietary pattern could be described as a "Western pattern", which compared to so called "prudent pattern" can predict CVD risk [70],[131] An unhealthy diet is usually linked with an unhealthy lifestyle (drinking alcohol, smoking, lack of activity) plus obesity, are correlated to one another [132],[133] What is more to a socioeconomic status as well. [134],[135],[136],[137] All of the above factors are described as CVD risk factors [5],[138] The coexistence of numerous risk factors and their correlations should be taken into account in the primary prevention of CVD.

First - a healthy diet. In the primary prevention of heart disease, low in saturated fat, trans fat and cholesterol diet, but rich in MUFAs, PUFAs and fiber is recommended [22] These recommendations are met in a Mediterranean diet. Several other studies have indicated a lower rate of all-causes and cause-specified mortality among the elderly by the intake of Mediterranean diet [139] Moreover, an inverse correlation of this type of diet with CVD risk factors was found as well [140],[141],[142] The above results, according to Estruch et al. [142] in a great extent, were caused by a high contain of olive oil in the Mediterranean diet. A beneficial impact on CHD risk associated with consumption of olive oil was observed in the other study [143] For this reason olive oil, instead of animal fat, is good for meal preparation and frying. Moreover, a Mediterranean-like dietary pattern is rich in vegetables and fruit, which intake is recommended by AHA [22] A high consumption of them is correlated with lower CHD [144] and an ischemic stroke risk [145] Vegetables and fruit are the part of parcel of the Mediterranean-like diet - a DASH diet, which in the primary prevention of the ischemic stroke, is also recommended [146]

The Mediterranean diet consists of whole-grain products, which its cardioprotective effect was described beforehand (especially for the elderly diet rich in cereals). Studies have found that a higher intake of whole-grain food in a diet increases vegetables and fruit as well as decrease of red meat consumption [147],[148] Healthy dietary pattern among elderly (mean age 72 years) were noted in the other study [76] The results showed a lower risk of a cardiovascular incident, associated with a greater amount of fish, and a lower meat and SFAs intake, as well as correlated with healthier lifestyle and greater education. It is common that the intake of fish could be a potential exposure to some contaminants, but according to AHA, for middle-aged and older people, the benefit from the fish intake is far outweigh the risk when they consume fish accordingly with the recommendation.

In the prevention of CVD, besides reduction of saturated fat in a diet, more important is a balanced calorie intake [22] Generally, the low-fat diet is recommended with references for people with obesity. For that reason, compared if a low-fat diet is the same profitable as the Mediterranean one. In the study, a 15% reduction in CVD risk, based on the Mediterranean diet, and only 9% based on the low-fat diets, were predicted [149] In the randomized trial by Estruch et al. [142] it was indicated that the Mediterranean diet, supplemented with nuts or olive oil vs. the low-fat diet is more effective for improvement of risk factors for participants aged 50-80 years at high CHD risk.

Nutritional habits are related to age. It was proved that age may be a more important determinant of dietary pattern efficiency [150] It was indicated that the promotion of an impact of the Mediterranean diet in reduction of overall mortality was only suitable for people below 80 years in comparison to the elderly. Moreover, nutritional patterns vary across the countries. The longitudinal Survey in Europe on Nutrition and the Elderly: a Concerted Action study (SENECA) [132] proved, that a dietary intake is varied even across Europe. In the above study no effect on a healthy, Mediterranean-like diet in case of the deterioration of health status was indicated. [151]. Other prospective studies made in nine European countries, showed that an adherence to the modified Mediterranean diet is associated with a longer life expectancy among elderly Europeans [152]

Secondly – a dietary supplementation. Nowadays, there is no convincing evidence that in the primary prevention of CVD, a diet should be supplemented by antioxidants (C, E, beta-carotene) and B-group vitamin as well as long chain fatty acids omega-3 [22] Moreover, use of isoflavones supplements in food or pills is not recommended by AHA [86] Because older people have decreased energy needs while their vitamins (similar like minerals) requirements are constant or increase, they should choose food groups selected and supplied by the above-mentioned ingredients from a casual diet.

Thirdly – healthy lifestyle, consisting of: physical activity, giving up smoking, moderation in alcohol drinking and maintaining suitable body weight. A cardioprotective role and benefits for longevity of the above presented lifestyle factors were proved in numerous studies [151],[153],[154],[155] These studies found that a moderate alcohol intake compared to an abstention of heavy drinking, is correlated with lower mortality from all the causes among the elderly and the middle-aged people [156] Profitable influences of flavones are contained in red wine [157],[158] AHA [22] recommended a limited drinking alcohol (no more than 2 drinks per day for men, 1 drink for women) to point that at the same time, if people never drink alcohol, they will not start it.

Fourthly – personality. A high level of hostility, anxiety and susceptibility to stress, which are included in the "type A behavior" [159] are linked to increased risk of a coronary heart disease, myocardial infarction and cardiovascular death [160],[161],[162],[163] Adopting or maintaining healthy lifestyles may be helpful in stress reduction and a good start in the subject of preventing of CVD.

Conclusion

Aging of population is related to an increasing risk of chronic diseases such as cardiovascular disease. Despite of health status, declined with time among the elderly, the independence of other lifestyle factors is much more important in the process of increase of public awareness about the benefits coming from a lower exposure of the potential risk factors of CVD. Coexistence of numerous risk factors and their mutual correlations should be taken into account in the primary prevention of heart diseases. In this group, a significant role is player by a healthy diet. Numerous studies showed that Mediterranean-like pattern, based on a large amount of olive oil, vegetables, fruit, fish and whole-grain products, could be suitable for older people in the prevention of CVD. With references for the elderly, we do not forget that they often have a few accompanying diseases, generally alimentary canal disorders or lack of dentition. That is why a dietary recommendation should be based on it. Moreover, the elderly nutritional habits are frequently related to their financial status and education. Older people usually prefer easy preparation and not time-consuming meals based on available products. The nutritional recommendation for the elderly should include all the above-presented factors. Nutritional education with a program improving an activity level among the elderly is considered as helpful to understand the fact, that even people above 60 are not too late to change nutritional habits for healthy ageing.

References

[1]   Thom, T; Haase, N; Rosamond, W; Howard, VJ; Rumsfeld, J; Manolio, T; Zheng, Z-J; Flegal, K; O'Donnell, Ch; Kittner, S; Lloyd-Jones, D; Goff, DC; Hong, Y; Adams, R; Friday, G; Furie, K; Gorelick, P; Kissela, B; Marler, J; Meigs, J; Roger, V; Sidney, S; Sorlie, P; Steinberger, J; Wasserthiel-Smoller, S; Wilson, M; Wolf, P. Heart Disease and Stroke Statistics-2006 Update. A Report From the American Heart Association Statistics Committee and Stroke Statistics Subcommittee. *Circulation*, 2006, 113, 85-151.

[2]   Diet, nutritional and the prevention of chronic diseases. Report of Joint WHO/FAO Expert Consultation. World Health Organization Geneva 2003.

[3]   Forman, D; Bulwer, BE. Cardiovascular diseases: Optimal Approaches to risk factors modification of diet and lifestyle. *Curr Treat Options Cardiovasc Med*, 2006, 8, 47-57.

[4]   Wojtyniak, B; Goryński, P; Seroka, W. Stan zdrowia ludności Polski na podstawie danych o umieralności. Przedwczesna umieralność w Polsce na tle sytuacji w Unii Europejskiej. W: Wojtyniak B., Goryński P. (red): Sytuacja zdrowotna ludności Polski. Warszawa: PZH - Zakład Statystyki Medycznej; 2003; 47-55.

[5]   Pyorala, K; De Backer, G; Graham, I; Poole-Wilson, P; Wood, D. Prevention of coronary heart disease in clinical practice. Recommendations of the Task Force of the European Society of Cardiology, European Atherosclerosis Society and European Society of Hypertension. *Eur Heart J*, 1994, 15, 1300-1331.

[6]   Okrainec, K; Banerjee, D; Eisenberg, M. Coronary artery disease in the developing world. *Am Heart J*, 2004, 148, 7-15.

[7]   Holme, I; Hjermann, I; Helgeland, A; Leren, P. The Oslo Study: diet and antismoking advice - additional results from a 5-year primary prevention trial in middle aged men. *Prev Med*, 1985, 14, 279-292.

[8]   Stampfer, NJ; Hu, FB; Mason, JE; Rimm, EB; Willet, WC. Primary prevention of coronary heart disease in woman through diet and lifestyle. *N Engl J Med*, 2000, 343, 16-22.

[9]   German, JB; Dillard, CJ. Saturated fats: what dietary intake? *Am J Clin Nutr*, 2004, 80, 550-559.

[10]   Knopp, RH; Retzlaff, BM. Saturated fat prevents coronary artery disease? An American paradox. *Am J Clin Nutr*, 2004, 80, 1102-1103.

[11]   Masson, LF; McNeill, G; Avenell, A. Genetic variation and the lipid response to dietary intervention: a systematic review. *Am J Clin Nutr*, 2003, 77, 1098-1111.

[12]   *Adult Treatment Panel III: Third Report of the National Cholesterol Education Program Expert Panel on Detection, Evaluation, and Treatment of High Blood Cholesterol in Adults. Final Report (ATP III). National Institute of Health, 2002.*

[13]   Grundy, SM. Small LDL, atherogenic dyslipidemia, and the matabolic syndrome. *Circulation*, 1997, 95, 1-4.

[14]   Kromhout, D; Menotti, A; Kesteloot, H; Sans, S. Preention of coronary heart disease by diet and lifestyle. Evidence from prospective cross-cultural, cohort, and intervention studies. *Circulation*, 2002, 105, 893-898.

[15]   de Lorgeril, M; Salen, P; Defaye, P; Mabo, P; Paillard, F. Dietary prevention of sudden cardiac death. *Eur Heart J*, 2002, 23, 277-285.

[16]   Mensink, RP; Zock, PL; Kester, ADM; Katan, MB. Effects of dietary fatty acids and carbohydrates on the ratio of serum total to HDL cholesterol and on serum lipids and alipoproteins: meta-analysis of 60 controlled trials. *Am J Clin Nutr*, 2003, 77, 1146-1155.

[17]   Schaefer, EJ. Lipoproteins, nutrition, and heart disease. *Am J Clin Nutr*, 2002, 75, 191-212.

[18]   Fernandez, ML; West, KL. Mechanisms by which dietary fatty acids modulate plasma lipids. *J Nutr*, 2005, 135, 2075-2078.

[19]   Kelly, FD; Sinclair, AJ; Mann, NJ; Turner, AH; Abedin, LLiD. A stearic acid-rich diet improves thrombogenic and atherogenic risk factor profiles in healthy males. *Eur J Clin Nutr*, 2001, 55, 88-96.

[20]   Hu, FB; Stampfer, MJ; Manson, JE; Rimm, E; Colditz, GA; Rosner, BA; Hennekens, ChH; Willett, WC. Dietary fat intake and the risk of coronary heart disease in women. N Engl J Med, 1997, 337, 1491-149.

[21]   Ascherio, A; Rimm, EB; Giovannucci, EL; Spiegelman, D; Stampfer, M; Willett, WC. Dietary fat and risk of coronary heart disease in men: cohort follows up study in the United States. *Brit Med J*, 1996, 313, 84-90.

[22]   American Heart Association Nutrition Committee, Lichtenstein, AH; Appel, LJ; Brands, M; Carnethon, M; Daniels, S; Franch, HA; Franklin, B; Kris-Etherton, P; Harris, WS; Howard, B; Karanja, N; Lefevre, M; Rudel, L; Sacks, F; Van Horn, L; Winston, M; Wylie-Rosett, J. Diet and lifestyle recommendations revision 2006: a scientific statement from the American Heart Association Nutrition Committee. *Circulation*, 2006, 114, 82-96.

[23] Sjogren, P; Rosell, M; Skoglund-Andersson, C; Zdravkovic, S; Vessby, B; Faire, U De; Hamsten, A; Hellenius, M-L; Fisher, RM. Milk-derived fatty acids are associated with a more favorable LDL particle size distribution in healthy men. *J Nutr*, 2004, 134, 1729-1735.

[24] Samuelson, G; Bratteby, LE; Mohsen, R; Vessby, B. Dietary fat intake in healthy adolescents: inverse relationships between the estimated intake ,of saturated fatty acids and serum cholesterol. *Br J Nutr*, 2001, 85, 333-341.

[25] Ness, AR; Smith, GD; Hart, C. Milk, coronary heart disease and mortality. *J Epidemiol Community Health*, 2001, 55, 379-382.

[26] Elwood, PC; Strain, JJ; Robson, PJ; Fehily, AM; Hughes, J; Pickering, J; Ness, A. Milk consumption, stroke, and heart attack risk: evidence from the Caerphilly cohort of older men. *J Epidemiol Community Health*, 2005, 59, 502-505.

[27] Parodi, PW. Milk fat in human nutrition. *Austr J Dairy Technol*, 2004, 59, 3.

[28] Faulconnier, Y; Arnal, MA; Patureau, MP; Chardigny, JM; Chilliard, Y. Isomers of conjugated linoleic acid decrease plasma lipids and stimulate adipose tissue lipogenesis without changing adipose weight in post-prandial adult sedentary or trained wistar rat. *J Nutr Biochem*, 2004, 15, 741-748.

[29] Kritchevsky, D; Tepper, SA; Wright, S; Czarnecki, SK; Wilson, TA. Conjugated linoleic acid isomer effects in atherosclerosis: Growth and regression of lesions. *Lipids*, 2004, 39, 611-616.

[30] Lock, AL; Horne, CAM; Bauman, DE; Salter, AM. Butter naturally enriched in conjugated linoleic acid and vaccenic acid alters tissue fatty acids and improves the plasma lipoprotein profile in cholesterol-fed hamsters. *J Nutr*, 2005, 135, 1934-1939.

[31] McGee, DL; Reed, DM; Yano, K; Kagan, A; Tillotson, J. Ten-Year incidence of coronary heart disease in the Honolulu Heart Program: Relationship to nutrient intake. *Am J Epidemiol*, 1984, 119, 667-676.

[32] Shekelle, RB; Shyrock, AM; Paul, O; Lepper, M; Stamler, J; Liu, S; Raynor, WJ. Diet, serum cholesterol, and death from coronary heart disease: the Western Electric Study. *N Engl J Med*, 1981, 304, 65-70.

[33] de Lorgeril, M; Salen, P; Monjaud, I; Delaye, J. The diet heart hypothesis in secondary prevention of coronary heart disease. *Eur Heart J*, 1997, 18, 14-18.

[34] McNamara, DJ. The impact of egg limitations on coronary heart disease risk: do the numbers add up? *J Am Coll Nutr*, 2000, 19, 540-548.

[35] Kritchevsky, SB; Kritchevsky, D. Egg consumption and coronary heart disease: an epidemiologic overview. *J Am Coll Nutr*, 2000, 19, 549-555.

[36] Song, WO; Kerner, JM. Nutritional contribution of eggs to American diets. *J Am Coll Nutr*, 2000, 19, 556-562.,

[37] Hu, FB; Stampfer, MJ; Rimm, EB; Manson, JE; Ascherio, A; Colditz, GA; Rosner, BA; Spiegelman, D; Speizer, FE; Sacks, FM; Hennekens, CH; Willett, WC. A prospective study of egg consumption and risk of cardiovascular disease in men and women. *J Am Med Assoc*, 1999, 281, 1387-1394.

[38] Fernandez, ML; West, KL. Mechanisms by which dietary fatty acids modulate plasma lipids. *J Nutr*, 2005, 135, 2075-2078.

[39] Kris-Etherton. P. Monosaturated fatty acids and risk of cardiovascular disease. *Circulation*, 1999, 100, 1253-1258.

[40] Stampfer, MJ; Hu, FB. Nut consumption and risk of coronary heart disease: a review of epidemiologic evidence. *Current Atherosclerosis Reports*, 1999, 1, 204-209.

[41] Sheridan, MJ; Cooper, JN; Erario, M; Cheifetz, CE. Pistachio Nut Consumption and Serum Lipid Levels. *J Am Coll Nutr*. 26, 141-148.

[42] Mukuddem-Petersen, J; Oosthuizen, W; Jerling, JC. A Systematic Review of the Effects of Nuts on Blood Lipid Profiles in Humans. *J Nutr*, 2005, 135, 2082-2089.

[43] Iwamoto, M; Sato, M; Kono, M; Hirooka, Y; Sakai, K; Takeshita, A; Imaizumi, K. Walnuts lower serum cholesterol in Japanese men and women. *J Nutr*, 2000, 130, 171-176.

[44] Zambon, D; Sabate, J; Munoz, S; Campero, B; Casals, E; Merlos, M; Laguna, JC; Ros, E. Substituting walnuts for monounsaturated fat improves the serum lipid profile of hypercholesterolemic men and women. A randomized crossover trial. *Ann Intern Med*, 2000, 132, 538-546.

[45] Morgan, WA; Clayshulte, BJ. Pecans lower low-density lipoprotein cholesterol in people with normal lipid levels. *J Am Diet Assoc*, 2000, 100, 312-318.

[46] Bes-Rastrollo, M; Sabaté, J; Gómez-Gracia, E; Alonso, A; Martínez, JA; Martínez-González, MA. Nut Consumption and Weight Gain in a Mediterranean Cohort: The SUN Study. *Obesity*, 2007, 15, 107-116.

[47] Oh K; Hu, FB; Manson, JE; Stampfer, M; Willett, W. Dietary fat intake and risk of coronary heart disease in women: 20 years of follow-up of the nurses' health study. *Am J Epidemiol*, 2005, 161, 672-679.

[48] Eritsland, J. Safety considerations of polyunsaturated fatty acids. *Am J Clin Nutr*, 2000, 71, 197-201.

[49] Nordoy, A. Dietary fatty acids and coronary heart disease. *Lipids*, 1999, 34 (suppl), 19-22.

[50] von Shacky, C. n-3 Fatty acids and the prevention of coronary atherosclerosis. *Am J Clin Nutr*, 2000, 71 (suppl), 224–227.

[51] Leaf, A; Albert, CM; Josephson, M; Steinhaus, D; Kluger, J; Kang, JX; Cox, B; Zhang, H; Schoenfeld, D. Prevention of fatal arrhythmias in high-risk subjects by fish oil n-3 fatty acid intake. *Circulation*, 2005, 112, 2762-2768.

[52] Mozaffarian, D; Fried, LP; Burke, GL; Fitzpatrick, A; Siscovick, DS. Lifestyles of older adults: can we influence cardiovascular risk in older adults? *Am J Geriatr Cardiol*, 2004, 13, 153-160.

[53] GISSI-Prevenzione Investigators. Dietary supplementation with n-3 polyunsaturated fatty acid and vitamin E after myocardial infarction: result of the GISSI-Prevenzione trial. Gruppo Italiano per lo Studio della Sopravvivenza nell`Infarto miocardico. *Lancet*, 1999, 354, 447-455.

[54] Singh, RB; Niaz, MA; Sharma, JP; Kumar, R; Rastogi, V; Moshiri, M. Randomized, double-blind, placebo-controlled trial of fish oil and mustard oil in patients with suspected acute myocardial infarction: the Indian experiment of infarct survival-4. *Cardiovasc Drugs Ther*, 1997, 11, 485–491.

[55] Hu, FB; Willett, WC. Optimal Diets for Prevention of Coronary Heart Disease. *J Am Med Assoc*, 2000, 288, 2569-2578.

[56] Hu, FB, Cho, E; Rexrode, KM; Albert, CM; Manson, JE. Fish and long-chain omega-3 fatty acid intake and risk of coronary heart disease and total mortality in diabetic women. *Circulation*, 2003, 107, 1852-1857

[57] Burr, ML; Fehily, AM; Gilbert, JF; Rogers, S; Holliday, RM; Sweetnam, PM; Elwood, PC; Deadman, NM. Effects of changes in fat, fish, and fibre intakes on death and myocardial reinfarction: diet and reinfarction trial (DART). *Lancet*, 1989, 2, 757-761.

[58] Hu, FB; Bronner, L; Willet, WC; Stampfer, MJ; Rexrode, KM; Albert, CM; Hunter, D; Manson, JE. Fish and omega-3 fatty acid intake and risk of coronary heart disease in women. *J Am Med Assoc*, 2002, 287, 1815-1821.

[59] Sun, Q; Ma, J; Campos, H; Hankinson, SE; Manson, JE; Stampfer, MJ; Rexrode, KM; Willett, WC; Hu, FB. A Prospective Study of Trans Fatty Acids in Erythrocytes and Risk of Coronary Heart Disease. *Circulation*, 2007, 115, 1858-1865.

[60] Oomen, CM; Ocke, MC; Feskens, EJ; van Erp-Baart, MA; Kok, FJ; Kromhout, D. Association between trans fatty acid intake and 10-year risk of coronary heart disease in the Zutphen Elderly Study: a prospective population-based study. *Lancet*, 2001, 357, 746-751.

[61] Meksawan, K; Pendergast, DR; Leddy, JJ; Mason, M; Horvath, PJ; Awad, AB. Effects of low and high fat diets on nutrient intake and selected cardiovascular risk factors in sedentary men and women. *J Am Coll Nutr*, 2004, 23, 131-140.

[62] Williams, PT; Blanche, PJ; Rawlings, R; Krauss, RM. Concordant lipoprotein and weight responses to dietary fat change in identical twins with divergent exercise levels. *J Am Coll Nutr*, 2005, 82, 181-187.

[63] Hodson, L; Skeaff, CM; Chisholm, W-AH. The effect of replacing dietary saturated fat with polyunsaturated or monounsaturated fat on plasma lipids in free-living young adults. *Eur J Clin Nutr*, 2001, 55, 908-915.

[64] Beulens, JWJ; de Bruijne, LM; Stolk, RP; Peeters, PHM; Bots, ML; Grobbee, DE; van der Schouw, YT. High Dietary Glycemic Load and Glycemic Index Increase Risk of Cardiovascular Disease Among Middle-Aged Women: A Population-Based Follow-Up Study. *J Am Coll Cardiol*, 2007, 50, 14 - 21.

[65] Hu, Y; Block, G; Norkus, EP; Morrow, JD; Dietrich, M; Hudes, M. Relations of glycemic index and glycemic load with plasma oxidative stress markers. *Am J Clin Nutr*, 2006, 84, 70-76.

[66] Hu, FB; Willett, WC. Diet and coronary heart disease: findings from the Nurses' Health Study and Health Professionals' Follow-Up Study. *J Nutr Health & Aging*, 2001, 5, 132-138.

[67] Pyramid Food Guidelines by United States Department of Agriculture http://www.mypyramid.gov

[68] Liu, S; Sesso, HD; Manson, JE; Willett, WC; Buring, JE. Is intake of breakfast cereals related to total and cause-specific mortality in men? *Am J Clin Nutr*, 2003, 77, 594-599.

[69] Truswell, AS. Cereal grains and coronary heart disease. *Eur J Clin Nutr*, 2002, 6, 1-14.

[70] Hu, FB; Rimm, EB; Stampfer, MJ; Ascherio, A; Spiegelman, D; Willett, WC. Prospective study of major dietary patterns and risk of coronary heart disease in men. *Am J Clin Nutr*, 2000, 72, 912-921.

[71] Meyer, KA; Kushi, LH; Jacobs, DR; Slavin, J; Sellers, TA; Folsom, AR. Carbohydrates, dietary fiber, and incident type 2 diabetes in older women. *Am J Clin Nutr*, 2000, 71, 921-930.

[72]   Liu, S; Manson, JE; Stampfer, MJ; Hu, FB; Giovannucci, E; Colditz, GA; Hennekens, CH; Willett, WC. A prospective study of whole-grain intake and risk of type 2 diabetes mellitus in US women. *Am J Public Health*, 2000, 90, 1409-1415.

[73]   Liu, S; Manson, J. Dietary carbohydrates, physical activity, obesity, and the 'metabolic syndrome' as predictors of coronary heart disease. *Curr Opin Lipidol*, 2001, 12, 395-404.

[74]   Anderson, JW; Hanna, TJ; Peng, X; Kryscio, RJ. Whole grain foods and heart disease risk. *J Am Coll Nutr*, 2000, 19, 291-299.

[75]   Davy, BM, Davy, KP; Ho, RC; Beske, SD; Davrath, LR; Melby, CL. High-fiber oat cereal compared with wheat cereal consumption favorably alters LDL-cholesterol subclass and particle numbers in middle-aged and older men. *Am J Clin Nutr*, 2002, 76, 351-358.

[76]   Mozaffarian, D; Kumanyika, SK; Lemaitre, RN; Olson, JL; Burke, GL; Siscovick, DS. Cereal, fruit, and vegetable fiber intake and the risk of cardiovascular disease in elderly individuals. *J Am Med Assoc*, 2003, 289, 1659-1666.

[77]   Rimm, EB; Ascherio, A; Giovannucci, E; Spiegelman, D; Stampfer, MJ; Willett, WC. Vegetable, fruit, and cereal fiber intake and risk of coronary heart disease among men. *J Am Med Assoc*, 1996, 275, 447-451.

[78]   Wolk, A; Manson, JE; Stampfer, MJ; Colditz, GA; Hu, FB; Speizer, FE; Hennekens, CH; Willett, WC. Long-term intake of dietary fiber and decreased risk of coronary heart disease among women. *J Am Med Assoc*, 1999, 281, 1998-2004.

[79]   Ascherio, A; Rimm, EB; Hernan, MA; Giovannucci, EL; Kawachi, I; Stampfer, MJ; Willett, WC. Intake of potassium, magnesium, calcium, and fiber and risk of stroke among US men. *Circulation*, 1998, 98, 1198-1204.

[80]   Moreyra, AE; Wilson, AC; Koraym, A. Effect of combining psyllium fiber with simvastatin in lowering cholesterol. *Arch Intern Med*, 2005, 165, 1161-1166.

[81]   Anderson, JW. Whole-grains intake and risk for coronary heart disease. In: Marquart, L; Slavin, JL; Fulcher, G. (eds.): Whole grains in health and diseae. St Paul, MN: *Am Assoc Cereal Chem*, 2002, 100-114.

[82]   Liu, S; Willett, WC; Stampfer, MI; Hu, FB; Franz, M; Sampson, L; Hennekens, CH; Manson, JE. A prospective study of dietary glycemic load, carbohydrate intake, and risk of coronary heart disease in US women. *Am J Clin Nutr*, 2000, 71, 1455-1461.

[83]   Lawrence, JA. The effects of protein intake on blood pressure and cardiovascular disease. *Curr Opin Lipidol*, 2003, 14, 55-59.

[84]   Anderson, JW; Johnstone, BM; Cook-Newell, M.E.: Meta-analysis of the effects of soy protein intake on serum lipids. *N Engl J Med*, 1995, 333, 276-282.

[85]   Food labeling: health claims: soy protein and coronary heart disease. Food and Drug Administration, HHS: final rule: soy protein and coronary heart disease. *Fed Reg*, 1999, 64, 57700–57733.

[86]   Sacks, FM; Lichtenstein, A; Van Horn, L; Harris, W; Kris-Etherton, P; Winston, M. Soy Protein, Isoflavones, and Cardiovascular Health. An American Heart Association Science Advisory for Professionals. *Circulation*, 2006, 113, 1034-1044.

[87]   Ford, ES; Smith, SJ; Stroup, DF; Steinberg, KK; Mueller, PW; Thacker, SB. Homocysteine and cardiovascular disease: a systematic review of the evidence with special emphasis on case-control studies and nested case-control studies. *Int J Epidemiol*, 2002, 31, 59-70.

[88] Durga, J; van Tits, LJH; Schouten, EG; Kok, FJ; Verhoef, P. Effect of lowering of homocysteine levels on inflammatory markers. *Arch Intern Med*, 2005, 165, 1388-1394.

[89] Schnyder, G; Roffi, M; Flammer, Y; Pin, R; Hess, OM. Effect of homocysteine-lowering therapy with folic acid, vitamin B (12), and vitamin B(6) on clinical outcome after percutaneus coronary intervention: the Swiss Heart Study, a randomized controlled trial. *J Am Med Assoc*, 2002, 288, 973-979.

[90] Lange H., Suryapranata H., De Luca, G; Borner, C; Dille, J; Kallmayer, K; Pasalary, MN; Scherer, E; Dambrink, J-HE. Folate therapy and in-stent restenosis after coronary stenting. *N Engl J Med*, 2004, 350, 2673-2681.

[91] Robertson, J; Iemolo, F; Stabler, SP; Allen, RH; Spence, JD.Vitamin B12, homocysteine and carotid plaque in the era of folic acid fortification of enriched cereal grain products. *Can Med Assoc J*, 2005, 172, 1569-1573.

[92] Rimm, EB; Willett, WC; Hu, FB; Sampson, L; Colditz, GA; Manson, JE; Hennekens, C; Stampfer, MJ. Folate and vitamin B6 from diet and supplements in relation to risk of coronary heart disease among women. *J Am Med Assoc*, 1998, 279, 359-364.

[93] Toole, JF; Malinow, MR; Chambless, LE; Spence, JD; Pettigrew, LC; Howard, VJ; Sides, EG; Wang, CH; Stampfer, M. Lowering homocysteine in patients with ischemic stroke to prevent recurrent stroke, myocardial infarction, and death: the Vitamin Intervention for Stroke Prevention (VISP) randomized controlled trial. *Am Med Assoc*, 2004, 291, 565-575.

[94] Bonaa, KH; Njalstad, I; Ueland, PM; et al. For the NORVIT Trial Investigators. Homocysteine lowering and cardiovascular events after myocardial infarction. *N Engl J Med*, 2006, 345, 1578-1588.

[95] Lonn, E; Yusuf, S; Arnold, MJ; et al. Homocysteine lowering with folic acid and B vitamins in vascular disease. The Heart Outcomes Prevention Evaluation (HOPE) 2 Investigators. *N Engl J Med*, 2006, 354, 1567-1577.

[96] Zoungas, S; McGrath, BP; Branley, P; Kerr, PG; Muske, C; Wolfe, R; Atkins, RC; Nicholls, K; Fraenkel, M; Hutchison, BG; Walker, R; McNeil, JJ. Cardiovascular morbidity and mortality in the Atherosclerosis and Folic Acid Supplementation Trial (ASFAST) in chronic renal failure. *J Am Coll Cardiol*, 2006, 47, 1108-1116.

[97] Mulligan, JE; Greene, GW; Caldwell, MC. Sources of folate and serum folate levels in older adults. *J Am Diet Assoc*, 2007, 107, 495-499.

[98] Foote, JA; Giuliano, AR; Harris, RB. Older adults need guidance to meet nutritional recommendations. *J Am Coll Nutr*, 2000, 19, 628-640.

[99] Ting, HH; Timimi, FK; Haley, EA; Roddy, MA; Ganz, P; Creager, MA. Vitamin C improves endothelium-dependent vasodilation in forearm resistance vessels of humans with hypercholesterolemia. *Circulation*, 1997, 95, 2617-2622.

[100] Levine, GN; Frei, B, Koulouris, SN; Gerhard, MD; Keaney, FJ; Vita, JA..Ascorbic acid reverses endothelial vasomotor dysfunction in patients with coronary artery disease. *Circulation*, 1996, 93, 1107-1113.

[101] Diaz, MN; Frei, B; Vita, JA; Keaney, JrJF. Antioxidants and atherosclerotic heart disease. *N Eng J Med*, 1997, 337, 408-416.

[102] Rimm, EB; Stampfer, MJ; Ascherio, A; Giovannucci, E; Colditz, GA; Willett, WC. Vitamin E consumption and the risk of coronary heart disease in men. *N Engl J Med*, 1993, 328, 1450-1456.

[103] Gaziano, JM; Manson, JE; Branch, LG; Colditz, GA; Willett, WC; Buring, JE. A prospective study of consumption of carotenoids in fruits and vegetables and decreased cardiovascular mortality in the elderly. *Ann Epidemiol*, 1995, 5, 255-260.

[104] Tavani, A; Negri, E; D'Avanzo, B; La Vecchia, C. Beta-carotene intake and risk of nonfatal acute myocardial infarction in women. *Eur J Epidemiol*, 1997, 13, 631-637.

[105] Kritchevsky, SB; Tell, GS; Shimakawa, T; Dennis, B; Li, R; Kohlmeier, L; Steere, E; Heiss, G. Provitamin A carotenoid intake and carotid artery plaques: the Atherosclerosis Risk in Communities Study. *Am J Clin Nutr*, 1998, 68, 726-733.

[106] Virtamo, J; Rapola, JM; Ripatti, S; Heinonen, OP; Taylor, PR; Albanes, D; Huttunen, JK. Effect of vitamin E and beta carotene on the incidence of primary nonfatal myocardial infarction and fatal coronary heart disease. *Arch Intern Med*, 1998, 158, 668-675.

[107] Omenn, GS; Goodman, GE; Thornquist, MD; Balmes, J; Cullen, MR; Glass, A; Keogh, JP; Meyskens, FL; Valanis, B; Williams, JH; Barnhart, S; Hamma, S. Effects of a combination of beta carotene and vitamin A on lung cancer and cardiovascular disease. *N Engl J Med*, 1996, 334, 1150-1155.

[108] Blot, WJ; Li, JY; Taylor, PR; Guo, W; Dawsey, S; Wang, GQ; Yang, ChS; Zheng, S-F; Gail, M; Li, G-Y; Yu, Y; Liu, B; Tangrea, J; Sun, Y; Liu, F; Fraumeni, JF; Zhang, Y-H; Li, JrB. Nutrition intervention trials in Linxian, China: supplementation with specific vitamin/mineral combinations, cancer incidence, and disease-specific mortality in the general population. *J Natl Cancer Inst*, 1993, 85, 1483-1492.

[109] Hennekens, CH; Buring, JE; Manson, JE; Stampfer, M; Rosner, B; Cook, NR; Belanger, C; LaMotte, F; Gaziano, JM; Ridker, PM; Willett, W; Peto, R. Lack of effect of long-term supplementation with beta-carotene on the incidence of malignant neoplasm and cardiovascular disease. *N Engl J Med*, 1996, 334, 1145-1149.

[110] Dietary reference intakes for vitamin C, vitamin E, selenium, and carotenoids. Institute of Medicine, August 3, 2000.

[111] Cutler, JA; Follmann, D; Allender, PS. Randomized trials of sodium reduction: an overview. *Am J Clin Nutr*, 1997, 65, 643-651.

[112] Stamler J. The INTERSALT Study: background, methods, findings. *Am J Clin Nutr*, 1997, 65 (suppl 2), 626-642.

[113] Zhou, BF; Stamler, J; Dennis, B; Moag-Stahlberg, A; Okuda, N; Robertson, C; Zhao, L; Chan, Q; Elliott, P. for the INTERMAP Research Group. Nutrient intakes of middles-aged men and women in China, Japan, United Kingdom, and United States in the late 1990s: The INTERMAP study. *J Hum Hypertens*, 2003, 17, 623-630.

[114] Sacks, FM; Svetkey, LP; Vollmer, WM; Appel, LJ; Bray, GA; Harsha, D; et al. DASH Sodium Collaborative Research Group. Effects on blood pressure of reduced dietary sodium and the Dietary Approaches to Stop Hypertension (DASH) diet. *N Engl J Med*, 2001, 344, 3-10.

[115] Vollmer, WM; Sacks, FM; Ard, J; Appel, LJ; Bray, GA; Simons-Morton, DG; et al. DASH-Sodium Collaborative Research Group. Effects of dietary patterns and sodium intake on blood pressure: subgroup results of the DASH-Sodium Trial. *Ann Intern Med*, 2001, 135, 1019-1028.

[116] He, FJ; MacGregor, GA. Universal Salt Reduction. *Hypertension*, 2004, 43, 12-13.

[117] Reddy, KS; Katan, MB. Diet, nutrition and the prevention of hypertension and cardiovascular disease. *Public Health Nutr*, 2004, 7, 167-186.

[118] Mink, PJ; Scrafford, CG; Barraj, LM; Harnack, L; Hong, C-P; Nettleton, JA; Jacobs, DR. Flavonoid intake and cardiovascular disease mortality: a prospective study in postmenopausal women. *Am J Clin Nutr*, 2006, 85, 895-909,

[119] Lamuela-Raventós, RM, Romero-Pérez, AI; Andrés-Lacueva, C; Tornero, A. Review: Health effects of cocoa flavonoids. *Food Sci Technol Int*, 2005, 11, 159-176.

[120] Geleijnse, JM; Launer, LJ; Van der Kuip, DA; Hofman, A; Witteman, JC. Inverse association of tea and flavonoid intakes with incident myocardial infarction: the Rotterdam Study. *Am J Clin Nutr*, 2002, 75, 880-886.

[121] Lee, KW; Kim, YJ; Lee, HJ; Lee, CY. Cocoa has more phenolic phytochemicals and a higher antioxidant capacity than teas and red wine. *J Agric Food Chem*, 2003, 51, 7292-7295.

[122] Strandberg, TE; Strandberg, AY; Pitka`la`, K; Salomaa, VV; Tilvis, RS; Miettinen, TA. Chocolate, well-being and health among elderly Men. *Eur J Clin Nutr*, 2007, 1–7.

[123] Ding, EL; Hutfless, SM; Ding, X; Girotra, S. Chocolate and Prevention of Cardiovascular Disease: A Systematic Review. *Nutr Metab*, 2006, 3, 2.

[124] Franco, OH; Bonneux, L; de Laet, C; Peeters, A; Steyerberg, EW; Mackenbach, JP. The Polymeal: a more natural, safer, and probably tastier (than the Polypill) strategy to reduce cardiovascular disease by more than 75%. *Br Med J*, 2004, 329, 1147-1150.

[125] Huxley, RR; Neil, HA. The relation between dietary flavonol intake and coronary heart disease mortality: A meta-analysis of prospective cohort studies. *Eur J Clin Nutr*, 2003, 57, 904-908.

[126] Lin, J; Rexrode1, KM; Hu, F; Albert, CM; Chae, CU; Rimm, EB; Stampfer, MJ; Manson, J E. Dietary Intakes of Flavonols and Flavones and Coronary Heart Disease in US Women. *Am J Epidemiol*, 2007, 165, 1305-1313.

[127] Sesso, HD; Gaziano, JM; Liu, S; Buring, JE. Flavonoid intake and the risk of cardiovascular disease in women. *Am J Clin Nutr*, 2003, 77, 1400-1408.

[128] Foote, JA; Murphy, SP; Wilkens, LR; Hankin, JH; Henderson, BE; Kolonel, LN. Factors associated with dietary supplement use among healthy adults of five ethnicities: the Multiethnic Cohort Study. *Am J Epidemiol*, 2003, 157, 888-897.

[129] Vitolins, MZ; Tooze, JA; Golden, SL; Arcury, TA; Bell, RA; Davis, C; Devellis, RF; Quandt, SA. Older Adults in the Rural South Are Not Meeting Healthful Eating Guidelines. *J Am Diet Assoc*, 2007, 107, 265-272.

[130] Zizza, CA; Tayie, FA; Lino, M. Benefits of Snacking in Older Americans. *J Am Diet Assoc*, 2007, 107, 800-?

[131] Kerver, JM; Yang, EJ; Bianchi, I; Song, WO. Dietary patterns associated with risk of factors for cardiovascular disease in healthy US adults. *Am J Clin Nutr*, 2003, 78, 1103-1110.

[132] de Groot, LCPMG; Verheijden, MW; de Henauw, S; Schroll, M; van Staveren, WA for the Seneca investigators. Lifestyle, Nutritional Status, Health, and Mortality in Elderly People Across Europe: A Review of the Longitudinal Results of the SENECA Study The Journals of Gerontology Series A: Biological Sciences and Medical Sciences, 2004, 59, 1277-1284.

[133] Belmin, J. Prevention of cardiovascular disease in the elderly. *Presse Med*, 2000, 29, 1234-1239.

[134] Popkin, BM; Siega-Riz, AM; Haines, PS; Jahns, L. Where's the fat? Trends in U.S. diets 1965–96. *Prev Med*, 2001, 32, 245–254.

[135] van Rossum, CT; van de Mheen, H; Witteman, JC; Grobbee, E; Mackenbach, JP. Education and nutrient intake in Dutch elderly people. The Rotterdam Study. *Eur J Clin Nutr*, 2000, 54, 159-165.

[136] Cai, H; Zheng, W; Xiang, YB; Hong, XuW; Yang, G; Li, H; Ou Shu, X. Dietary patterns and their correlates among middle-aged and elderly Chinese men: a report from the Shanghai Men's Health Study. *Br J Nutr*, 2007, 25, 1-8.

[137] Galobardes, B; Costanza, MC; Bernstein, MS; Delhumeau, C; Morabia, A. Trends of risk factors for lifestyle-related diseases by socioeconomic position in Geneva, Switzerland, 1993-2000: Health Inequalities Persist. *Am J Public Health*, 2003, 93, 1302-1309.

[138] de Backer, G; Ambrosioni, E; Borch-Johnsen, K; Brotons, C; Cifkova, R; Dallongeville, J; et al. European guidelines on cardiovascular disease prevention in clinical practice. Third Joint Task Force of European and Other Societies on Cardiovascular Disease Prevention in Clinical Practice. *Eur J Cardiovasc Prevention Rehab*, 2003, 10 (Suppl 1), 1-78.

[139] Knoops, KTB; de Groot, LCPGM; Kromhout, D; Perrin, A-E; Moreiras-Varela, O; Menotti, A; van Staveren, WA. Mediterranean Diet, Lifestyle Factors, and 10-Year Mortality in Elderly European Men and Women The HALE Project. *J Am Med Assoc*. 2004, 292, 1433-1439

[140] Esposito, K; Marfella, R; Ciotora, M; et al. Effect of Mediterranean-style diet on endothelial dysfunction and markers of vascular inflammation i the metabolic syndrome: a randomized trial. *J Am Med Assoc*, 2004, 292, 1440-1446.

[141] Psaltopoulou, T; Naska, A; Orfanos, P; Trichopoulos, D; Mountokalakis, T; Trichopoulou, A. Olive oil, the Mediterranean diet, and arterial blood pressure: the Greek European Prospective Investigation into Cancer and Nutrition (EPIC) study. *Am J Clin Nutr*, 2004, 80, 1012-1018.

[142] Estruch, R; Martinez-Gonzales, MA; Corella, D; Salas-Salvado, J; Ruiz-Gutierrez, V; Covas, MI; Fiol, M; Gomez-Gracia, E; Lopez-Sabater, MC; Vinyoles, E; Aros, F; Conde, M; Lahoz, C; Lapetra, J; Saez, G; Ros, E. for the PREDIMED Study Investigators. Effects of a Mediterranean-Style Diet on Cardiovascular Risk Factors. A Randomized Trial. *Ann Intern Med*, 2006, 145, 1-11.

[143] Fernández-Jarne, E; Martínez-Losa, E; Prado-Santamaría, M; Brugarolas-Brufau, C; Serrano-Martínez, M; Martínez-González, MA. Risk of first non-fatal myocardial infarction negatively associated with olive oil consumption: a case-control study in Spain. *Int J Epidemiol*, 2002, 31, 474-480.

[144] Joshipura, KJ; Hu, FB; Manson, JE; Stampfer, MJ; Rimm, EB; Speizer, FE; Colditz, G; Ascherio, A; Rosner, B; Spiegelman, D; Willett, W C. The Effect of Fruit and Vegetable Intake on Risk for Coronary Heart Disease. *Ann Intern Med*, 2001, 134, 1106-1114.

[145] Joshipura, KJ; Ascherio, A; Manson, JE; Stampfer, MJ; Rimm, EB; Speizer, FE; Hennekens, CH; Spiegelman, D; Willett, WC. Fruit and Vegetable Intake in Relation to Risk of Ischemic Stroke. *J Am Med Assoc*, 1999, 282, 1233-1239.

[146] Goldstein, LB; Adams, R; Alberts, MJ; Appel, LJ; Brass, LM; Bushnell, CD; Culebras, A; DeGraba, TJ; Gorelick, PB; Guyton, JR; Hart, RG; Howard, G; Kelly-Hayes, M; Nixon, JV; Sacco, RL. American Heart Association; American Stroke Association Stroke Council. Primary prevention of ischemic stroke: a guideline from the American

Heart Association/American Stroke Association Stroke Council: cosponsored by the Atherosclerotic Peripheral Vascular Disease Interdisciplinary Working Group; Cardiovascular Nursing Council; Clinical Cardiology Council; Nutrition, Physical Activity, and Metabolism Council; and the Quality of Care and Outcomes Research Interdisciplinary Working Group. *Circulation*, 2006, 113, 873-923.

[147] Jacobs, DR; Meyer, KA; Kushi, LH; Folsom, AR. Is whole grain intake associated with reduced total and cause-specific death rates in older women? The Iowa Women's Health Study. *Am J Public Health*, 1999, 89, 322-329.

[148] Liu, S; Stampfer, MJ; Hu, FB; Giovannucci, E; Rimm, E; Manson, JE; Hennekens, CH; Willett, WC. Whole - grain consumption and risk of coronary heart disease: results from the Nurses' Health Study. *Am J Clin Nutr*, 1999, 70, 412-419.

[149] Vincent-Baudry, S; Defoort, C; Gerber, M; Bernard, M-Ch; Verger, P; Helal, O; Portugal, H; Planells, R; Grolier, P; Amiot-Carlin, M-J; Vague P; Lairon, D. The Medi-RIVAGE study: reduction of cardiovascular disease risk factors after a 3-mo intervention with a Mediterranean-type diet or a low-fat diet. *Am J Clin Nutr*, 2005, 82, 964-971.

[150] Lasheras, C; Fernandez, S; Patterson, AM. Mediterranean diet and age with respect to overall survival in institutionalized, nonsmoking elderly people. *Am J Clin Nutr*, 2000, 71, 987-992.

[151] Haveman-Nies, A; de Groot LCPGM; van Staveren, WA for the Seneca investigators. Relation of Dietary Quality, Physical Activity, and Smoking Habits to 10-Year Changes in Health Status in Older Europeans in the SENECA Study. *Am J Public Health*, 2003, 93, 318-323.

[152] Trichopoulou, A; Orfanos, P; Norat, T; Bueno-de-Mesquita, B; Ocke, MC; Peeters, PH; et al. Modified Mediterranean diet and survival: EPIC-elderly prospective cohort study. Br Med J, 2005, 33, 1325-1332.

[153] Thompson, PD; Buchner, D; Pina, IL; Balady, GJ; Williams, MA; Marcus, BH; Berra, K; Blair, SN; Costa, F; Franklin, B; Fletcher, GF; Gordon, NF; Pate, RR; Rodriguez, BL; Yancey, AK; Wenger, NK. Exercise and physical activity in the prevention and treatment of atherosclerotic cardiovascular disease: a statement from the Council on Clinical Cardiology (Subcommittee on Exercise, Rehabilitation, and Prevention) and the Council on Nutrition, Physical Activity, and Metabolism (Subcommittee on Physical Activity). *Circulation*, 2003, 107, 3109-3116.

[154] Hambrecht, R; Wolf, A; Gielen, S; Linke, A; Hofer, J; Erbs, S; Schoene, N; Schuler, G. Effect of exercise on coronary endothelial function in patients with coronary artery disease. *N Engl J Med*, 2000, 342, 454–460.

[155] Kiechl, S; Willeit, J; Rungger, G; Egger, G; Oberhollenzer, F; Bonora, E. Alcohol consumption and atherosclerosis: what is the relation? Prospective results from the Bruneck Study. *Stroke*, 1998, 29, 900-907.

[156] Grønbæk, M; Becker, U; Johansen, D; Tønnesen, H; Jensen, G; Sørensen, TIA; et al. Alcohol and mortality: is there a U-shaped relation in elderly people? *Age Ageing*, 1998, 27, 739-744.

[157] Dufour, MC. If you drink alcoholic beverages do so in moderation: what does this mean? *J Nutr*, 2001, 131 (suppl), 552-561.

[158] Broustet, JP. Wine and health. *Heart*, 1999, 81, 459-460.

[159] Friedman, M; Roseman, RH. Type A behaviour and your heart. New York: Knopf, 1974.

[160] Csef, H; Hefner, J. Stress and myocardial infarction. *MMW Fortschr Med*, 2005, 147, 33-35.

[161] Das, S; O`Keefe, KH. Behavioral cardiology: Recognizing and addressing the profound impact of psychosocial stress on cardiovascular health. *Curr Atheroscler Rep*, 2006, 8, 111-118.

[162] Steptoe, A; Whitehead, DL. Depression, stress, and coronary heart disease: the need for more complex models. *Heart*, 2005, 91, 419-420.

[163] Penninx, BWJH; Beekman, ATF; Honig, A; Deeg, DJH; Schoevers, RA; van Eijk, JTM; van Tilburg, W. Depression and cardiac mortality: results from a community-based longitudinal study. *Arch Gen Psychiatry*, 2001, 58, 221-227.

In: Research Trends in Nutrition…
Editor: Johan P. Urster, pp. 171-185

ISBN: 978-1-60456-147-0
© 2008 Nova Science Publishers, Inc.

Chapter 5

Prevention of Obesity in Older Adults

Danuta Gajewska, Anna Harton and Joanna Myszkowska-Ryciak

Chair of Dietetics, Faculty of Human Nutrition and Consumer Sciences,
Warsaw University of Life Sciences, Poland

Abstract

Obesity in adults is an increasing health problem. The increasing prevalence of obesity in many developing countries can be due to adoption of Western-style diet. In some countries obesity has reached epidemic levels and obesity related complications are the most important problems globally. It seems that in current strategy to stop obesity escalation too little attention has been given to the prevention of this disease. In the prevention of obesity three components: total energy intake, diet composition and portion size play a crucial role. Management of older, obese patients is difficult, and it is not obvious whether weight reduction is associated with beneficial health effect. Therefore prevention in earlier ages, rather than intervention in late life, is the recommended, most cost-effective strategy for successful aging. General nutritional strategies for obesity prevention include promotion of fruit, vegetables and whole grain product intake, restriction of energy-dense (salty, fatty and sugary), micronutrients-poor foods intake, and reduction of consumption of sugars-sweetened beverages. These strategies can result in improving the quality of diet.

This chapter focuses on energy and nutrients intake as well as on portions sizes as possible causative factors for unhealthy weight gain. Topics include epidemiology information as well as nutrients and recommendations. Special attention is paid on energy intake and density of food in weight gain prevention. Dietary fat, carbohydrates and selected micronutrients intakes are also discussed. The paper has been written based on research and epidemiological data.

Introduction

Significant changes in body composition are known to occur with age during adulthood. Successful aging defined as maintenance of good health and functional status over time, could be achieved by applying a healthy diet. A well-balance diet with adequate amount of calories and nutrients is the key factor to maintain an ideal body weight and fat-free mass.

Management of older, obese patients is difficult, and it is not obvious whether weight reduction is associated with beneficial health effect. Therefore prevention in earlier ages, rather than intervention in late life, is the recommended, most cost-effective strategy for successful aging. It seems that in current strategy to stop escalation in obesity too little attention has been given to the prevention of this disease. It is essential to treat obesity now and to prevent next generation becoming obese. Direction for future obesity prevention, identified by the National Institutes of Health was published in 2003 [[1]] and 2004 [[2]].

Epidemiology

In some countries obesity has reached epidemic levels and obesity related complications are the most important problems globally. According to the World Health Organization [WHO] more than 300 million people are obese worldwide [[3],[4]]. Recent estimates indicate that 64% of United States adults are overweight or obese and obesity rates have increased from 12.8% in 1962 to 30% in 2000 [[5]]. For the first time in America the next generation may live shorter than their parents [[6]].

The prevalence of obesity among adults in Europe tends to be lower than in US and is estimated to be in the range of 10-20% in men and 10-25% in women [[6]]. In UK obesity is currently estimated to affect just over one fifth of population while two thirds of that population are estimated overweight [[8]]. In France 11.3% of adults were obese in 2003 compared with 8.2% in 1997 [[9]]. In China the prevalence of overweight and obesity increased from 14.6% in 1992 to 21.8% in 2002 (and to 29.9% according to Chinese obesity standard) [[10]]. Some ethics groups, such as African American and Mexican American, have a higher prevalence of obesity [[6]].

The increasing prevalence of obesity in many developing countries can be due to adoption of Western-style diet. Prevention of weight gain should be a primary therapeutic target for reducing several obesity-related healthy problems including hypertension, type 2 diabetes mellitus, insulin resistance or nonalcoholic fatty liver disease [[11], [12],[13], [14]].

The Healthy People 2010 goal is to reduce the percentage of adults with BMI greater than 30 by one third, from 23% to 15% [[15]]. Is still realistic?

Obesity Definition and Measurement

Obesity is defined as a very high amount of body fat in relation to lean body mass [[3], [16]]. To achieve optimum health, for the adult population WHO [[4]] consider body mass index (BMI) in the range 21-23 kg/m^2, while the goals for individuals should be to maintain BMI in the range 18.5-24.9 kg/m^2. The cut-off criterion of 30 kg/m^2 is set to define obesity in adults, whereas a BMI between 25.0 and 29.9 kg/m^2 meets a definition of overweight. These conventional BMI categories may not be appropriate in individuals of all populations groups (e.g. Asian populations), and may be too restrictive for older adults [[17], [18]]. It has been suggested that in healthy adults over age 65 moderately higher BMI (between 25 to 27 kg/m^2) is not a risk factor for cardiovascular mortality and death. Dolan et al. [[19]] in 8 years of follow-up study found that the lowest mortality rates, among women aged 65 and older, were in the range 24.6 to 29.8 kg/m^2, and the optimal value was estimated as 29.2 kg/m^2.The U-shaped or J-shaped relations between BMI and mortality were found in several studies in adults [[17],[19],[20], [21], [22]]. A low BMI was associated with increased risk of death and stroke in the Systolic Hypertension [SHEP] in the Elderly Program [[23]] and there was a negative correlation between BMI and pulse pressure in older adults using NHANES III data [[24]]. Data from the Nurses' Health Study revealed that the risk of diabetes was 20-fold greater in women with BMI 30-35 kg/m^2 as compared to those with BMI <23 kg/m^2 [[25]].

Waist circumference and ratio of waist-to-hip circumference (reflecting abdominal or visceral adiposity), correlate closely with BMI, and provide additional information on the nature of obesity. Abdominal obesity is linked with metabolic disturbance including hyperinsulinemia, insulin resistance, dyslipidemia, and chronic inflammatory and prothrombotic clinical states [[4], [26], [27], [28]]. Changes in waist circumferences reflect changes in risk for metabolic complications. In longitudinal study Chuang and colleagues [[29]] found that abdominal obesity (and its progression) was a predictor to future hypertension incidence, independent of general obesity. Lakka et al. [[30]] also found that visceral obesity was an independent risk factor for coronary hearth disease in middle-age men. Adipose tissue is a metabolically active endocrine organ secreting hormones, cytokines, and polypeptides and these secretory products (including inflammatory cytokines interleukin-6 (IL-6), tumor necrosis factor-α (TNF-α), leptin, angiotensinogen) may influence on regulation of numerous coronary risk factor [[30], [31]].

BMI, waist circumference and waist-to-hip ratio are useful, simple to measure population-level of overweight and obesity, and they have been recommended for the assessment of obesity in population [[30]] and predicting mortality in older person [[19]]. Computed tomography (CT), magnetic resonance imaging (MRI) or dual-energy X-ray absorptiometry (DXA) can also be useful to measure visceral adiposity, but such techniques are expensive and difficult to apply in practice [[6]].

Nutrients and Recommendation

In the prevention of obesity three components: total energy intake, diet composition and portion size (food volume) play a crucial role. Between macronutrients fat is the most energy dense and low-fat diets are often considered in the obesity management. Some studies confirmed that prevalence of obesity is highly related to fat intake [[32], [33]] while others established that saturated fat, rather that total fat intake or energy density leads to obesity [[16]]. However fat intake is not associated with body weight independently of total energy intake [[34]]. Current opinions are that different diets might work better for some individuals than others, but simply reducing fat intake (without calorie restriction) is not the best practice to prevent obesity [[34],[35]]. It is worth to underline than there is an important difference between preventing weight gain and achieving weight loss. A multidisciplinary team approach is required to ensure long-term success of treatment [[16]].

Because the slow and persistent overconsumption of energy relative to individuals needs leads to obesity, the control of total energy intake, and diet macro- and micronutrient composition seems to be a reasonable strategies to weight gain prevention. Consume excessive calorie results in negative health consequences [[16]] and eating behaviors include snacking, binge-eating patterns, eating out have been also linked to overweight and obesity [[4]].

According to current WHO recommendations the potential nutritional protective factors related to unhealthy weight gain are high dietary intake of dietary fiber, low glycemic index foods and increasing eating frequency. In contrast, factors that might promote weight gain, overweight and obesity are high intake of energy-dense, micronutrient-poor foods, high intake of sugars-sweetened soft drinks and fruit juices, large portion size, high proportion of food prepared outside the home (developed countries), high intake of alcohol and sedentary lifestyles [[4]].

Caterson and Gill [[6]] underline than our contemporary environment is very obesogenic and only few individuals are able to avoid moving into positive energy balance. In such environment is very easy to increase weight and very hard to loose it. Some authors suggest that implementation of increased tax on unhealthy food (like high-fat, high-sugar, high-salt, soft drinks, snack foods and junk food) could enhance food industry to produce healthy food and consumers to make better choice [[36], [37]]. However special group interest could be a major barrier to implementation of junk food taxes [[37]].

Energy Intake, Portion Size and Energy Density

The weight set point hypothesis has emerged that holds that "individuals posses a desired weight set point under the control of tightly regulated feedback system. Those genetically predisposed to obesity are believed have a thrifty phenotype, which defaults to storing calories. In contrast, individuals predisposed to thinness have a wasteful phenotype, which promotes burning calories. Regardless of whether or not individuals possesses a thrifty or wasteful metabolism, a thermodynamic model of obesity holds that weight gain via increased accumulation of body fat represents an excess of energy intake compared to energy expenditure" [[38]].

Consuming excess of calories slowly leads to increased weight gain. Reducing energy intake by an amount equal to100 kcal/d and increasing physical activity could prevent weight gain in most of the population [[39]]. In US daily average caloric intake between 1971 and 2001 increased by 168 kcal among men and by 355 kcal among women [[40]], and this could be only one possible explanation for weigh gain. Between 1977 and 1996 soft drink consumption among US adults aged 49 to 59 years increased by 111% and salty snack by 171% [[37]] Consumption of sugar-sweetened beverages has also been linked to increasing rates of obesity in US [[41]].

Energy intake depends on sex, age, weight, height and activity level, and can be calculated using the National Academy of Sciences/Institute of Medicine (NAS/IOM) total energy expenditure (TEE) prediction equitation and physical activity coefficient (PA). PA coefficients are grouped into four categories: sedentary, low active, active and very active. [[42],[43]]. The resting or basal energy expanditure (REE) should be also calculated using classic Harris-Benedict formula [[44]]. Heymsfield et al. [[42]] underline that these equitations were developed as a means of predicting group energy requirements and are suitable for group TEE estimates.

Body weight remains stable over long time when energy intake balance TEE. In adults the energy requirement for weight maintenance decreases with each decade increase in age as a result of decline in metabolically active tissue (lean tissue) relative to body weight [[42]].

This reduction in energy requirement coexists with increased requirements for nutrients such as vitamin B_{12}, vitamin D, vitamin B_6 or calcium. It is difficult for older adults to meet their nutrients requirements from food, thus consumption of fortified food or supplementation should be necessary [[45]].

To prevent weight gain total energy intake could be limited by reducing density of foods/diet. This can be achieved by increasing the water content or reducing the fat content in consuming food. Some authors suggested that a high consumption of energy-dense foods promotes weight gain [[46], [47]]. Energy density of food is defined "as available energy per unit weight". These foods are usually highly processed, poor in micronutrients, often high in fat and sugar and also relatively cheap. What is more, these foods tend to be more palatably [[48], [49]]. High energy-dense diets can destabilize normal appetite regulation leading to passive overconsumption [[50]]. However consumption of high-energy density nuts is associated with lower BMI in adults and higher satiety [[57]].

The most energy-dense and micronutrient-poor foods are dry and usually high in fat and/or sugar: for example potato chips (23 kJ/g), chocolate (22 kJ/g). Low energy-dense (or energy-dilute) foods, such as raw vegetables, fruit, legumes, and whole grain cereals, are high in dietary fiber and water. Energy density of beverages such as regular Cola or orange juice is 1.8 kJ/g, skim milk 1.0 kJ/g and water 0 kJ/g [[4]]. There is a hypothesis that energy-dense diet (high in added sugar and added fat) is low-priced and palatable, while diet high in fruit and vegetables [[48]], so this could be an obstacle for healthy food choice.

The physiological effects of energy intake on satiation and satiety appear to be quite different for energy in solid foods as opposed to energy in fluids. Mattes [[58]] estimated that consumption of each additional can or glass of sugar-sweetened drink that children consume every day increases the risk of becoming obese by 60%. In United States on average 56 gallons of Coca-Cola is consumed per person per year [[16]] meanwhile WHO [[4]] considers the evidence implicating a high intake of sugar-sweetened drinks in promoting weight gain as moderately strong.

Large portions sizes are a possible causative factor for unhealthy weight gain [[4], [52]]. In many countries super-sized meals are often offered by fast-food outlets as well as by food markets. Expectations for a larger portion size and habituation to portion sizes have grown. People weakly estimates portion size and that subsequent energy compensation for a large meal is imperfect [[4]]. Tendency to eat more when larger portion is offered provide to raising total calorie intake.

For the past 50 yr portion size has been increasing progressively [[35]]. Condrasky et al. [[51]] determining chefs' opinions of restaurant' portion size found that the real portions of steak and pasta served in restaurants were 2 to 4 times larger than sizes recommended by the US government. Moreover, restaurant usually served food that is highly palatable. Nielsen and Popkin [[52]] highlighted that in US sweetened beverages portion sizes (at home as well as at fast food and restaurants) increased significantly and in contrast very small decreases in milk portion sizes was observed.

Snacking is an important dietary habit among older adults. It may promote energy overconsumption resulting in weight gain and obesity. However Zizza et al.[[53]] suggest that snacking may ensure older adults consume diets adequate in energy. For the reason that reduction in appetite is observed with increasing age, older adults should be advised to consume nutritious and appetizing snacks [[45]]. For younger adults fruits and vegetables should be encouraged for snacks.

Several studies have indicated that high intake of protein was positively related to BMI in adults [[54]] and fatness in children [[55]]. McCarthy [[56]] concluded that high animal protein and starchy food might be a strong factor in the origins of Western obesity epidemic. Noakes et al. [[59]] summarizing research on dietary protein and effects on obesity and type 2 diabetes mellitus concluded that this macronutrient is more satiating than CHO or fat, and higher-protein lower carbohydrates dietary patterns could be considered for weight management as well as for individuals with insulin resistance. According to "protein-leverage" hypothesis intake of low-protein diet inevitably requires the ingestion of additional energy. The consumption of diet that is relatively high in protein content requires the ingestion of lower levels of energy, creating the potential for weight loss [[60]].

Older adults, over the age of 70 years have an approximate 20% higher daily requirement for protein compared with younger adults. Higher protein intakes from food with a high biological value, such as meat, eggs or dairy product would be beneficial for the elderly [[45]].

Dietary Fat, and Low-Fat Substitutes

Dietary fat consists of various fatty acids (FA) and cholesterol, and different type of FA have different metabolic effects [[61]]. Limiting intake of saturated fats, trans fatty acids, and dietary cholesterol is recommended. The traditional recommendation for saturated fatty acids (SFA) in the diets are less than 10% of total energy, and less than 7% of daily energy intake for high-risk groups (if there is an inadequate serum cholesterol response) [[4], [61]]. Fat foods are highly palatable, less satiating and easily consumed in excess [[62]]. When energy excess becomes a potential problem, the FA composition of the fat source should be monitored and restriction of certain food (e.g. chips, frits, and snack) should be considered. Recommendations for total fat intake may be based on current levels of population consumption in different regions/countries.

The daily energy intake from fats should be limited to 30%-35% [[4]] of total energy. A further reduction in fat intake may have some additional cardiovascular benefits, but adherence to such diet for most individuals may be difficult [[61]]. A 10% reduction in the proportion of fat in the diet can result in a related decrease of 238 kcal/d of total energy intake [[33]]. Fat reduction could be achieved by limiting the intake of fat from meat and dairy high-fat products, avoiding the use of hydrogenated oils, using appropriate edible vegetable oils in small amounts, and ensuring a regular intake of fish or plant sources of α-linolenic acid. Preferences should be given to food preparation practices that employ non-frying methods [[3]].

The data showed that the ability to reduce food intake to compensate for the food eaten earlier is impaired when the subsequent foods are high in fat [[63]] and especially when they are high in both sugar and fat [[64]]. It is possible that energy from fat may have a greater effect on body weight than energy from nonfat sources [[35]] especially in individuals genetically predisposed to the obesity. However reducing in fat intake alone should not be the best way to prevent weight gain. Ingestible fat substitutes such as sucrose polyester (e.g., Olestra), are used to replace conventional fat. Moderate use of fat replacers by adults can be safe and useful in decreasing total calorie and fat intake [[34]].

Carbohydrates, and Dietary Fiber

Besides obesity, diet high in sugar can be associated with additional health problems including dyslipidemia, bone loss and dental caries [[16]]. Diet high in carbohydrates (CHO) can cause an increase in triglycerides, and the effect may be greater in overweight subjects and those with insulin resistance [[65]]. CHO quality plays a critical role in stimulating de novo lipogenesis. Consumption of high amount of simple sugars has been reported to be more effective in stimulating hepatic de novo lipogenesis than complex CHO [[69]].

A high dietary intake of dietary fiber (soluble and insoluble fraction) as well as fiber consumed as supplements promote weight loss [[4], [66]]. High-fiber foods may increase satiation through delayed gastric emptying and decreasing of postprandial glucose and insulin responses [[70]]. Adequate intakes of fiber should be achieved by regular consumption of wholegrain cereals, legumes, fruits and vegetables. To minimize undesirable gastrointestinal symptoms, high-fiber food should be added gradually to diet and consumption of higher amount of water is suggested. A minimum daily intake of 20 g is recommended, however most authorities recommend an intake in the range of 25 to 30 g/day or 10 to 13 g/ 1000 kcal [[61], [67]].

Low-glycemic foods consumption has been proposed as a potential protective factor against weight gain, obesity, diabetes, and CVD [[68]]. This hypothesis was supported by several studies and several mechanisms have been proposed to explain how glycemic index contribute to weight changes [[71], [72]].

Vitamins and Minerals

Overweight and obese older adults may be at nutritional risk due to the persistent consumption of high-energy, low-micronutrients food. On the other hand, decrease in secretion of gastric acid, pepsin and intrinsic factor which can reduce the bioavailability of iron, calcium, vitamin B_6, vitamin B_{12} and folate is associated with process of aging [[45]].

Table 1. Daily vitamins and minerals recommendation for older adults

Vitamin A (µg retinols eqvivalents)	600-700
Vitamin B2 (mg)	1.3 for men/1.1 for women
Vitamin B12 (µg)	2.5
Vitamin D (µg)	10-15
Vitamin C (mg)	60-100
Vitamin E (IU)	100-400
Iron (mg)	10
Zinc (mg)	14 for men/9.8 for women*
Calcium (mg)	800-1200
Folate (µg)	400
Magnesium (mg)	225-280
Selenium (mg)	50-70
Cooper (mg)	1.3-1.5
Chromium (µg)	50

Adopted from[[74]], * low zinc availability (15%)

Older adults may be at risk for inadequate folate intake especially if their total energy intake is low, and if they do not take a supplement. However, individuals consuming supplement and folate-fortified cereals may at risk for excess folic acid intake [[73]]. Vitamins and minerals recommended for older adults are presented in table 1.

Antioxidants, and Bioactive Component of Diet

Some authors suggest that obesity is independently associated with oxidative stress [[75]], therefore antioxidant therapy with vitamin E or vitamin C supplementations might be beneficial [[76]].

Some food ingredients have been shown to stimulate thermogenesis, to enhance satiety, to increase sympathetic nervous system (SNS) activity, to increase fat oxidation and to decrease appetite and fat accumulation [[77], [78]]. Catechines from green tea [[79], [80]], capsaicin from hot pepper, caffeine from coffee or tea [[80], [81]], glucomannan from Konjac root [[82]], chitosan from exoskeleton of crustaceans and psyllium, water-soluble fiber from the seeds of *Platago ovata* have been reported to use in weight loss management [[83]].

Belza and colleagues [[84]] using a combination of bioactive food ingredients such as tyrosine, capsaicine, catechine, caffeine and calcium observed body fat mass significantly decreasing in the supplement group compared with placebo. They also found that the bioactive supplement increase 4-h thermogenesis by 90 kJ more than placebo. Because this effect was maintained after an 8 weeks supplementation, authors concluded than mentioned above bioactive components may be used for weight maintenance support.

Calcium containing low-fat dairy products may be also useful for weight management. High levels of dietary calcium stimulate lypolyisis while inhibiting lipogenesis, resulting in weight loss [[83]].

Alcohol

Alcohol is a source of energy (7 kcal/g), and alcoholic beverages containing carbohydrates are more caloric, so alcohol overconsumption might be associated with excess weight gain. It is an example of food contains so-called "empty calories". However some studies showed that alcohol intake has an inverse association with BMI [[85],[86]].

It has been recognized that moderate (or low) alcohol consumption has cardio protective effect [[87]]. In type 2 diabetes moderate alcohol consumption was associated with lower risk of cardiovascular disease by improving HDL-C and increasing in insulin sensitivity [[88], [89], [90]].

Diet for Obesity Management

People have tried to loose weight by eating specific foods such as cabbage soup, avoiding particular food group like CHO or fat, or else by adding some bioactive ingredient such as vinegar or cinnamon [[83]]. Traditionally low-calorie diets have been recommended for obesity management. The efficiency of most dietary strategies for weight reduction, including low-carbohydrates and low-fat diets, over the long term remains uncertain [[92]]. A variety of popular weight-loss diets that restrict food choices may result in reduced energy intake and short-term weight loss in individuals but most do not have trial evidence of long-term effectiveness and nutritional adequacy and therefore cannot be recommended for population [[4]]. Some of diet may even cause adverse health effects [[92]].

The National Heart, Lung and Blood Institute, North American Association for the Study of Obesity recommend a low-calorie diet containing 1000-1200 kcal/d for women and diet between 1200 and1600 kcal/d for men. Diets lower that 800 kcal/d are not considered [[91]].

Low-Fat versus Low-Carbohydrates Diets

Low-fat and low-carbohydrates diet work by reducing total calorie intake. Both diets are often considered for weight loss, and both can be safe and effective. However there is lack of convincing data which diets is more effective.

Low-carbohydrate diets can lead to weight loss in a short time, but the long-term effects on weight loss and CHD risk factors are uncertain. Low-fat diets have been shown to lower total cholesterol and LDL-C, but HDL-C level reduction in many dieters has been also observed [[92], [65]]. Low-fat, high-carbohydrates diet increase de novo lipogenesis and triacylglycerol concentrations [[69]]. These diets may be effective only when total energy intake is low. In conclusion, the right combination of food and macronutrient content for weight loss therapy depends on an individual's health status and genetic susceptibility. Lowering daily energy intake from CHO to 50-55% might be appropriate for people with metabolic syndrome and type 2 diabetes, while total fat limitation (to 20%) may be beneficial to control dyslipidemia and hypercholesterolemia [[83]]. Weight loss is considered the most effective nonpharmacological therapy for lowering blood pressure in obese hypertension [[93], [94]].

Lifestyle Changes

Lifestyles modification is the basis of both prevention and treatment of obesity. Health education has been the primary tool to encourage the general public to fight "obesogenic behaviors" [[95]]. A preventive program should begin with a detailed assessment of food intake and physical activity. Most attention should be focused on relationship with diet (as a measure of energy intake) and physical activity (as a measure of energy expenditure [[8]]. The most challenging issues in education involve helping patients to make long-term lifestyle changing, but which educational strategy is most effective is not clear.

Conclusion

Malnutrition posses two hands (and many fingers), one is undernutrition (insufficient energy and/or nutrients intake) and the second is overnutrition (excessive energy and/or nutrients intake). Both result in negative health consequences. As many authorities emphasize changes in lifestyle are the major contributor to the current epidemic of overweight and obesity. General nutritional strategies for obesity prevention include promotion of fruit, vegetables and whole grain product intake, restriction of energy-dense (salty, fatty and sugary), micronutrients-poor foods intake, and reduction of consumption of sugars-sweetened beverages. These strategies can result in improving the quality of diet [[3], [4]]. It is well known than adults' habits are very difficult to change on a permanent basis, so application of recommendation is more cost effective when applied to the young persons.

Physical activity is the most variable component of energy expenditure. Exercise in addition to healthy diet may help to maintain weight, thus physical activity at moderate level of intensively (e.g. brisk walking) for at least 30 min per day on most days of the week is also considered. Reduction in the time spent in sedentary behaviors should be important strategy for weight gain prevention in younger people.

Consumption of vegetables, fruits, whole grain cereals, and adequate quantity of fiber, monounsaturated fats, calcium should be recommended. Intake of total fat, saturated fatty acids, trans fatty acids, sodium, and refined CHO should be limited. Thus "ideal diet" is a combination of different dietary components and synergy of interaction between them can generate beneficial health effect.

References

[1]   Kumanyika, SH; Obarzanek, E. Pathways to obesity prevention: report of a National Institutes of Health Workshop. *Obes Res*, 2003, 11, 10, 1263-1274

[2]   NIH. Strategic plan for NIH obesity research. A report of the NIH obesity Task Force. US Department of Health and Human Services, National Institutes of Health. 2004, *NIH Publication* No 04-5493,

[3]   WHO. Obesity: preventing and managing the global epidemic. Report of a WHO Consultation. Geneva, World Health Organization, 2000 WHO Technical Report Series, No. 894

[4]   WHO. Diet, nutritional and the prevention of chronic diseases. Report of Joint WHO/FAO Expert Consultation. Geneva, World Health Organization, 2003 *WHO Technical Report Series*, No. 916.

[5]   www.cdc.gov/nchs/products/pubs/pubd/hestats/obese/obse99.htm

[6]   Olshansky, SJ; Passoro, DJ; Hershow, RD; Layden, J; Carnes, BA; Brody, J; Hayflick, L; Butler, RN; Allison DB; Ludwig DS. A potential decline ih the life expectancy in the United States in the 21st century. *N Engl J Med*, 2005, 352, 1138-1145

[7]   Caterson, JD; Gill, TP. Obesity: epidemiology and possible prevention. *Best Prac Res Clin Endocrin Metab*, 2002, 16 (4), 595-610

[8]   Moon, G; Quarendon, G; Barnard, S; Twigg, L; Blyth, B. Fat nation: Deciphering the distinctive geographies of obesity in England. *Soc Science Med*, 2007, 65, 20-31

[9]   ObEpi 2003. L'obesite et le surpoids en France. Available at : www.tns-sofres.com/etudes/sante/190603_obesite.htm

[10]   Wang, Y; Mi, J; Shan, X-y; Wang, QJ; Ge, X-y. Is China facing an obesity epidemic and the consequences? The trends in obesity and chronic disease in China. *Int J Obes*, 2007, 31, 177-188

[11]   Davy, KP; Hall, JE. Obesity and hypertension: two epidemics or one? *Am J Physiol Regul Integr Comp Physiol*, 2004, 286, R803-R813

[12]   Charlton, M. Nonalcoholic fatty liver disease: a review of current understanding and future impact. *Clin Gastroenterol Hepatol*, 2004, 2, 1048-1058

[13]   Schwimmer, JB; Deutsch, R; Kahen, T; Lavine, JE; Stanley, C; Behling, C. Prevalence of fatty liver in children and adolescents. *Pediatrics*, 2006, 118, 1388-1393

[14] Fu, JF; Liang, L; Zou, CC; Hong, F; Wang, CL; Wang, XM; Zhao, ZY. Prevalence of the metabolic syndrome in Zhejiang Chinese obese children and adolescents and the effect on metformin combined with lifestyle intervention. *Int J Obes*, 2007, 31, 15-22

[15] www.healthypeople.gov/datamidcourse/html/focusareas/FA19objectives.htm

[16] Boogerd, A; Alvredy, J; Kumar, S; Olson, DL; Schwenk, WF. Part. III. Obesity. *Dis Mon*, 2002, 48, 725-742

[17] Corrada, MM; Kawas, CH; Mozaffar, F; Paganini-Hill, A. Association of body mass index and weight change with all-cause mortality in elderly. *Am J Epidemiol*, 2006, 163, 938-949

[18] Heiat, A; Vaccarino, V; Krumholz, HM. An evidence-based assessment of federal guidelines for overweight and obesity as they apply to elderly persons. *Arch Intern Med*, 2001, 161, 9, 1194-1203

[19] Dolan, CM; Kraemer, H; Browner, W; Ensrud, K; Keesley, JL. Association between body composition, anthropometry, and mortality in women aged 65 years and older. *Am J Public Health*, 2007, 97, 913-918

[20] Calle, EE; Thun, MJ; Petrelli, JM; Rordiguez, C; Heath, CW. Body-mass index and mortality in a prospective cohort of US adults. *N Eng J Med*, 1999, 341, 1097-1105

[21] Durazo-Arvizu, RA; McGee, DL; Cooper, RS; Liao, Y; Luke, T. Mortality and optimal body mass index in sample of the US population. *Am J Epidemiol*, 1998, 147, 739-749

[22] Flegal, KM; Graudbard, BI; Williams, DF; Gail, HM. Excess deaths associated with underweight, overweight, and obesity. *J Am Med Assoc*, 2005, 293, 1861-1867

[23] Wassertheil-Smoller, S; Fann, C; Allman, RM; Black, HR; Camel, GH; Davis, B; Masaki, K; Preseel, S; Prineas, RJ; Stamler, J; Vogt, TM; Relation of low body mass to death and stroke in the systolic hypertension in the elderly program. The SHEP Cooperative Research Group. *Arch Intern Med*, 2000, 160, 4, 494-500

[24] Martins, D; Tareen, N; Pan, D; Norris, K. The relationship between body mass index and pulse pressure in older adults with isolated systolic hypertension. *Am J Hypertens*, 2002, 15, 538-543

[25] Hu, FB; Manson, JE; Stampfer, MJ; Colditz, G; Liu, S; Solomon CG; Willet, WC. Diet, lifestyle, and risk of type 2 diabetes mellitus in women. *N Eng J Med*, 2001, 345, 790-797

[26] Sowers, JR; Obesity as a cardiovascular risk factor. *Am J Med*, 2003, 115(8A), 37S-41S

[27] Litwin, SE. the growing problem of obesity and the heart. The plot "thickens". Editorial comments. *J Am Coll Cardiol*, 2006, 47, 3, 617-6619

[28] Nicklas, BJ; Cesari, M; Penninx, BWJH; Kritchevsky, SB; Ding, J; Newman, A; Kitzman, DW; Kanaya, AM; Pahor, M; Harris, TB. Abdominal obesity is an independent risk factor for chronic heart failure in older people. *J Am Geriatr Soc*, 2006, 54, 3, 413-420

[29] Chuang, SH; Chou, P; Hsu, PF; Cheng, HM; Tsai, ST; Lin, IF, Chen, CH. Presence and obesity progression of abdominal obesity are predictors of future high blood pressure and hypertension. *Am J Hypertens*, 2006, 19, 788-795

[30] Lakka, HM; Lakka, TA; Tuomilehto, J; Salonen, JT. Abdominal obesity is associated with increased risk of acute coronary events in men. *Eur Heart J*, 2002,23, 706-713

[31] Kopelman, P. Health risk associated with overweigh and obesity. *Obes Rev*, 2007, 8 (Suppl. 1), 13-17

[32] Bray, GA; Popkin, BM. Dietary fat intake does affect obesity rate. *Am J Clin Nutr*, 1998, 68, 1157-1173

[33] Astrup, A; Grunwald, GK; Melanson, EL; Saris, WH; Hill, JO. The role of low-fat diets in body weight control: a meta-analysis of ad libitum dietary intervention studies. *Int J Obes Relat Metab Disord*, 2000, 24, 1545-1551

[34] ADA Reports. Position of American Dietetic Association: fat replacers. *J Am Diet Assoc*, 2005, 105, 266-275

[35] Paeratakul, S; Bray, GA; Popkin, BM. Diet in the prevention and treatment of obesity. In: Temple, NJ; Wilson, T; Jacobs, DR (eds). Nutritional health, Totowa, New Jersey, Humana Press, 2006, 223-238

[36] Elrick, H; Samaras, TT; Demas, A. Missing links in the obesity epidemic. *Nutr Res*, 2002, 22, 1101-1123

[37] Kim, D; Kawachi, I. Food taxation and pricing strategies to "thin out" the obesity epidemic. *Am J Prev Med*, 2006, 30, 5, 430-437

[38] Chia, DJ; Boston, BA. Childhood obesity and the metabolic syndrome. *Advance Ped*, 2006, 53, 23-53

[39] Hill, JO; Reeg, GW; Peters, JC. Obesity and the environment: where do we go from here? Science, 2003, 299, 853-855

[40] Williams, DF. Weight change in middle-age Americans. *Am J Prev Med*, 2004, 27, 1 81-82

[41] Drewnowski, A; Bellisle, F. Liquid calories, sugar, and body weight. *Am J Clin Nutr*, 2007, 85, 651-661

[42] Heymsfield, SB; Harp, JB; Rowell, PN; Nguyen, AM; Pietrobelli, A. How much may I eat? Calorie estimates based upon energy expenditure prediction equations. *Obesity Rev*, 2006, 7, 361-370

[43] James, WPT; Schofield, EC. *Human energy requirements*. Oxford Medical Publications, Oxford, New York, Tokyo 1990

[44] Harris, JA; Benedict, FG.A biometric study of basal metabolism in man. Publication No. 279, Carnegie Institute of Washington, Washington DC, 1919

[45] Nowson, C. Nutritional challenges for the elderly. *Nutrition & Dietetics*, 2007, 64, (Suppl. 4), S150-S153

[46] Kral, TV; Roe, LS; Rolls, BJ. Combined effects of energy density portion size on energy intake in women, *Am J Clin Nutr*, 2004, 79, 962-968

[47] Devitt, AA; Mattes, RD. Effect of food unit size and energy density on intake in humans. *Appetite*, 2004, 42, 213-220

[48] Drewnowski, A. Obesity and the food environment. *Am J Prev Med*, 2004, 27, (3S), 154-162

[49] Drewnowski, A; Darmon, N; Briend, A. Replacing fats and sweets with vegetables and fruit – a question of cost. *Am J Public Health*, 2004, 94, 1555-1559

[50] Brown, T; Kelly, S; Summerbell, C. Prevention of obesity: a review of interventions. *Obes Rev*, 2007, 8, (Suppl. 1), 127-130

[51] Condrasky, M; Ledikwe, JH; Flood, JE; Rolls, BJ. Chefs' opinion of restaurant portion sizes. *Obesity*, 2007, 15, 2086-2094

[52] Nielsen, SJ; Popkin, BM. Changes in beverage intake between 1977 and 2001. *Am J Prev Med*, 2004, 27, 3, 205-210

[53] Zizza, CA; Tayie, FA; Lino, M. Benefits of snacking in older Americans. J Am Diet Assoc, 2007, 107, 5, 800-806

[54] Trichopoulou, A; Gnardellis, C; Benetou, V; Lagiou, P; Bamia, C; Trichopoulos, D. Lipid, protein and carbohydrate intake in relation to body mass index. Eur J Clin Nutr, 2002, 56, 1, 37-43

[55] Rolland-Cachera, MF; Deheeger, M; Akrout, M; Bellise, F. Influence of macronutrients on adiposity development: a follow up study of nutrition and growth from10 month to 8 years of age. Int J Obes, 1995, 19, 573-578

[56] McCarty, MF. The origins of Western obesity: a role for animal protein? Med Hyp, 2000, 54, 3, 488-494

[57] Sabate, J. Nut consumption and body weight. Am J Clin Nutr, 2003, 78 (Suppl.), S647-S650

[58] Mattes, RD. Dietary compensation by humans for supplemental energy provided as ethanol or carbohydrate in fluids. Physiol Beh, 1996, 59, 179-187

[59] Noakes, M; Keogh, J; Clifton, P. Obesity and type 2 diabetes mellitus. Section 4: The role of red meat in the prevention and management of chronic disease. Nutrition & Dietetics, 2007, 64, (Suppl. 4), S156-S161

[60] Simpson, SJ; Raubenheimer, D. Obesity: the protein leverage hypothesis. Obes Rev, 2005, 6, 133-142

[61] Shikany, JM; White, GL Jr. Dietary guidelines for chronic disease prevention. South Med J, 2000, 93, 12, 1157-1161

[62] Astrup, A; Toubro, S; Raben, A; Skov AR. The role of low-fat diets and fat substitutes in body weight management: what have we learned from clinical studies? J Am Diet Assoc, 1997, 97, (Suppl.7), S82-S87

[63] Sparti, A; Windhauser, MM; Champagne, CM; Bray, GA. Effect of an acute reduction in carbohydrate intake on subsequent food intake in healthy men. Am J Clin Nutr, 1997, 66, 1144-1150

[64] Green, SM; Blundell, JE. Effect of fat-and sucrose containing food on the size of eating episodes and energy intake in lean dietary restrained and unrestrained females: potential for causing overconsumption. Eur J Clin Nutr, 1996, 50, 625-635

[65] Parks, EJ; Hellerstein, MK. Carbohydrate induced hypertriglyceridemia: historical perspective and biological mechanisms. Am J Clin Nutr, 2000, 71, 412-433

[66] Pereira, MA; Ludwig, DS. Dietary fiber and body –weight regulation. Observations and mechanisms. Ped Clin North Am, 2001, 48, 969-980

[67] ADA Reports. Position of American Dietetic Association: Health implications of dietary fiber. J Am Diet Assoc, 2002, 102, 7, 993-1000

[68] Foster-Powell, K; Holt, SHA; Brand-Miller, JC; International table of glycemic index and glycemic load values: 2002, Am J Clin Nutr, 2002, 76, 5-56

[69] Schwartz, JM; Linfoot, P; Dare, D; Aghajanian, K. Hepatic de novo lipogenesis in normoinsulinemic and hyperinsulinemic subjects consuming high-fat, low-carbohydrate and low-fat, high-carbohydrate isoenergetic diets. Am J Clin Nutr, 2003, 77, 43-50

[70] Jebb, SA. Dietary determinants of obesity. Obes Rev, 2007, 8, (Suppl.1), 93-97

[71] Ludwig, D. The glycemic index: physiological mechanisms relating to obesity, diabetes and cardiovascular disease. J Am Med Assoc, 2002, 287, 2414-2423

[72] Brand-Miller, J; Holt, SHA; Pawlak, DB; McMillan, J. Glycemic index and obesity. Am J Clin Nutr, 2002, 76 (suppl), 218S- S285

[73] Mulligan, JE; Greene, GW; Caldwell, M. Sources of folate and serum folate levels in older adults. *J Am Diet Assoc*, 2007, 107, 3, 495-499

[74] WHO. Keep fit for life. Meeting the nutritional needs of older person. World Health Organization, Tufts University Consultation on Nutritional Guidelines for   elderly, 2002

[75] Keaney, JF JR; Larson, MG; Vasan, RS; Wilson, PWF; Lipinska, I; Corey, D; Massaro, JM; Sutherland, P; Vita, JA; Benjamin, EJ. Obesity and systemic oxidative stress: clinical correlates of oxidative stress in Framingham Study. *Arterioscler Thromb Vasc Biol*, 2003, 23, 434-439

[76] Higdon, JV; Frei, B. Obesity and oxidative stress a direct link to obesity? Editorial, *Arterioscler Thromb Vasc Biol*, 2003, 23, 365-367

[77] Belza, A; Jessen, AB. Bioactive food stimulants of sympathetic activity: effect on 24-h energy expenditure and fat oxidation. *Eur J Clin Nutr*, 2005, 59, 733-741

[78] Pittler, MH; Ernst, E. Dietary supplements for body-reduction: a systematic review. *Am J Clin Nutr*, 2004, 79, 529-536

[79] Kovacs, EM; Lejeune, MP; Nijs, I; Westerterp-Plantenga, MS. Effects of green tea on weight maintenance after body-weight loss. *Br J Nutr,* 2004, 91, 431-437

[80] Zheng, G; Sayama, K; Okubo, T; Juneja, LR; Oguni, I. Anti-obesity effects of three major components of green tea, catechins, caffeine and theanine, in mice. *In Vivo*, 2004, 18, 55-62

[81] Dulloo, AG. Herbal stimulation of ephedrine and caffeine in treatment of obesity. *Int J Obes*, 2002, 26, 590-592

[82] Walsh, DE; Yaghoubian, V; Behforooz, A. Effect of glucomannan on obese patients: a clinical study. *Int J Obes*, 1983, 8, 289-293

[83] Mermel, VL. Old paths new directions: the use of functional foods in the treatment of obesity. *Trends Food Scie Technol*, 2004, 15, 532-540

[84] Belza, A; Frandsen, E; Kondrup, J. Body fat loss by stimulation of thermogenesis by a combination of bioactive food ingredients: a placebo controlled, double-blind 8-week intervention in obese subjects. *Int J Obesity*, 2007, 31, 121-130

[85] Williamson, DF; Forman, MR; Binkin, NJ; Gentry, EM; Remington, PL; Trowbridge, FL. Alcohol and body weight in United Stated adults. *Am J Public Health* 1987, 7, 1324-1330

[86] Hellersted, WL; Jeffery, RW; Murray, DM. The association between alcohol intake and adiposity in the general population. *Am J Epidemiol*, 1990, 132, 549-611

[87] Rimm, EB, Klatsky, A; Grobbee, D; Stampfer, MJ. Review of moderate alcohol consumption and reduced risk of coronary heart disease: is effect due to beer, wine, or spirits? *Br Med J*, 1996, 312, 731-736

[88] Valmadrid, CT; Klein, R; Moss, SE, Klein, BE; Cruickshanks, KJ. Alcohol intake and the risk of coronary heart disease mortality in persons with older-onset diabetes mellitus. *J Am Med Assoc*, 1999, 282, 239-246

[89] Solomon, CG; Hu, FB; Stampfer, MJ; Colditz, GA; Speizer FE; Rimm, EB; Willet, WC, Manson, JE. Moderate alcohol consumption and risk of coronary heart disease among women with type 2 diabetes mellitus. *Circulation*, 2000, 102, 494-499

[90] Tanasescu, M; Hu, FB; Willet, WC; Stampfer, MJ; Rimm, EB. Alcohol consumption and risk of coronary heart disease among men with type 2 diabetes mellitus. *J Am Coll Cardiol*, 2001, 38, 1836-1842

[91] NIH/NHLBI The practical guide, identification, evaluation, and treatment of overweight and obesity in adults. National Institutes of Health, National Hearth, Lung, and Blood Institute, North American Association for the study of obesity. 2000, NIH Publication number 00-4084

[92] Freedman, MR; King, J; Kennedy, Popular diet: a scientific review. *Obes Res*, 9, (Suppl. 1), S1-S40

[93] Hall, JE; Jones, DW. What we can do about the "epidemic" of obesity. *Am J Hypertens*, 2002, 15, 657-659

[94] Stevens, VJ; Obarzanek, E; Cook, NR; Lee, IM; Appel, LJ; Smith West, D; Millas, NC; Mattfeldt-Beman, M; Belden, L; Bragg, C; Millstone, M; Raczynski, J; Brewer, A; Singh, B; Cohen, J. Long-term weight loss and changes in blood pressure: results of the Trials of Hypertension Prevention Group, phase II. *Ann Intern Med*, 2001,134, 1-11

[95] Brug, J; van Lenthe, FJ; Kremers, SP. How to gain insight into environmental correlates of obesogenic behaviors. *Am J Prev Med*, 2006, 31, 6, 525-52

In: Research Trends in Nutrition...
Editor: Johan P. Urster, pp. 187-206

ISBN: 978-1-60456-147-0
© 2008 Nova Science Publishers, Inc.

Chapter 6

Nutritional Considerations in Older Persons with Diabetes Mellitus

Ali A. Rizvi[*]

Division of Endocrinology, Diabetes, and Metabolism, University of South Carolina
School of Medicine, Two Medical Park, Suite 502, Columbia, SC 29203, USA

Abstract

Adults age 60 and older will comprise two-thirds of the diabetic population by the year 2025. Nutritional needs and patterns change with age, especially in the presence of a chronic metabolic disease such as diabetes. More than any other factor, the process of aging defines the daily requirements of protein, fat, carbohydrate, vitamins, and trace elements. It is expected that the prevalence of overweight and obesity will increase in the elderly and be a significant contributory factor to insulin resistance, hyperglycemia, and comorbid health conditions like hypertension and dyslipidemia. The issue of attainment and maintenance of an optimal body weight in elderly diabetic persons may not be as straightforward as in other age groups, and the risk-benefit ratio may be different as well. On the other hand, older inhabitants of long-term care facilities who suffer from diabetes tend to be underweight, which may signify malnutrition and be a risk factor for increased morbidity and mortality. The attendant problems of appetite changes, palatability of food, dietary restrictions, loneliness, and depression may affect the type and quantity of food consumed by elderly persons. Any involuntary change of greater than 10 pounds or 10% of body weight within a short time-frame may be nutrition-related and warrants further investigation from this standpoint. Overall, there is a paucity of information on the nutritional aspects of older patients with diabetes. This area would benefit from ongoing research because of the enormous increase in diabetes underway in the elderly population.

[*] E-mail address: arizvi@gw.mp.sc.edu; Tel: 803-540-1000 ; Fax: 803-540-1050;

Introduction – The Status of Nutrition in the Elderly with Diabetes

The Framingham Heart Study data shows that men and women with diabetes 50 years and older lived on average 7.5 and 8.2 years less than individuals without diabetes [1]. Most of the increased mortality from diabetes stems from associated cardiovascular causes. Diet and nutritional factors play a significant role in modulating all the traditional risk factors for atherosclerotic disease. For example, the total amount of calories and carbohydrate affects the propensity to glucose intolerance and lipid profile, while sodium and potassium intake influences blood pressure levels. Appropriate dietary changes in the setting of diabetes is a critical task in the pursuit of healthy aging in this subgroup. Minorities living in urban areas are prone to suboptimal nutrition and have increased rates of obesity, which increases the risk of glucose intolerance and diabetes [2]. Diabetes in older persons increases the risk of hospitalizations, suboptimal nutrition, nursing home admissions, and physical disability that substantially impairs their quality of life [3][4]. Community-dwelling older adults with diabetes are treated less vigorously than younger persons with diabetes, and many of them do not achieve targets for glucose control that are generally advocated by professional organizations [5].

Optimal nutrition is an important factor in determining the quality of life of older people. The reality, however, is that malnutrition in older people is not only common, but frequently overlooked. The prevalence increases with frailty and physical infirmity, and the institutionalized elderly are at highest risk. In the U.S., about 16% of elderly persons living in the community are undernourished and these figures rise up to 59% in long-term care institutions and 65% in acute care hospitals [6]. Malnutrition encompasses both under-nutrition, due to a deficiency of nutrients, and over-nutrition, resulting from overeating and lack of physical activity. Protein-energy malnutrition is a significant cause of weight loss among older people, while "failure to thrive" refers to a state of decline in functional status disproportional to disease burden, manifested by a weight loss greater than 5 percent of baseline. Although the prevalence of failure to thrive increases with age, it should not be considered a normal consequence of the aging process. It may result from a variety of causes including protein-energy deficiency, loss of muscle mass and endurance, problems with balance and equilibrium, cognitive impairment, and depression. The latter is a particularly prevalent cause in the elderly with diabetes [7].

Many physical and clinical factors lead to malnutrition. The rate of metabolism slows down with advancing age due to a decrease in lean body mass and sedentary lifestyle, resulting in a reduced daily energy requirement (figure 1). Other age-related complications like digestive, oral, and dental problems, functional disability, dementia, acute or chronic diseases and medication-related issues add to the burden. Altered absorption of nutrients and declining renal function may compound the scenario. Many elderly experience social, family and economic changes, which are apt to be more common if the elderly individual suffers from chronic medical conditions such as diabetes. To accurately recognize and treat malnutrition among older adults, comprehensive assessment is often necessary. Quick assessment and screening tools as well as interventions manuals that identify adults of all ages who are malnourished or at risk of malnutrition are available [8][9]. In addition, lifestyle and social change issues are also important. Housing conditions and hygiene, availability of affordable meal services - delivered for individuals who are housebound - and a variety of networks that help with food shopping and meal preparations should all be part of comprehensive nutritional care. Nutrition services need to be well coordinated across acute, home, community and long-term care sites.

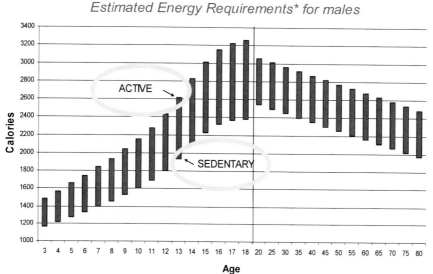

Figure 1. Estimated energy requirements for males in relation to age. From: *The National Academy of Sciences, Institute of Medicine Dietary Reference Intakes Macronutrient Report.* Available at www.iom.edu/CMS/3708.aspx, accessed 8-15-07).

The Triumvirate of Diet, Ageing, and Glucose Metabolism

The prevalence of diabetes increases with advancing age, and is highest in the above-60 age group (figure 2). Underlying pathophysiologic mechanisms include an increase in insulin resistance related to weight gain and physical inactivity. A factor that is being increasingly appreciated as a significant cause leading to the ultimate manifestation of clinical hyperglycemia is the progressive failure of insulin production from the pancreatic beta cells; this may be a pre-programmed genetic defect, a natural concomitant of the ageing process, or possibly a combination of both [10]. A diagrammatic representation of these processes and the resultant emergence of postprandial followed by fasting hyperglycemia is shown in figure 3. Note also the fairly long time interval leading from the metabolic syndrome and pre-diabetes to frank diabetes, and the inexorable march from normoglycemia to increasingly severe degrees of glucose intolerance.

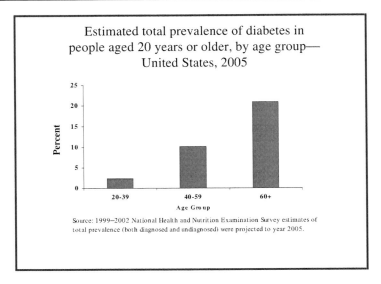

Figure 2. Estimated prevalence of diabetes in the U.S. is highest in persons 60 years of age and above (available at www.diabetes.niddk.nih.gov/dm/pubs/statistics/, accessed 8-15-07).

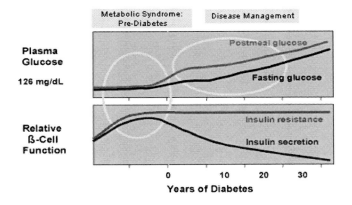

Figure 3. A diagrammatic representation of the natural history of type 2 diabetes. From: *Cefalu T. New options in exogenous insulin therapy.* Available at: http://www.diabetesroundtable.com/courses/update/options.asp, accessed 8-15-07.

Insulin resistance, referred to as a reduction in the in-vivo rate of insulin-mediated glucose disposal, is central to the pathophysiology of type 2 diabetes and the metabolic syndrome [11]. The mechanisms underlying the development of insulin resistance are multifactorial, and likely involve alterations of the insulin signaling pathway. Several hormones and regulatory factors affect insulin action and may contribute to the insulin resistance observed in overweight and aging. Recent research suggests that abnormal free fatty acid metabolism plays an important role in insulin resistance and carbohydrate metabolism seen in individuals who are obese or diabetic. Obesity and increased age are thought to be risk factors that worsen insulin resistance. The basis for this statement comes from the observation that the aging process is associated with an increase in body weight and fat mass in most individuals. Abdominal fat and visceral adiposity are associated with hyperinsulinemia and correlate with insulin resistance. It follows that modifications of the changes in body composition with aging by diet and exercise could delay the onset or progression of insulin resistance [12][13]. It is well-known that weight loss and exercise training result in loss of total and abdominal fat, resulting in increased insulin sensitivity and improved glucose tolerance. The deterioration in insulin sensitivity observed in older persons can be modified by physical training. Longitudinal studies indicate significant improvements in glucose metabolism with aerobic exercise in middle-aged and older men and women. Moreover, the improvements in insulin sensitivity with resistance training are similar in magnitude to those achieved with aerobic activity [14]. The improvements in glucose metabolism after weight loss and increased physical activity may be partially attributed to changes in body composition, including reductions in total and central body fat. Lifestyle modifications that include efforts at weight loss and physical activity lead to improved insulin sensitivity and prevent glucose intolerance and type 2 diabetes mellitus in older adults. These changes should be promoted at the community level for enhancing health benefits and functional status.

Although the exact mechanisms underlying normal ageing are not fully understood, there is generally an associated increase in chronic conditions such as cardiovascular disease, diabetes, cancer and osteoporosis. It is becoming clear that it is possible to prevent, slow or reverse the onset of many these by modifying lifestyle factors such as diet. No aspect of health is this more applicable than the specter of progressive deterioration in glucose tolerance with age. The challenge in the area of diet and healthy ageing relates to both an obvious need to improve the diet of older adults and to encourage other age groups to adapt their diet so they can enter old age in a healthier overall condition. Studies of older adults in many areas of the world have highlighted a number of arenas in which diet composition could be improved. In this respect, it is important to identify dietary patterns in addition to specific dietary components that offer protection against chronic disease [15].

The aging process alters body composition that impact changes in nutritional status as we grow older. There is individual variability in its rate of development determined mostly by genetic factors. Premature aging of cells and tissues is due to interplay of genetic factors and long-term exposure to physical or chemical environments that cause irreversible tissue damage. Early aging as well as geriatric disease impact lifespan, but both can be prevented to some extent by diet and exercise. Diseases that can be nutritionally prevented include nutritional deficiency states and chronic diet-related diseases such as type 2 diabetes, hypertension, coronary artery disease, and cancer. Disabilities resulting from these diseases and from degenerative arthritis are also subject to modulation by diet. The nutritional requirements of the elderly are mostly similar to those of younger people, with some key differences. The elderly usually need fewer calories, but some groups like the homebound or institutionalized who lack sunlight exposure have higher needs for specific nutrients like vitamin D. Nutritional requirements to promote longer life expectancy and freedom from disabilities that result from chronic disease include restriction of food energy and fat. Nutritional assessment of the elderly is aimed at identifying not only the presence of deficiency states but also states of nutrient excess and chronic diet-related diseases [16]. There are obstacles in doing accurate nutritional assessment in the elderly, but techniques are now available which make valid assessments possible. In general, those who live longest have less genetic risk of premature aging, but factors such as education, coping skills, and higher socioeconomic status also furnish them with a greater likelihood of consuming a diet that best meets their long-term nutritional needs. Those most at risk for developing malnutrition as they get older lack food access because of poverty, or have disability resulting from chronic ill-health. Malnutrition is more likely to be found in the elderly in our society if the reasons that they reside in their own homes include indigence or social isolation, and because of homebound status stemming from physical disability.

Interestingly, recent evidence suggests that the rate of carbohydrate digestion and absorption may influence the development of type 2 diabetes in the older individual. The Health, Aging and Body Composition Study [17] was a prospective, cohort analysis of 2248 adults aged 70-80 years that evaluated cross-sectional relations of dietary glycemic index and glycemic load with measures of glucose metabolism and body fat distribution in participants. In men, dietary glycemic index was positively associated with 2-hour glucose (p = 0.04) and fasting insulin (p = 0.004), inversely associated with thigh intramuscular fat (p = 0.02), and not significantly associated with fasting glucose, glycosylated hemoglobin (HbA1c), or visceral abdominal fat. Notably, dietary glycemic load was inversely associated with visceral abdominal fat (p = 0.02) and not significantly associated with fasting glucose, 2-hour glucose, HbA1c, fasting insulin, or thigh intramuscular fat. In women, although dietary glycemic index and load were not significantly related to any measures of glucose metabolism or body fat distribution, the association between dietary glycemic index and 2-hour glucose was nearly significant (p = 0.06). Thus, an association between dietary glycemic index and selected predictors of type 2 diabetes in older adults was seen, particularly in men.

Nutritional Challenges in the Older Diabetic Patient

It is evident that healthy eating habits is important for optimal diabetes management. However, it is possible that the amount of food sufficiency and affordability influences the degree of adherence to dietary self-care behaviors. The Nutrition and Function Study (NAFS) [18] examined whether homebound older adults with diabetes were at greater risk for heightened food insufficiency over one year, despite regular receipt of home-delivered meals. This longitudinal study followed a randomly recruited sample of 268 homebound older adults who regularly received home-delivered meals and completed baseline and 1-year in-home assessments. Based on an economic context model, self-reported data were collected and determinants of increased food insufficiency were examined with multivariate logistic regression models. Not only did food-sufficiency status diminish over time in this sample, but it became or remained worse for older adults with diabetes. In addition to diabetes status, heightened food insufficiency was associated with perceived inadequacy of economic resources. The investigators concluded that health care providers and nutrition programs should attempt to identify high-risk older adults, especially those who have diabetes and are at risk of food insufficiency. This information can be utilized to develop community links and strategies that integrate nutrition with diabetes care plans, thus supporting a multidisciplinary, chronic care model to improve diabetes management and outcomes in the older population.

Individuals with diabetes receive more nutrition advice than other population segment. However, very little is known about how well they comply or differ in nutrient intake from the rest of the population. An Australian study [19] determined the mean macronutrient intake, glycemic index (GI), and glycemic load (GL) of a cohort of 3654 older persons, with and without diabetes. Fasting blood tests including plasma glucose were drawn, and a 145-item semi-quantitative food-frequency questionnaire was completed by the residents. 6 % of participants had diagnosed diabetes. Only seven individuals with diabetes (4.3 %) met all macronutrient recommendations while only four (2.4 %) had adequate fiber intake. These older individuals with diabetes chose a diet that had significantly more protein and less sugars than those without diabetes. This difference led to a moderate reduction in the average GL but had little impact on the average GI. The significant finding was that only a small percentage was able to meet nutritional recommendations for optimal diabetes management.

In order to investigate the benefits of weight loss in the overweight elderly, Hsieh and colleagues [20] compared cardiovascular risk factors in both younger and older patients with type 2 diabetes who had elevated body mass index (BMI) and percentage of body fat. Participants were enrolled in a one-year weight-reduction and lifestyle management program. While changes in BMI and lipids were similar in both age groups, raw figures for change in body fat, fasting plasma glucose, HbA1c, leptin, high sensitivity C-reactive protein (hs-CRP), and adiponectin values were significantly greater in the older group (p-value: 0.02, 0.01, 0.03, 0.04, 0.02, 0.01, 0.03 respectively). This indicated that weight loss was beneficial for older overweight patients with type 2 diabetes, mainly through reduced body fat. Simple diet and life-style modification of adding 20-min daily aerobic exercise and an adequate but restricted calorie diet appears effective in elderly diabetic patients.

Alcohol intake may influence the occurrence of new-onset diabetes in older persons. A study from the Netherlands [21] aimed to investigate the relation between alcohol consumption and type 2 diabetes among older women. Between 1993 and 1997, 16,330 women aged 49-70 years and free from diabetes were enrolled in one of the Dutch Prospect-EPIC (European Prospective Study Into Cancer and Nutrition) cohorts and followed for an average of 6.2 years (range 0.1-10.1). At enrollment, women filled in questionnaires and blood samples were collected. 760 cases of type 2 diabetes were documented, and data showed a linear inverse association (P = 0.007) between alcohol consumption and type 2 diabetes risk after adjusting for potential confounders. Compared with non-drinkers, the hazard ratio for type 2 diabetes was 0.86 (95% CI 0.66-1.12) for women consuming 5-30 g alcohol per week, 0.66 (0.48-0.91) for 30-70 g per week, 0.91 (0.67-1.24) for 70-140 g per week, 0.64 (0.44-0.93) for 140-210 g per week, and 0.69 (0.47-1.02) for >210 g alcohol per week. Lifetime alcohol consumption was associated with type 2 diabetes in a U-shaped fashion. The authors concluded that their findings supported the evidence of a decreased risk of type 2 diabetes with moderate alcohol consumption in a population of older women.

Some studies have provided further insights into the dietary habits and nutrient intakes of older individuals with diabetes. One study compared 151 Australian persons with diabetes with those without diabetes through a survey of 3,000 individuals aged 65 years and older residing in Adelaide, South Australia [22]. A semi-quantitative food frequency questionnaire by mail was used. In the 77% of individuals who responded, only 64% of individuals with diabetes reported following a diabetic diet, and only 6% were consuming a high-carbohydrate, low-fat diet (defined as greater than or equal to 50% energy intake from carbohydrate and less than or equal to 30% from fat). Individuals with diabetes had lower intakes of refined carbohydrate but were just as likely as those without diabetes to eat high-fat foods. Eggs and cheese were consumed more frequently by those with diabetes, and they were no more likely than those without diabetes to consume the recommended complex-carbohydrate and fiber-rich foods. The extent of adherence to current dietary recommendations for the management of diabetes was found to be independent of sex, age, occupational status, educational attainment, marital status, living arrangements, and source of income. In the investigators' conclusion, the dietary habits of elderly persons with diabetes in the population surveyed suggested an awareness of the need to limit simple sugars; however, adherence to the latest recommendations concerning dietary fat and fiber was inadequate.

In this context, it is worth mentioning the diet and exercise practices obtained from a nationally representative sample of U.S. adults with type 2 diabetes, many of whom were older than age 50 [23]. Data from 1,480 adults with a self-reported diagnosis of type 2 diabetes from the Third National Health and Nutrition Examination Survey (NHANES III) was analyzed. Thirty-six percent of the sample were overweight and another 46% were obese. 31% reported no regular physical activity and another 38% reported less than recommended levels of physical activity. Sixty-two percent of respondents ate fewer than five servings of fruits and vegetables per day. Almost two thirds of the respondents consumed >30% of their daily calories from fat and >10% of total calories from saturated fat. Lower income and increasing age were associated with physical inactivity. In conclusion, the majority of individuals with type 2 diabetes were overweight, did not engage in recommended levels of physical activity, and did not follow dietary guidelines for fat and fruit and vegetable consumption.

Diet and Lifestyle Interventions for Diabetes Management in Older Persons

Overweight and obesity are among the most common nutrition-related disorders in older people. A plant-based diet is associated with reduced risk of chronic diseases such as obesity, cardiovascular disease, cancer, and diabetes. Vitamin B12 deficiency is prevalent in older adults, but there are misconceptions about the causes, consequences, and treatments. Diminished synthesis of vitamin D in the skin that occurs with aging and poor dietary intake contribute to the high prevalence of poor vitamin D status in older adults. Vitamin D deficiency is associated with chronic disorders beyond poor bone health. Supplements containing vitamin B12 and vitamin D will help older adults meet their needs for these key nutrients. Practical advice about foods and dietary supplements that are beneficial for the health of older people is available [24].

Dye et al. [25] conducted a research study with the purpose of identifying factors that affect the nutrition and exercise behaviors of persons over the age of 55 with type 2 diabetes. They conducted focus groups interviews to determine primary health concerns and health behaviors, favored learning modalities, barriers to learning, food preferences, and exercise preferences. The following major themes were identified: some risk factors for diabetes and heart disease seemed more pertinent than others; perceived susceptibility for serious outcomes of diabetes could occur through vicarious learning; willpower, often obtained through faith, was necessary for successful behavior change; effective modification of behavior and building self-efficacy started with small steps; and intrinsic reinforcement was necessary for behavior change. These data were used to identify strategies to enhance adherence to nutrition and activity recommendations for persons with type 2 diabetes and cardiovascular risk factors.

Another study examined the effects of a nutrition education intervention on improving the intake and behaviors related to whole grain foods in congregate meal recipients in senior centers in north Georgia [26]. A sample of 84 participants with a mean age of 77 years completed a pretest, an educational intervention, and a post-test. They were 88% female and 24% African-American. Most participants were knowledgeable that eating more whole grain foods would help reduce their risk of cancer (69%), heart disease (76%), type 2 diabetes (65%), and bowel disorders (82%). However, consumption of 11 whole grain foods was low (10.5 times/week). Following the intervention, participants were more likely to suggest one or more correct ways to identify whole grain foods, and to report an increased intake of whole grain bread, cereal, and crackers. The intervention improved several aspects of the consumption of whole grain foods; however, the authors felt that additional interventions that target the individual and the congregate meal program were necessary to increase intakes to the recommended three servings daily.

When high-intensity progressive resistance training was combined with moderate weight loss through diet manipulation, the result was effective in improving glycemic control in 36 sedentary, overweight patients aged 60-80 years with type 2 diabetes [27]. This intervention demonstrated that high-intensity resistance training can be a feasible and effective component in the management program for older patients with type 2 diabetes.

Miller and others [28] evaluated a randomized intervention to improve food label knowledge and skills in diabetes management among 98 adults aged 65 years and older with diabetes mellitus. The intervention program included 10 weekly group sessions led by a dietitian, incorporating information processing, learning theory, and social cognitive theory principles. The experimental group had greater improvement in total knowledge scores, positive outcome expectations, promoters of diabetes management, and decision-making skills, and a greater reduction in barriers to diabetes management. Older adults with diabetes can benefit, at least in an intent-to-treat research setting, from nutrition education designed to improve knowledge and skills necessary for diabetes management.

Older adults with diabetes need structured nutrition education to achieve metabolic control. In spite of the plethora of advice available, very few diabetes education programs have been designed specifically for older adults. One such study evaluated the impact of a nutrition intervention on the blood glucose and lipoprotein levels of 98 adults 65 years of age and older without functional limitations but with type 2 diabetes for one or more years [29]. The 10-week intervention incorporated principles from information processing, learning theory, and social cognitive theory targeted to meet the needs of older adults. The experimental group had greater improvements in fasting plasma glucose ($P = 0.05$), HbA1c ($P < 0.01$) and total cholesterol ($P < 0.05$) than the control group.

In older adults there are many correctable health factors that can be assessed through screening protocols [30]. The use of a variety of adult education theories and models will enhance behavior changes that lead to more healthful habits and enable a health educator to be successful in effecting change. There is a reluctance to develop nutrition promotion programs for older adults exists because of a perception that they would not adhere to such plans or be able to change their lifestyles. However, longitudinal studies have shown that health promotion activities extend the number of years of health in older people although the relationship weakens somewhat in older age. Changes in diet and exercise patterns are most effective in the prevention of nutrition-related conditions when they are instituted early in life, but positive effects can occur at any age. If nutritional interventions are instituted early, a substantial reduction in health care expenditures may result from a decrease in the incidence or the delayed onset of these conditions.

The American Dietetic Association advocates that the public should consume adequate amounts of dietary fiber from a variety of plant foods [31]. The recommended intake of 20-35 grams/day for healthy adults is not usually met because of low intakes fruits, vegetables, whole and high-fiber grain products, and legumes. Consumption of insoluble dietary fiber lowers blood cholesterol levels and reduces blood glucose and insulin levels. A diet adequate in fiber-containing foods usually has fewer calories, fat, and refined sugar, and is also usually rich in micronutrients and nonnutritive ingredients that have additional health benefits. A fiber-rich meal is processed more slowly in the gastrointestinal tract, thus promoting satiety. These salubrious features of a high-fiber diet promote the treatment and prevention of overweight, obesity, cardiovascular disease, and type 2 diabetes. By increasing variety in the daily food pattern, older adults can achieve adequate dietary fiber intakes. Maintenance of body weight in the inactive older adult with diabetes is accomplished in part by decreasing food intake. Even with a fiber-rich diet, though, a supplement may be needed to bring fiber intakes into a range adequate to prevent constipation.

A central element of glucose management and the achievement and sustaining of ideal body weight is the amount and composition of diet in elderly persons. In this respect, the experience and qualifications of the educator delivering the educational components would intuitively seem important. One study looked at differences between non-certified diabetes educator registered dietitians (non-CDE-RDs) and certified diabetes educator registered dietitians (CDE-RDs) in the design and content of programs to promote physical activity in older adults with type 2 diabetes [32]. The knowledge, design and content scores were significantly higher (p value < .001) in the CDE-RDs compared to those of the non-CDE-RDs. The results of this study indicate that education and experience play a key role in the design and content of programs to improve diet patterns and promote physical activity in older adults, and highlight the role of the dietitian and nutrition educator in this process.

The dietitian, therefore, working with other members of the health care team, plays a very important role in developing a care plan for the older person with diabetes [33]. Individuals in this age group put nutritional changes low on their list of priorities since they often have so many health care needs that consume their time and resources. They need an emphasis on the prevailing wisdom that optimum nutrition is essential to maintain health and well-being and to keep blood glucose levels in the target range. Nutrition education should be individually tailored and should incorporate patience, kindness, humor, understanding, and above all a respect for the differences that make each older person an individual. The dietitian working with this population must be skilled at multifaceted assessment, be able to pinpoint challenges in nutritional care, and be ready to offer solutions on an individual and domestic level. Further, he/she must be able to synthesize all the information obtained in order to creatively design a workable dietary intervention, and be able to adapt instruction techniques and tools for a wide variety of educational needs and abilities. Some important attributes to possess for successful outcomes are knowledge, skill, experience, astute judgment, and sincere caring.

The United States Department of Agriculture (USDA) released a new food guidance system in 2005, replacing the former Food Guide Pyramid. The new system, called "MyPyramid," provides a set of tools based on caloric requirements to help Americans make healthy food choices. It also encourages regular physical activity. A "Food Guide Pyramid for Older Adults" developed by Tufts University, Boston, MA, is also available for use in the elderly population (figure 4).

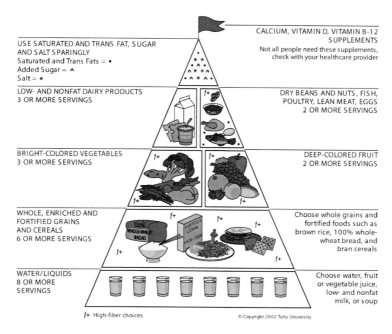

Figure 4. The Food Guide Pyramid for Older adults. From: *Tufts University, 2002: TUFTS Food Guide Pyramid for Older Adults*. Available at http://nutrition.tufts.edu/docs/pyramid.pdf, accessed 8-15-07.

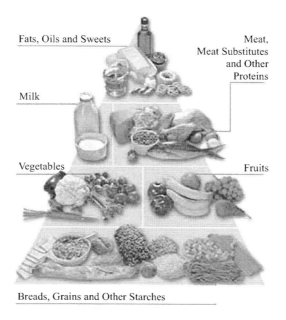

Figure 5. The Diabetes Food Pyramid. From: *The American Diabetes Association*. available at http://www.diabetes.org/nutrition-and-recipes/nutrition/foodpyramid.jsp, accessed 8-15-07.

For people with diabetes, the American Diabetes Association (ADA) recommends an individualized meal plan as an important aspect of managing diabetes and weight. The ADA supports the USDA's effort to emphasize the importance of balancing food intake with daily physical activity, advocating that such a balance is essential in promoting health including the prevention of diabetes and its complications, such as cardiovascular disease. In order to formulate a meal plan tailored to the individual goals, the ADA recommends that individuals with diabetes consult a registered dietitian (RD) or certified diabetes educator (CDE). The ADA's Diabetes Food Pyramid (figure 5) divides food into six groups. These groups or sections on the pyramid vary in size. The largest group consisting of servings of grains, beans, and starchy vegetables forms the base. The smallest group comprising of fats, sweets, and alcohol is at the top of the pyramid; patients with diabetes are advised to consume sparingly from this food group.

Psychosocial Support, Economic Factors, and Structured Educational Interventions

One of the most challenging diabetes-related behavior changes is adhering to a healthful diet. Drawing on the social cognitive theory and social support literature, a qualitative study explored how spousal support influences dietary changes following a diagnosis of type 2 diabetes in middle-aged and older adults [34]. The purpose of this study was to determine how aspects of the spousal relationship translate into behavior changes, specifically adherence to a healthful diet. Analyses revealed five core themes related to dietary adherence: control over food, dietary competence, and commitment to support, spousal communication, and coping with diabetes. The themes can be categorized within two key social cognitive theory constructs: reinforcement and self-efficacy. Implications from the focus group data can inform the development of more effective, targeted nutrition messages and programs to provide specific knowledge and skills.

Low income individuals with diabetes are at particularly high risk for poor health outcomes. What about the confluence of low socioeconomic status and old age? A cross-sectional study was conducted using an urban, diabetes education center database in Canada [35]. The findings demonstrated that low income patients presenting to the diabetes clinic were older and heavier lipid profile than do high income patients. Overall medication use was higher among the lower income group. This suggested that differences in clinical profiles were not the result of under-treatment and implicated lifestyle factors as potential contributors.

Should education and income level be used as a criterion for targeted screening for diabetes in older adults? This question was investigated utilizing measures of diabetes status, fasting plasma glucose, socio-economic status, and demographic characteristics from the National Health and Nutrition Examination Survey (NHANES III) [36]. Socio-economic status, as measured by education and income, was not associated with whether or not individuals are likely to have undiagnosed diabetes. This finding suggests that screening for type 2 diabetes should focus on those adults who are at risk for diabetes in general (based on age, racial/ethnic groups, obesity and other clinical risk factors) and that socio-economic characteristics are unlikely to provide further information.

Examination of the relationship between diabetes-specific family support and other psychosocial factors with regard to diet and exercise self-care behavior was the focus of a survey in older Mexican Americans with type 2 diabetes in order to assess family support specific to diabetes, barriers to self-management, self-efficacy, and diabetes self-care activities [37]. Higher levels of perceived family support and greater self-efficacy were associated with higher reported levels of diet and exercise self-care. The results reinforce the notion that family dynamics self-care activities in the elderly, and diabetes educators and healthcare providers should consider involving the entire family in the management of older patients with type 2 diabetes. Data also validate the Transtheoretical Model, where those in the action stages displayed healthier eating [38]. They also indicate that demographic and psychosocial factors may mediate readiness to change diet. Precontemplators were a heterogeneous group and may need individually tailored interventions.

A study was undertaken to evaluate an interventional weight loss and exercise program consisting of both individual and group sessions designed to improve diabetes management in older, overweight African-Americans [39]. The intervention program was effective in improving glycemic and blood pressure control. After the adjustment for changes in weight and activity, the intervention group was approximately twice as likely to have a one unit decrease in HbA1c value as those in usual care. The decrease in HbA1c values was generally independent of the relatively modest changes in dietary intake, weight, and activity and may reflect indirect program effects on other aspects of self-care.

Diabetes Medications, Meals, and Food-Related Glycemic Excursions

Whatever mechanisms eventually explain the emergence of impaired glucose tolerance during aging, the clinically important extrinsic modifiers of glycemic levels include diet, medications, activity, and chronic illness and stress. Although prospective studies are not available in the elderly, retrospective studies suggest that good blood glucose control reduces the likelihood and severity of stroke, cardiovascular disease, visual impairment, nephropathy, infections, and even cognitive dysfunction [40]. Good control also reduces the symptoms of hyperglycemia that disrupt quality of life in older persons, including nocturia, polyuria, polydipsia, hypovolemia, and fatigue.

The elderly segment of the population is more likely to develop coexisting illnesses that can predispose to the development of diabetes and complicate its management. Traditionally, providers have concentrated their therapeutic efforts at controlling fasting and average glucose values. Fasting glucose is, however, a crude index of glucose control in light of the fact that mealtime glucose excursions, such as those occurring in an absorptive state, are also responsible for overall glucose burden. Many mechanisms have been described by which mealtime glucose excursions could pose a potential risk factor for cardiovascular disease in diabetic patients. Recent work in the field of diabetes suggests that post-meal glucose elevations and glycemic variability carries an increased risk of endothelial dysfunction, oxidative stress, and possibly vascular complications, perhaps independently of the HbA1c level [41]. Acute elevations of plasma glucose concentrations trigger an array of tissue response that may contribute to the development of vascular complications, especially in the older person with diabetes [42]. The ominous finding is that post-prandial glucose may be a risk factor for cardiovascular disease and chronic diabetic complications [43]. Even among patients in apparently good glycemic control may have undetected post-meal elevations, and that simple clinical characteristics identify subsets of diabetic patients with frequent post-prandial hyperglycaemia. Thus in multivariate analysis adjusted for pre-prandial glucose levels, older age, longer duration of diabetes, absence of obesity, hyperlipidemia and hypertension, as well as treatment with sulfonylureas, were significantly associated with greater glucose excursions after meals [44]. With advancing age, post-meal glucose glycemic excursions are the initial abnormality that progress to fasting and pre-meal elevations.

Although no long-term studies have been conducted in this area in older adults with diabetes, it is clear from our previous discussion that this age group has a heightened predilection to uncontrolled postprandial glycemia. The American Geriatric Society's stance is that a person's functional capacity and not age should determine the best treatment modality individualized to each situation [45].

Diet and exercise form the cornerstone of therapy of older persons. Oral agents are the next step, although there may be contraindications to many of the medication classes currently available. The effect of aging on metabolism and pharmacokinetics also need to be taken into account. In general, treatment strategies follow a continuum over time from lifestyle modification to intensive management [46]. Intensive insulin therapy, through the use of either multiple daily injections (MDII) or continuous subcutaneous insulin infusion (CSII, or insulin pump therapy), has been demonstrated to be beneficial in the elderly [47][48]. Such insulin regimens, although complex, should not be withheld from older patients if they are otherwise capable of understanding and adhering to the treatment. General practitioners and patients alike have reluctance to initiating insulin, the so-called phenomenon of 'clinical inertia'. The expertise of diabetologists or endocrinologists may be highly desirable in this regard. A big advantage of tailoring insulin to patients' glucose profiles is a more precise control of meal-related hyperglycemia, as long as a physiologic 'basal-bolus' insulin regimen is used and timing of injections to food is achieved. In addition, the use of carbohydrate counting or exchange lists gives more flexibility to the older adult with diabetes. It must be kept in mind, however, that there is a lack of evidence-based outcomes regarding intensive management in older patients, and the risk-benefit ratio should always be calculated in the individual person. Hypoglycemia and hypoglycemia unawareness is more deleterious in the elderly and should be avoided. Properly conducted studies evaluating safe and effective use of diet and insulin treatment algorithms are needed.

Nutrition in the Management of Complications and Co-morbidities

Although a detailed review is beyond the scope of this chapter, certain salient points are worth mentioning. Maintenance of adequate hydration may be challenging in the elderly suffering from significant hyperglycemia, yet is an important parameter to monitor. Changes in thirst perception, cultural and eating habits, and cognitive of functional impairment may play a role. Hypertension is a common comorbid health condition in older patients with diabetes. Individuals with diabetic nephropathy may need both sodium and protein restriction.

Although protein needs for the aged are the same or slightly higher than other adults, a moderate reduction may be in order if advanced renal insufficiency is present. A survey of 742 individuals 55 years or older (representing 8.02 million U.S. adults) with self-reported diabetes in the 1999 to 2002 National Health and Nutrition Examination Survey [49]. showed low rates of diet and nutritional advice. The investigators found that although the entire non-institutionalized older population with diabetes had indications for angiotensin-converting enzyme and angiotensin-receptor blockers, only 43% of the population was receiving them. Diabetes is a "cardiac risk equivalent", and older persons with atherosclerotic cardiovascular disease need to adhere to a low-fat, step 1 or step 2 diet as advised by the National Cholesterol Education Program (NCEP) Adult Treatment Panel (ATP) III guidelines, updated in 2004 to include more aggressive targets in patients with diabetes [50]. The risk of peripheral vascular disease in persons with diabetes mellitus increases with advanced age, necessitating clinical vigilance [51]. Individualized and comprehensive prevention efforts are required to address the complicated and diverse nature of the diabetic foot in the elderly patient. A multidisciplinary management strategy, including promotion of lifestyle changes to offset the deleterious effects of hyperglycemia, provision of foot care education and management, emphasis on the need for appropriate foot wear yields the best results. Development of lower extremity ulcers and their clinical presentation and proper assessment, is dependent on physiologic and socioeconomic factors. To help ulcer-related complications and prevent lower leg amputations, clinicians must address diabetes management; the cost of supplies; the importance of offloading, nutrition, and exercise; and challenges inherent to impaired eyesight, dexterity, and ability to self-care. The role of optimal nutrition in preventing and managing foot problems remains paramount.

Group-based lifestyle and diet interventions are practical and produce positive health changes in middle-aged and older patients with schizophrenia and diabetes mellitus. The feasibility and preliminary efficacy of a lifestyle intervention was shown in middle-aged and older patients with schizophrenia and type-2 diabetes mellitus over the age of 40 were randomly assigned to either a 24-week "Diabetes Awareness and Rehabilitation Training" group or "Usual are Plus Information" comparison group [52].

Evidence is increasing that oral health has important impacts on systemic health. Data from the third National Health and Nutrition Examination Survey (NHANES III) describing the prevalence of dental caries and periodontal diseases in the older adult population has been published [53]. Periodontal infection is a risk factor for poor glycemic control in type 2 diabetes; however, studies on relationships among oral health status, chronic oral infections, and certain systemic diseases, specifically type 2 diabetes and aspiration pneumonia, need to be conducted. Both of these diseases increase in occurrence and impact in older age groups. There is evidence to support recommending oral care regimens in protocols for managing type 2 diabetes and preventing aspiration pneumonia [54].

More than a third of people over age 65 are edentulous, which makes maintenance of optimal nutrition and intake of adequate cellulose fiber difficult to achieve. Routine dental exams and a liberal fluid ingestion usually help to prevent the tendency to constipation in these circumstances [55]. Many diabetic individuals complain of dry mouth or xerostomia, a condition that can affect oral health, nutritional status, and diet selection. Older adults with poorly controlled diabetes may have impaired salivary flow in comparison with subjects with better controlled diabetes and nondiabetic subjects, yet they may not have concomitant xerostomic complaints [55]. Routine questioning may not uncover the problem, and maintaining a high index of suspicion and meticulous physical examination are necessary.

Maintaining Optimal Nutrition for Older Diabetic Persons in the Community

As the epidemic of diabetes rages on, ensuring proper nutritional intake is an important challenge facing communities world wide. The presence of senility and frailty in the elderly person suffering from diabetes makes this task even more difficult. Community nurses will have increasingly larger caseloads of elderly patients with diabetes [56]. Home visits and interactions with family members will require special attention. It is important that visiting nurses assess the patient's understanding of the disease and its treatment. The aim of good diabetic control in the elderly person may not be the same as in other age groups. Amelioration of symptoms is foremost, although reducing morbidity from complications is a worthy long-term goal [57]. The degree of glycemic control should be decided on an individual basis. Factors that affect the patients' quality of life and their ability to manage their condition should be assessed. Providing education and support for both the patients and caregivers on an ongoing basis cannot be ignored. The importance of diet, blood glucose monitoring and adherence to prescribed medications are important aspects of care for the frail elderly with diabetes [58].

The principles of sound nutrition remain as true in the older person with diabetes as in younger ones [59]. Occasionally, however, financial considerations have to be taken into account. The social dynamics that affect lifestyle changes include retirement, widowhood, or moving into an assisted living facility, all of which can cause emotional instability and impact the quantity and quality of food consumed. Anticipation of the cost of food and the provision of low-cost alternatives should be routinely recommended. Fortunately, numerous resources are available for adequate short- and long-term nutritional supplementation; these include adult day care centers, social services, "meals-on-wheels", in-home personal aides, aging centers, food stamps, and community nutritional sites [60]. Food palatability and consistency as well as cultural preferences and life-long culinary habits are important considerations in the diabetic patient for optimal weight maintenance and glucose control.

Conclusion

Abnormal glucose tolerance is present in more than 60% of adults older than 60 years of age as a result of a decrease in glucose tolerance as a result of decreased insulin sensitivity and impairment of pancreatic beta-cell function. Because the population in Western societies is aging and the prevalence of obesity is going up world wide, the incidence of diabetes mellitus continues to increase. Current diet and lifestyle recommendations for patients with diabetes mellitus mainly focus on young and middle-aged persons. It is imperative to understand the role of dietary factors in the genesis and progression of glucose intolerance and diabetes in the older individual. There is a paucity of definitive, long-term studies examining the part that nutrition plays in the overall health and metabolism of older people.

The elderly diabetic population stands to benefit enormously from streamlining and optimizing diet planning in order to enhance longevity, minimize complications, and improve quality of life.

References

[1] Franco OH, Steyerberg EW, Hu FB, Mackenbach J, Wilma Nusselder W. Associations of Diabetes Mellitus With Total Life Expectancy and Life Expectancy With and Without Cardiovascular Disease. *Arch Intern Med* 2007; 167:1145-1151.

[2] Jen KL, Brogan K, Washington OG, Flack JM, Artinian NT. Poor nutrient intake and high obese rate in an urban African American population with hypertension. *J Am Coll Nutr* 2007;26(1):57-65.

[3] Russell LB, Valiyeva E, Roman SH, Pogach LM, Suh DC, Safford MM. Hospitalizations, nursing home admissions, and deaths attributable to diabetes. *Diabetes Care*. 2005;28(7):1611-7.

[4] Gregg EW, Beckles GL, Williamson DF, Leveille SG, Langlois JA, Engelgau MM, Narayan KM. Diabetes and physical disability among older U.S. adults. *Diabetes Care* 2000;23(9):1272-7.

[5] Shorr RI, Franse LV, Resnick HE, Di Bari M, Johnson KC, Pahor M. Glycemic control of older adults with type 2 diabetes: findings from the Third National Health and Nutrition Examination Survey, 1988-1994. *J Am Geriatr Soc* 2000;48(3):264-7.

[6] Beers MH, M.D., Berkow R., M.D. eds. (2000-2004). The Merck Manual of Geriatrics. Medical Services, USMEDSA, USHH. Section 1. Nutritional Disorders. Chapter 2. Malnutrition. Available at www.merck.com/mrkshared/mmanual/section/chapter2/2a.jsp, accessed 8-15-07.

[7] Markson EW. Functional, social, and psychological disability as causes of loss of weight and independence in older community-living people. *Clin Geriatr Med* 1007;13:639-652.

[8] *Malnutrition Universal Screening Tool (MUST)*. British association for Parenteral and Enteral Nutrition (BAPEN) Advancing Clinical Nutrition, Malnutrition Advisor Group (MAG), 2003. Nutricia Ltd., UK. Available at: http://www.bapen.org.uk/pdfs/must/must_full.pdf, accessed 8-20-07.

[9] Nutrition Screening Initiative. Nutrition Interventions Manual for Professionals Caring for Older Americans. Washington DC;1992.

[10] Barbara A. Ramlo-Halsted BA, Edelman SV. The natural history of type 2 diabetes: practical points to consider in developing prevention and treatment strategies. Clinical *Diabetes* 2000;18(2):80-84.

[11] Reaven GM. Banting lecture 1988. Role of insulin resistance in human disease. *Diabetes* 1988;37(12):1595-1607.

[12] Kohrt WM, Kirwan JP, Staten MA, Bourey RE, King DS, and Holloszy JO. Insulin resistance in aging is related to abdominal obesity. *Diabetes* 1993;42: 273-281.

[13] Kevin R. Short KR, Janet L, el al. Impact of Aerobic Exercise Training on Age-Related Changes in Insulin Sensitivity and Muscle Oxidative Capacity. *Diabetes* 2003;52: 1888-1896.

[14] Holten MK, Zacho M, Gaster M, et al. Strength Training Increases Insulin-Mediated Glucose Uptake, GLUT4 Content, and Insulin Signaling in Skeletal Muscle in Patients With Type 2 Diabetes. *Diabetes* 2004;53: 294-305.

[15] Joint WHO/FAO Expert Consultation on Diet, Nutrition and the Prevention of Chronic Diseases (2002 : Geneva, Switzerland). Diet, nutrition and the prevention of chronic diseases: report of a joint WHO/FAO expert consultation, Geneva, 28 January -- 1 February 2002. Available at: http://whqlibdoc.who.int/trs/WHO_TRS_916.pdf, accessed 8-26-07.

[16] Vellas B, Lauque S, Andrieu S, et al. Nutrition assessment in the elderly. *Curr Opin Clin Nutr Metab Care* 2001;4(1):5-8.

[17] Sahyoun NR, Anderson AL, Kanaya AM, Koh-Banerjee P, Kritchevsky SB, de Rekeneire N, et al. Dietary glycemic index and load, measures of glucose metabolism, and body fat distribution in older adults. *Am J Clin Nutr* 2005;82(3):547-52.

[18] Sharkey JR. Longitudinal examination of homebound older adults who experience heightened food insufficiency: effect of diabetes status and implications for service provision. *Gerontologist.* 2005 Dec;45(6):773-82.

[19] Barclay AW, Brand-Miller JC, Mitchell P. Macronutrient intake, glycaemic index and glycaemic load of older Australian subjects with and without diabetes: baseline data from the Blue Mountains Eye study. *Br J Nutr* 2006;96(1):117-23.

[20] Hsieh CJ, Wang PW. Effectiveness of weight loss in the elderly with type 2 diabetes mellitus. *J Endocrinol Invest* 2005;28(11):973-7.

[21] Beulens JW, Stolk RP, van der Schouw YT, Grobbee DE, Hendriks HF, Bots ML. Alcohol consumption and risk of type 2 diabetes among older women. *Diabetes Care* 2005;28(12):2933-8.

[22] Horwath CC, Worsley A. Dietary habits of elderly persons with diabetes. *J Am Diet Assoc* 1991;91(5):553-7.

[23] Nelson KM, Reiber G, Boyko EJ. NHANES III. Diet and exercise among adults with type 2 diabetes: findings from the third national health and nutrition examination survey (NHANES III). *Diabetes Care* 2002;25(10):1722-1728.

[24] Johnson MA. Nutrition and aging--practical advice for healthy eating. *J Am Med Womens Assoc* 2004;59(4):262-9.

[25] Dye CJ, Haley-Zitlin V, Willoughby D. Insights from older adults with type 2 diabetes: making dietary and exercise changes. *Diabetes Educ* 2003;29(1):116-27.

[26] Ellis J, Johnson MA, Fischer JG, Hargrove JL. Nutrition and health education intervention for whole grain foods in the Georgia older Americans nutrition programs. *J Nutr Elder* 2005;24(3):67-83.

[27] Dunstan DW, Daly RM, Owen N, Jolley D, De Courten M, Shaw J. High-intensity resistance training improves glycemic control in older patients with type 2 diabetes. *Diabetes Care* 2002;25(10):1729-36.

[28] Miller CK, Edwards L, Kissling G, Sanville L. Evaluation of a theory-based nutrition intervention for older adults with diabetes mellitus. *J Am Diet Assoc* 2002;102(8):1069-81.

[29] Miller CK, Edwards L, Kissling G, Sanville L. Nutrition education improves metabolic outcomes among older adults with diabetes mellitus: results from a randomized controlled trial. *Prev Med* 2002;34(2):252-9.

[30]   Chernoff R. Nutrition and health promotion in older adults. *J Gerontol A Biol Sci Med Sci* 2001;56 Spec No 2:47-53.

[31]   Marlett JA, McBurney MI, Slavin JL; American Dietetic Association. Position of the American Dietetic Association: health implications of dietary fiber. *J Am Diet Assoc* 2002;102(7):993-1000.

[32]   George VA, Stevenson J, Harris CL, Casazza K. CDE and non-CDE dietitians' knowledge of exercise and content of exercise programs for older adults with type 2 diabetes. *J Nutr Educ Behav* 2006;38(3):157-62.

[33]   Templeton CL. Nutrition education: the older adult with diabetes. *Diabetes Educ* 1991;17(5):355-6, 358.

[34]   Beverly EA, Miller CK, Wray LA. Spousal Support and Food-Related Behavior Change in Middle-Aged and Older Adults Living With Type 2 Diabetes. *Health Educ Behav* 2007.

[35]   Rabi DM, Edwards AL, Svenson LW, et al. Clinical and medication profiles stratified by household income in patients referred for diabetes care. *Cardiovasc Diabetol.* 2007 Mar 30;6:11.

[36]   Wilder RP, Majumdar SR, Klarenbach SW, Jacobs P. Socio-economic status and undiagnosed diabetes. *Diabetes Res Clin Pract* 2005;70(1):26-30.

[37]   Wen LK, Shepherd MD, Parchman ML. Family support, diet, and exercise among older Mexican Americans with type 2 diabetes. *Diabetes Educ* 2004;30(6):980-93.

[38]   Vallis M, Ruggiero L, Greene G, Jones H, Zinman B, Rossi S, et al. Stages of change for healthy eating in diabetes: relation to demographic, eating-related, health care utilization, and psychosocial factors.

[39]   Agurs-Collins TD, Kumanyika SK, Ten Have TR, Adams-Campbell LL. A randomized controlled trial of weight reduction and exercise for diabetes management in older African-American subjects. *Diabetes Care* 1997;20(10):1503-11.

[40]   Samos LF, Roos BA. Diabetes mellitus in older persons. *Med Clin North Am.* 1998;82(4):791-803.

[41]   Brownlee M, Hirsch IB. Glycemic Variability: A Hemoglobin A_{1c}–Independent Risk Factor for Diabetic Complications. *JAMA* 2006;295:1707-1708.

[42]   Abbatecola AM, Paolisso G. Plasma glucose excursions in older persons with Type 2 diabetes mellitus. *J Endocrinol Invest* 2005;28(11 Suppl Proceedings):105-7.

[43]   Gerich JE. Postprandial hyperglycemia and cardiovascular disease. *Endocr Pract* 2006;12 Suppl 1:47-51.

[44]   Bonora E, Corrao G, Bagnardi V, Ceriello A, Comaschi M, Montanari P, Meigs JB. Prevalence and correlates of post-prandial hyperglycaemia in a large sample of patients with type 2 diabetes mellitus. *Diabetologia* 2006;49(5):846-54.

[45]   Hainer TA. Managing older adults with diabetes. *J Am Acad Nurse Pract.* 2006;18(7):309-17.

[46]   Oiknine R, Mooradian AD. Drug therapy of diabetes in the elderly. *Biomed Pharmacother* 2003;57(5-6):231-9.

[47]   Raskin P, Bode BW, Marks JB, et al: Continuous subcutaneous insulin infusion and multiple daily injection therapy are equally effective in type 2 diabetes. A randomized, parallel group, 24-week study. *Diabetes Care.* 2003:26(9);2598-2603.

[48]   Rizvi AA. Benefits of insulin pump therapy in the elderly. *Geriatric Times* 2002; 3(4):23-30.

[49]   Rosen AB. Indications for and utilization of ACE inhibitors in older individuals with diabetes. Findings from the National Health and Nutrition Examination Survey 1999 to 2002. *J Gen Intern Med* 2006;21(4):315-9.

[50]   Grundy SM, Cleeman JI, Merz CNB, et al. NCEP Report: Implication of recent clinical trials for the National Cholesterol Education Program Adult Treatment Panel III Guidelines. *Circulation* 2004;110:227-239.

[51]   Van Gils CC, Stark LA. Diabetes mellitus and the elderly: special considerations for foot ulcer prevention and care. *Ostomy Wound Manage.* 2006;52(9):50-2, 54, 56.

[52]   McKibbin CL, Patterson TL, Norman G, Patrick K, Jin H, Roesch S, Mudaliar S, Barrio C, O'Hanlon K, Griver K, Sirkin A, Jeste DV. A lifestyle intervention for older schizophrenia patients with diabetes mellitus: a randomized controlled trial. *Schizophr Res* 2006;86(1-3):36-44.

[53]   Taylor GW, Loesche WJ, Terpenning MS. Impact of oral diseases on systemic health in the elderly: diabetes mellitus and aspiration pneumonia. *J Public Health Dent* 2000;60(4):313-20.

[54]   Loesche W, Schork A, Terpenning M, Yin-Miao Chen, Dominguez L, Grossman N. Assessing the relationship between dental disease and coronary artery disease in elderly US veterans. *J Am Dent Assoc* 1998;129:301-311.

[55]   Chávez EM, Borrell LN, Taylor GW, Ship JA.A longitudinal analysis of salivary flow in control subjects and older adults with type 2 diabetes. *Oral Surg Oral Med Oral Pathol Oral Radiol Endod.* 2001 Feb;91(2):166-73.

[56]   Mayes M. Management of the older person with diabetes in the community. *Br J Community Nurs.* 2000;5(9):448-53.

[57]   Gallichan M. Promoting health in older people with diabetes. *Prof Nurse* 1997;13(2):96-100.

[58]   AADE: Special considerations for the education and management of older adults with diabetes. American Association of Diabetes Educators. *Diabetes Educ.* 1999 Nov-Dec;25(6):879-81.

[59]   Gilden JL. Nutrition and the older diabetic. *Clin Geriatr Med* 1999;15(2):371-90.

[60]   Stanley K. Assessing the nutritional needs of the geriatric patient with diabetes. *Diabetes Educ* 1998;24:29-36.

In: Research Trends in Nutrition...
Editor: Johan P. Urster, pp. 207-229

ISBN: 978-1-60456-147-0
© 2008 Nova Science Publishers, Inc.

Chapter 7

The Choice of Nutritional Strategy in Acute Pancreatitis

Maxim S. Petrov[*]
Department of Surgery,
Nizhny Novgorod State Medical Academy,
Nizhny Novgorod, Russia

Abstract

Acute pancreatitis is an acute inflammatory process of the pancreas with variable involvement of peripancreatic tissues or remote organ systems, usually caused by gallstones or alcohol. Supportive care rather than specific therapy characterizes the current management of acute pancreatitis and the arsenal of valuable options is pretty scarce. Thereby, the role of artificial nutrition as a novel therapeutical modality in acute pancreatitis should be carefully explored.

While the concept of "pancreatic rest" and a nil-per-mouth regimen dominated throughout the 20th century, the latest studies demonstrate unequivocal benefits of enteral over parenteral nutrition in terms of better glucose tolerance as well as reduction in infectious complications and mortality in patients with severe acute pancreatitis. Now that the advantages of enteral feeding have become apparent, the next step would be to clarify the optimal timing of onset of nutritional support. Theoretically, enteral feeding can prevent mucosal barrier dysfunction, small bowel bacterial overgrowth, and bacterial translocation and, therefore, should be instituted as early as possible in the course of disease. However, this hypothesis should be tested in the randomized trial on early versus delayed enteral nutrition.

Furthermore, as two recent randomized controlled trials demonstrated no difference in morbidity and mortality between nasogastric and nasojejunal feeding, the potential cumbers with the positioning of feeding tube in the jejunum with the aid of endoscopy or interventional radiology might be solved. Apart from this, intermittent feeding may probably decrease the gastric retention in patients on nasogastric tube feeding. Thereby, the effect of intermittent versus continuous enteral tube feeding should be investigated in the setting of acute pancreatitis.

---

[*] E-mail address: max.petrov@gmail.com; Tel: +7-910-383-3963; Fax: +1-801-788-7383; PO Box 568, Nizhny Novgorod, 603000 Russia

Another important aspect for the optimizing of management of acute pancreatitis is observed in the modification in composition of enteral formula. Such immune-enhanced supplementations as glutamine, arginine and ώ-3 fatty acids are unlikely to be effective. At the same time, the use of enteral nutrition supplemented with pro- pre- and synbiotics may potentially bring benefits to the patients with acute pancreatitis. However, further adequately powered studies are warranted before implementing them in clinical practice.

To this end, enteral nutrition appears to be an indisputable tool in acute pancreatitis and further high-quality studies should focus on the ways to elaborate it.

Introduction

Acute pancreatitis (AP) is a common cause of acute abdominal pain and is the most frequent pancreatic disease, for which alcohol abuse and gallstone disease are the two most common causes [1]. In 1925, the famous British surgeon lord Berkeley Moynihan aptly described the dramatic nature of acute pancreatitis as "the most terrible of all calamities that occur in connection with abdominal viscera. The suddenness of its onset, the illimitable agony which accompanies it, and the mortality attendant upon it, all render it most formidable of catastrophes…" [2]. Nowadays mortality associated with severe AP can be as high as 40 per cent and follows biphasic distribution. About half the deaths occur within the first week of the attack, mostly from multiple organ dysfunction, which is not different from the systemic complications found in other diseases or injuries (e.g. major trauma, burns) [3-6]. The second phase ensues usually after the second week of onset and includes the formation of infected pancreatic necrosis or fluid collection with possible progression to sepsis, multiple organ dysfunction and death [6-8].

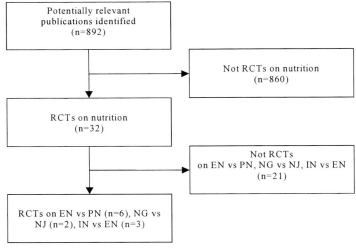

RCT=randomized controlled trial
EN=enteral nutrition
PN=parenteral nutrition
IN=immunonutrition
NG=nasogastric nutrition
NJ=nasojejunal nutrition

Figure 1. Identification of eligible randomized controlled trials.

Despite more than 100 years of experience and thousands of experimental and clinical studies, the treatment of AP is challenging. Application of the principles of evidence-based medicine, i.e. "conscientious, explicit and judicious use of current best evidence in making decisions about individual patients" [9], may help physicians to integrate their own individual clinical expertise with the best available evidence from systematic research. Patients with acute pancreatitis represents a wide range of medical problems while being treated in the hospital, such as requirement of intensive care unit treatment, infection problems, need of dialysis, surgical and radiological procedures, diabetes, symptoms of polyneuropathy, continual abdominal pain and recurrent pancreatitis. The present chapter focuses on the nutritional management as the modern and most dynamically evolving paradigm of treatment in acute pancreatitis. The effect of nutrition on main clinical outcomes is systematically assessed by 5 comparisons: enteral vs parenteral nutrition, nasogastric vs nasojejunal feeding, immunonutrition vs standard enteral nutrition, early vs delayed enteral nutrition, and continuous vs intermittent feeding.

A computerized literature cross-search on three databases (MEDLINE, EMBASE and Cochrane Central Register of Controlled Trials) from January 1, 1980 to June 30, 2007 was performed. The search strategy for MEDLINE was "acute pancreatitis"[Title/Abstract] AND ("nutrition"[Title/Abstract] OR "feeding" [Title/Abstract]). The search strategy for EMBASE was "acute pancreatitis" AND ("feeding" OR "nutrition") AND [humans]/lim. The search strategy in Cochrane library was "acute pancreatitis" AND ("nutrition" OR "feeding"). No language restrictions were applied.

To guarantee control of selection bias and provide the best quality evidence (level 1) only randomized controlled trials (RCTs) on nutrition in patients with acute pancreatitis were selected. A RCT was defined as a study in which participants were assigned to one of two interventions by random allocation. Figure 1 depicts the selection process. Methodological quality of included studies was assessed using a modification (Table 1) of the previously published quality score [10] with quality score range from 0 to 16 points. Study characteristics for the included RCTs are presented in Table 2. The data analysis was performed using the meta-analysis software (Bax L, Yu LM, Ikeda N, Tsuruta N, Moons KGM. MIX: Comprehensive Free Software for Meta-analysis of Causal Research Data - Version 1.51. 2006)). Data were aggregated to determine risk ratio (RR), with its 95% confidence interval (CI). The presence of heterogeneity was assessed using I^2 measure, with $I^2 > 0.2$ indicating significant heterogeneity. Irrespective of the degree of heterogeneity of effect among the included trials, a random-effects model was used. Statistical significance was accepted at a p value of less than 0.05.

Table 1. Methodological quality score

		Criteria	Score
Population	*Patient selection*	Consecutive patients/ random series	2
		Attempt made to enroll as such, but failure outlined	1
		Selected patients or not described	0
	Patient characteristics	Groups comparable ≥ 6 items	2
		Groups comparable 3 to 5 items	1
		Groups comparable ≤ 2 items • Age (mean differs < 10%) • Sex (proportion of men differs < 10%)) • Severity score (mean differs < 10%)) • Mean CRP (differs < 10%) • Pancreatic necrosis presence (differs < 10%) • Aetiology (differs < 10%) • Time between inclusion and onset of symptoms (differs < 10%)	0
Intervention	*Allocation sequence*	Computer-generated, random number table	2
		No more information	1
		Quasi-randomisation	0
	Concealment of allocation	Non-manipulable	2
		Potentially manipulable	1
		Open label	0
	Blinding	Double-blind	2
		Single-blind	1
		(Potentially) unblinded	0
	Protocol of nutrition	Reproducibly described	2
		Poorly described	1
		Not described	0
	Description of cointerventions	Described and equal between groups	2
		Described but not equal between groups	1
		Not described	0
	Missing data	No	2
		< 10%	1
		> 10%	0

Enteral vs Parenteral Nutrition (Part 1)

Severe acute pancreatitis elicits a stress response which leads to a hypercatabolic state promoting nutritional deterioration in the setting of a systemic inflammatory response. In turn, nutritional deterioration is associated with augmentative physiological instability and increased mortality. Malnutrition affects the immune response and renders patients with acute pancreatitis more susceptible to infection. Thereby, enteral or parenteral nutritional management is essential in acute pancreatitis and should be an integral part of patient care.

Table 2. Summary of study characteristics for the included trials

Study	Quality of studies§	Study group	Control group	Total number of patients*	Primary endpoint	Severity* (score)	Onset of symptoms*	Feeding start	Days on nutrition*
Kalfarentzos et al [18]	12	NJ	PN	18/20	Not stated	12.7±2.6/ 11.8±1.9 (APACHE II)	Not stated	<48 h of admission	34.8/32.8
Paraskeva et al [19]	5	NJ	PN	11/12	Need for surgery	>6 (APACHE II)	Not stated	<48 h of admission	Not stated
Gupta et al [20]	12	NJ	PN	8/9	C-reactive protein concentration	8 (6-12)/ 10 (7-14)	Not stated	<6 h of admission	2 (2-7)/ 4 (2-7)
Louie et al [21]	12	NJ	PN	10/18	Time to a 50% reduction in C-reactive protein	11.8±8.3/ 12.7±5.5 (APACHE II)	Not stated	>96 h of admission	13.1±10.5/ 14.6±10.3
Eckerwall et al [22]	14	NG	PN	23/25	Intestinal permeability	10 (8-13)/ 9 (8-10) (APACHE II)	25 (22-35)/ 30 (20-35) h	<24 h of admission	6 (5-9)/ 6 (5-9)
Petrov et al [23]	14	NJ	PN	35/34	Total infectious complications	12 (10-14)/ 12.5 (11-16) (APACHE II)	<72 h	<24 h of admission	14 (8-20)/ 14 (10-21)
Casas et al [24]	10	NJ	PN	11/11	C-reactive protein concentration	3 patients/ 5 patients (grade D-E, Balthazar)	Not stated	<72 h of admission	At least 15

Table 2. Continued.

Study	Quality of studies§	Study group	Control group	Total number of patients*	Primary endpoint	Severity* (score)	Onset of symptoms*	Feeding start	Days on nutrition*
Eatock et al [45]	14	NG	NJ	27/22	C-reactive protein concentration	10 (7-18)/ 12 (8-18) (APACHE II)	<72 h	72 (24-72) h after onset	5
Pandey et al [46]	13	NG	NJ	16/14	Not stated	10.5±3.8/ 9.6±5 (APACHE II)	7.8±6.5/ 5.7 ±4.7 d	48-72 h of admission	7
Hallay et al [58]	7	IN	NJ	11/8	Not stated	3.6 (3-5)/ 3.9 (3-6) (Ranson)	Not stated	<24 h of admission	5
Lasztity et al [59]	12	IN	NJ	14/14	Not stated	8 (5-12)/ 7.6 (5-13) (APACHE II)	Not stated	<24 h of admission	10.6±6.7/ 17.6±10.5
Pearce et al [60]	16	IN	NJ	15/16	C-reactive protein concentration	9 (8-19)/ 9.5 (8-16) (APACHE II)	<72 h	< 72 h after onset	3-15

§The range of the quality score is 0 to16.
* Study group/ Control group.

PN=parenteral nutrition
NG=nasogastric nutrition
NJ=nasojejunal nutrition
IN=immunonutrition

The feasibility of both routes of feeding in patients with acute pancreatitis was shown in the 1970s, but parenteral nutrition (PN) became the standard of nutritional management for many years due to the advocacy of nil-per-mouth conception. The rationale for this strategy was to rest the inflamed pancreas, thereby preventing the stimulation of exocrine function and release of proteolytic enzymes [11]. However, critics argue that, in addition to cost and catheter-related sepsis, PN may lead to electrolyte and metabolic disturbances, gut barrier alteration and increased intestinal permeability [12,13]. By contrast, enteral nutrition (EN) has been shown to be safe in patients with severe acute pancreatitis. Furthermore, it is known that failure of the intestinal barrier leads to development of sepsis and multiple organ failure in critically ill patients [14]. At present, sepsis remains the major factor in morbidity and late mortality in patients with severe acute pancreatitis, due to secondary bacterial infection of (peri-)pancreatic necrosis. Bacteria isolated from infected pancreatic tissue resemble common gastrointestinal flora, suggesting that they reach the pancreas by translocation from the gut. The mechanisms leading to bacterial translocation are not completely understood and may involve (1) disturbed enteric bacterial ecology with subsequent overgrowth of facultative pathogenic bacteria, (2) impaired local and systemic host immune defense, and (3) injured integrity of the gut mucosa, resulting in compromised intestinal barrier function [15-17]. In any case, preservation or restoration of the gut barrier function may have a beneficial impact on infectious morbidity from severe acute pancreatitis and may reduce mortality.

A total of 245 patients with severe acute pancreatitis from 7 RCTs [18-24] were included in the analysis, of whom 116 received EN and 129 received PN. The incidence of pancreatic infections (infected pancreatic necrosis and pancreatic abscess) was 10.3% (12 of 116) in the EN group and 23.3% (30 of 129) in the PN group. When meta-analysed, EN resulted in a statistically significant reduction in risk of pancreatic infectious complications (RR, 0.44; 95% CI, 0.25-0.80; p<0.01) (Fig. 2). There was no significant heterogeneity between trials ($I^2 = 0$).

The incidence of non-pancreatic infections was 10.5% in the EN group and 22.2% in the PN group. When meta-analysed, EN resulted in a statistically significant reduction in risk of pancreatic infectious complications (RR, 0.46; 95% CI, 0.23-0.88; p=0.02) (Fig. 3). There was no significant heterogeneity between trials ($I^2 = 0$).

The incidence of total infectious complications was 20.9% in the EN group and 44.4% in the PN group. When meta-analysed, EN resulted in a statistically significant reduction in risk of pancreatic infectious complications (RR, 0.44; 95% CI, 0.27-0.70; p<0.01) (Fig. 4). There was no significant heterogeneity between trials ($I^2 = 0.03$).

The mortality rate was 5.2% (6 of 116) in the EN group and 17.1% (22 of 129) in the PN group. When meta-analysed, EN resulted in a statistically significant reduction in risk of total infectious complications (RR, 0.38; 95% CI, 0.16-0.88; p=0.02) (Fig. 5). There was no significant heterogeneity between trials ($I^2 = 0$).

Despite the evident clinical benefits of EN over PN in terms of the risk reduction of infectious complications and mortality, the exact mechanism of its favourable effect remains unclear [25]. It is believed that EN may prevent or attenuate mucosal barrier breakdown and subsequent bacterial translocation that play a pivotal role in the development of infectious complications in the course of severe acute pancreatitis [26-28]. When monitoring mucosal barrier function, permeability of the structural mucosal barrier often is the main measured parameter. Unfortunately, there is no consistency in clinical studies with regard to the gut permeability. On the one hand, three clinical studies on acute pancreatitis showed increased intestinal permeability to both micromolecules and macromolecules in patients with severe acute pancreatitis when compared with mild acute pancreatitis and healthy volunteers [29-31]. On the other hand, the RCT by Powell et al [32], in which patients with predicted severe acute pancreatitis were randomized to receive either EN or no artificial nutritional support, showed significantly increased intestinal permeability by day 4 in patients allocated to the EN group. Similarly, the recent RCT on nasogastric versus parenteral feeding in predicted severe patients demonstrated impaired gut permeability on day 3 in the EN group [22]. However, in fact, both RCTs included a considerable number of patients with mild acute pancreatitis (11 of 27 and 26 of 48, correspondingly), in which it is unlikely that intestinal permeability changed considerably [25].

Furthermore, concentrations of anti-endotoxin core antibodies for immunoglobulin M (IgM) were also used as an indirect marker for intestinal permeability [25]. Results of the early RCT from the UK [33] showed that serum IgM antibodies decreased significantly following seven days of EN when compared with the PN group (p<0.05). Similarly, the RCT by Gupta et al [20] demonstrated that IgM antibodies fell significantly in the EN group (p=0.03) and tended to rise in the PN group over the week of treatment. Conversely, the recent RCT by Eckerwall et al [22] found decreasing level of IgM antibodies in both EN and PN groups with no significant difference at any time point within ten days of observation. The influence of EN on intestinal barrier function in severe acute pancreatitis has to be further investigated.

Enteral vs Parenteral Nutrition (Part 2)

For a long time hyperglycemia in patients without history of diabetes mellitus has often been viewed as an adaptive phenomenon, caused by increased insulin resistance during periods of stress [34]. It was referred to as "stress" hyperglycemia, and it was considered a marker of disease severity rather than a real medical entity that needs to be managed [35]. This postulate has been undermined by the RCT in surgical ICU patients from Belgium in 2001 [36]. This study, targeting blood glucose to lower levels (4.4-6.1 mmol/L) using intensive insulin therapy versus infusion of insulin only if the blood glucose level exceeded 12 mmol/L and maintenance of glucose at the level 10.0-11.1 mmol/L, demonstrated that hyperglycemia predispose patients to infectious complications and associated with increased mortality. Additionally, this study showed that parenterally-fed patients required a significantly higher dose of insulin in order to achieve normoglycemia than those receiving EN. This finding indicates the higher hyperglycemic potential of PN. Thereby, at least partially, the worse effect of PN versus EN in acute pancreatitis can be ascribed to hyperglycemia [35].

A total of 174 non-diabetic patients with severe acute pancreatitis from 4 RCTs [18,21-23] were included in the analysis, of whom 84 received EN and 90 received PN. Nine of 84 (10.7%) patients required insulin administration in the EN group and 25 of 90 (27.7%) in the PN group. When meta-analysed, EN resulted in a statistically significant reduction in need for insulin therapy (RR, 0.42; 95% CI, 0.21-0.83; p=0.01) (Fig. 6). There was no significant heterogeneity between trials ($I^2 = 0$).

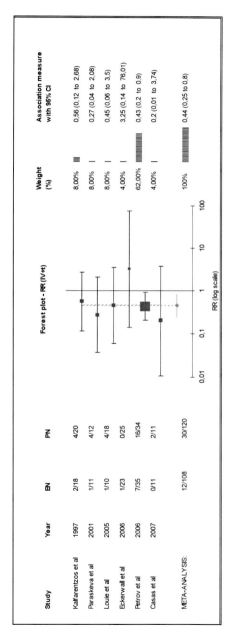

Figure 2. Relative risk of pancreatic infectious complications associated with enteral nutrition in comparison with parenteral nutrition in patients with severe acute pancreatitis.

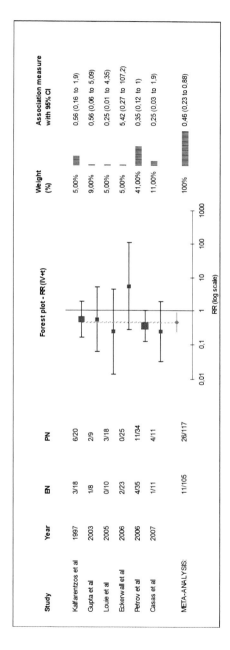

Figure 3. Relative risk of non-pancreatic infectious complications associated with enteral nutrition in comparison with parenteral nutrition in patients with severe acute pancreatitis.

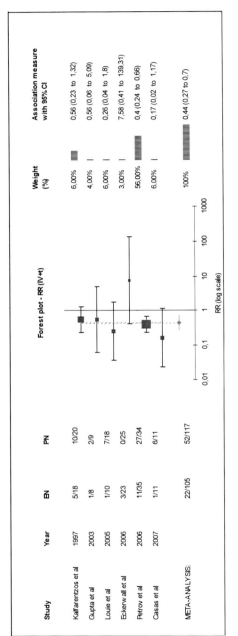

Figure 4. Relative risk of total infectious complications associated with enteral nutrition in comparison with parenteral nutrition in patients with severe acute pancreatitis.

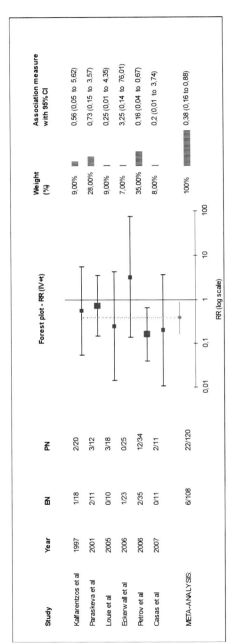

Figure 5. Relative risk of death associated with enteral nutrition in comparison with parenteral nutrition in patients with severe acute pancreatitis.

The incidence of hyperglycemia was 40.8% in the EN group and 78.8% in the PN group. When meta-analysed, EN resulted in a statistically significant reduction in risk of hyperglycemia (RR, 0.53; 95% CI, 0.29-0.98; p=0.04). There was a significant heterogeneity between trials (I^2 = 0.22) [35].

These results show that EN, in comparison with PN, is associated with statistically significant risk reduction in hyperglycemia and insulin requirement in previously non-diabetic patients with severe acute pancreatitis [35]. The findings are in line with the studies in other diseases. In particular, in the earlier study involving patients with traumatic head injuries or cerebral lesions undergoing emergency craniotomy, the group receiving EN had lower insulin requirements than those receiving PN, suggesting that tight glucose control may be more easily achieved with EN [37]. Similarly, the RCT by Moore et al [38] in abdominal trauma patients showed that the use of EN in comparison with PN results in reduction the incidence of hyperglycemia and the lower amount of insulin required.

The results of the present meta-analysis also indicate that hyperglycemia is a quite common in acute pancreatitis and is associated with increased risk of infectious complications and mortality. These data are in line with the RCT by Van den Berghe et al [36] proving that intensive insulin therapy and tight glucose control decrease infectious complications and mortality rates in surgical critically ill patients. However, some points of this trial should be taken into account before implementation of tight glucose control in practice. First of all, serious hypoglycemia was substantially more frequent in the intensive insulin group, which herein poses a question of the practical difficulty to maintain blood glucose in the range of 4.4-6.1 mmol/L in the community hospitals and the potential dangers associated with hypoglycemia. This goal may only be achievable in ICUs with a high nursing to patient ratio and close physician supervision [39]. Apart from this, there was no evidence of a threshold below which the glucose level was no longer associated with an increased risk of death [40].

Thereby, since the enteral route of feeding decreases the risks of hyperglycemia and insulin requirement, administration of EN in patients with severe acute pancreatitis may render the controversy regarding the maintenance of target level of blood glucose less relevant in the setting of acute pancreatitis [35].

Nasogastric vs Nasojejunal Feeding

Now when the benefits of intra-luminal nutritional therapy have become apparent, the next logical step is to define the most appropriate site of tube feeding administration. A systematic review of critically ill patients found no differences in complications, mortality and length of hospital stay between gastric and post-pyloric feeding [41]. Because the placement of nasojejunal tube requires special expertise of the physician, intra-hospital transfer of critically ill patients, and usually results in a delay in the initiation of enteral feeding, the administration of gastric feeding seems to be more reasonable. However, as to acute pancreatitis, there was a fear of reactivation of the inflammatory process with gastric feeding and for years enteral feeding instilled past the Treitz' ligament was recommended to avoid excessive pancreatic stimulation [11,42]. Indeed, a recent study [43] demonstrated that only mid-distal jejunal feeding had no influence on the pancreatic secretory response to enteral diet, whereas duodenal infusions of nutrients resulted in significantly increased rates

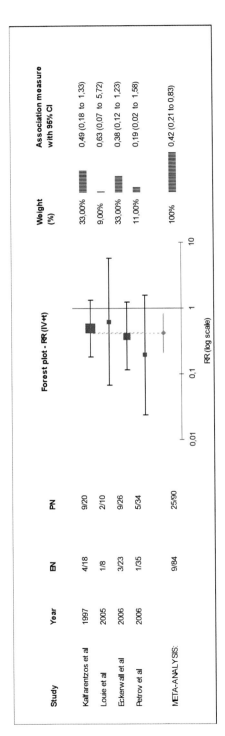

Figure 6. Relative risk of need in insulin therapy associated with enteral nutrition in comparison with parenteral nutrition in patients with severe acute pancreatitis.

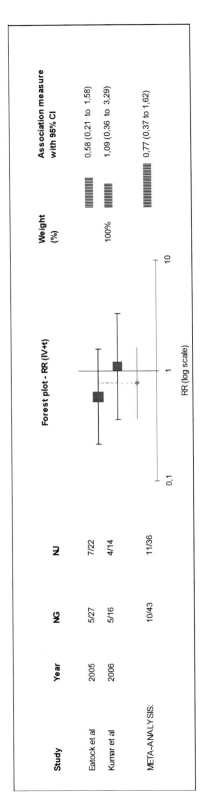

Figure 7. Relative risk of death associated with nasogastric in comparison with nasojejunal enteral feeding in patients with severe acute pancreatitis.

of trypsin and lipase secretion when compared with fasting. Nevertheless, while the majority of patients receiving enteral nutrition due to acute pancreatitis have received nasojejunal tube feeding, there are some studies of successful nasogastric administration of enteral nutritional formula [44,45].

A total of 79 patients with severe acute pancreatitis from 2 RCTs [45,46] were included in the analysis, of whom 43 received nasogastric tube feeding and 36 received nasojejunal tube feeding. The mortality rate was 23.3% (10 of 43) in the nasogastric group and 30.5% (11 of 36) in the nasojejunal group. When meta-analysed, EN did not result in a statistically significant reduction in risk of death (RR, 0.77; 95% CI, 0.37-1.62; p=0.50) (Fig. 7). There was no significant heterogeneity between trials (I^2 = 0). Proximal delivery of enteral nutritional formula appeared to be well-tolerated in 34 of 43 (79.1%) patients on nasogastric feeding. Pulmonary aspiration, which is considered to be the most serious complication of nasogastric feeding, was presented in no patient.

These results show that the rate of complications and mortality did not differ significantly between patients with severe acute pancreatitis who received nasogastric and nasojejunal feeding. In this context, probably the most important issue is a pancreatic enzyme response on feeding. It was shown by O'Keefe et al [47] that all forms of enteral nutrition stimulate pancreatic secretion. In particular, when compared with placebo-saline, oral diet resulted in significantly higher level of amylase (p=0.001) and lipase (p=0.006); duodenal polymeric enteral formula led to increased level of amylase (p=0.002), lipase (p=0.001) and trypsin (p=0.001); duodenal elemental feeding formula resulted in elevated level of lipase (p=0.04). The same research group also compared pancreatic secretory response to tube feeding delivered into the duodenum, mid (40-60 cm distal to the ligament of Trietz) and distal (100-120 cm distal to the ligament of Trietz) jejunum [43]. Authors demonstrated a significantly lower secretion of trypsin (p<0.01) and lipase (p<0.05) in response on the elemental formula delivered into the jejunum (40 cm or more distal to the ligament of Trietz) in comparison with duodenum. Moreover, trypsin and lipase secretory response in the mid-distal jejunum group was as low as in the fasting group.

At the same time, it is worth to mention that both of these studies [43,47] dealt with healthy subjects, whereas there is an evidence [48] that patients with acute pancreatitis, when compared with healthy volunteers have significantly lower rates of secretion of trypsin (p=0.005), amylase (p=0.03) and lipase (p=0.005) in response to duodenal administration of elemental nutritional formula. Surprisingly enough, a comparison of patients with mild/moderate and necrotizing acute pancreatitis revealed 6 times lower secretion rate of trypsin, 22 times lower rate of amylase and 42 times lower rate of lipase in the subgroup of patients with necrotizing acute pancreatitis. It means that the greater the severity of acute pancreatitis, the greater the reduction in pancreatic enzymes secretion as a response on elemental feeding. This is, likely, due to the loss of synthetic function of injured acinar cells as a consequence of pancreatic necrosis. The possible clinical implication of these findings is that nasogastric feeding may not aggravate the course of severe acute pancreatitis due to the pancreatic enzymes secretion in the duodenum.

On the other hand, because the zymogen stores were significantly lower in patients with severe acute pancreatitis compared with healthy subjects (p=0.015) in the same study [48], it is reasonable to assume that there is a compensative secretory hyperfunction of the surviving pancreatic acinar cells with two vectors of secretion – in the blood and in the duodenum. The latter hypothesis is confirmed by the earlier than in normal (p<0.05) appearance of newly synthesized trypsin in duodenal juice of patients with necrotizing pancreatitis as well as a significant increase of serum lipase concentration (p<0.01) in patients with severe versus mild acute pancreatitis [48].

To this end, nasogastric delivery of nutrients may be feasible in patients with severe acute pancreatitis. However, a well-designed and adequately powered randomized trial on gastric versus mid-jejunal feeding is needed before implementation of nasogastric nutrition into routine practice.

Immunonutrition vs Standard Enteral Nutrition

Because the gastrointestinal tract is the largest immune organ in the body, containing more than a half of immune tissue overall, the use of immune-enhanced enteral formulations may further amplify the beneficial effect of intra-luminal therapy in acute pancreatitis [49,50]. Of the various substances that thought to have immune-enhancing properties, glutamine, arginine, omega-3 fatty acids and nucleotides have been advocated for the use both separately and in combined preparations [51,52]. The nutritional formulas on the basis of these nutrients had positive effects on the rate of infectious complications in different experimental settings, including acute pancreatitis [53,54].

There were also a number of clinical studies, which suggested that immune-enhancing enteral nutrition may have a potential to modify the inflammatory response. The results of RCTs that compared the use of immunonutrition and non-enhanced enteral nutrition were statistically aggregated in 3 meta-analyses [55-57]. The most recent and comprehensive systematic review [57] found that the effect of immunonutrition may depend on the subset of the analyzed patients. In particular, there was no effect of immunonutrition on the risk of infectious complications or death within the subgroup of critically ill patients only. At the same time, administration of high-arginine-content formulas in a combined group of critically ill and elective surgery patients were associated with a statistically significant reduction in infectious complications. On the other hand, the use of high- and low-arginine-content enteral formulas was associated with a significantly lower risk of infectious complications in elective surgery patients when compared with critically ill patients. The heterogeneity of study population in this meta-analysis questioned the clinical applicability of "immunoactive" enteral formulations in patients with acute pancreatitis.

A total of 78 patients with acute pancreatitis from 3 RCTs [58-60] were included in the analysis, of whom 40 received enteral nutrition supplemented with glutamine, arginine and/or omega-3 fatty acids and 38 received standard enteral tube feeding. The incidence of total infectious complications was 37.5% (15 of 40) in the immunonutrition group and 34.2% (13 of 38) in the standard enteral nutrition group. When meta-analysed, enteral nutrition supplemented with immunoactive nutrients did not result in a statistically significant increase in risk of total infectious complications (RR, 1.05; 95% CI, 0.57-1.93; p=0.89) (Fig. 8). There was no significant heterogeneity between trials ($I^2 = 0$).

The mortality rate was 10% (4 of 40) in the immunonutrition group and 18.4% (7 of 38) in the standard enteral nutrition group. When meta-analysed, "immunoactive" enteral nutrition did not result in a statistically significant reduction in risk of death (RR, 0.64; 95% CI, 0.20-2.07; p=0.46) (Fig. 9). There was no significant heterogeneity between trials ($I^2 = 0$).

These results did not show any clinical beneficial effect of enteral nutrition enriched with glutamine, arginine and/or omega-3 fatty acids, when compared with standard enteral nutrition, in patients with acute pancreatitis. These findings are in accordance with the results of the meta-analysis of critically ill and elective surgery patients [57] which found a statistically significant benefit of "immunoactive" enteral nutrition (reduced risk of infectious complications) only in the subgroup of patients who received high-arginine-content formulas. However, supplementing arginine in excess could potentially lead to a pancreas damaging effect [61,62], probably due to the excessive production of nitric oxide [63]. It is also known that administration of omega-3 fatty acids decreases antioxidant capacity [64]. Thereby, it seems prudent to switch a vector of scientific thought to other substances which may modify enteral nutrition and potentially have a beneficial clinical implication in acute pancreatitis [65].

No doubts, the most investigated among them are probiotics (supplements containing potentially beneficial bacteria, usually lactic acid bacteria) [66,67]. A number of studies demonstrated the benefits of probiotics in experimental setting [68,69], but whether their administration is justifiable in patients with severe acute pancreatitis will be known from the PROPATRIA trial [70]. Meanwhile, a recent double-blind RCT from Turkey [71] compared enteral feeding with prebiotics (non-absorbable fibers that selectively induce intestinal microbial growth) versus standard enteral feeding. The study demonstrated that nasojejunal feeding with prebiotics decreases overall complications and length of hospital stay. Another research team demonstrated a favourable effect of enteral tube feeding supplemented with synbiotics (combined use of probiotics and prebiotics) over prebiotics in two double-blind RCTs [72,73]. Thereby, synbiotics have a potential to become an advanced supplement to enteral tube feeding in patients with acute pancreatitis.

Early vs Delayed Enteral Nutrition

It is believed that gut dysfunction contributes to the inflammatory response and organ failure in severe acute pancreatitis [14-16]. Theoretically, enteral feeding can prevent mucosal barrier dysfunction, small bowel bacterial overgrowth, bacterial translocation and, therefore, should be instituted as early as possible in the course of disease [26,27]. However, while some authors showed the clinical benefits of early enteral nutrition [20,23,76], others demonstrated the favourable effects of delayed enteral feeding [21,77,78]. Unfortunately, such a strategical question as the timing of EN in patients with acute pancreatitis has never been studied in RCTs. At the same time, some RCTs in critically ill patients suggest enteral feeding start time has to be within hours of onset of disease.

In particular, burn patients were studied in the RCT by Chiarelli et al [79]. Patients were randomized to receive early enteral feeding within 4.4±0.5 h postburn or delayed feeding administered a mean of 57.7±2.6 h after injury. It was shown that patients with very early start of nutrition had fewer infections as well as a significantly shortened length of hospital stay. Furthermore, Grahm et al [80] demonstrated with a RCT the benefits of early (<36 h) enteral feeding compared with delayed (3-5 d) in 32 patients after head injury. Infectious

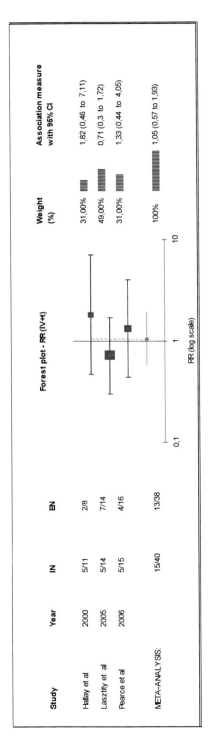

Figure 8. Relative risk of total infectious complications associated with immunonutrition in comparison with standard enteral nutrition in patients with acute pancreatitis.

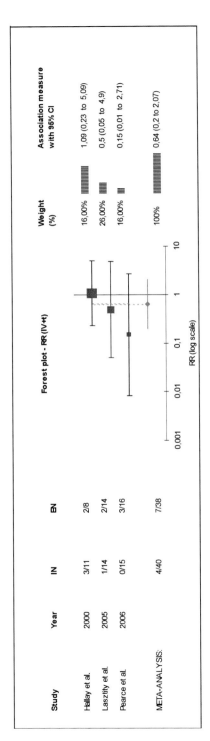

Figure 9. Relative risk of death associated with immunonutrition in comparison with standard enteral nutrition in patients with acute pancreatitis.

complications and length of hospital stay in the ICU were reduced significantly with early feeding into the jejunum. In a trial conducted by Peng et al [81], 22 patients with severe burns were randomized to either early enteral feeding (within 24 h) or delayed enteral feeding (after 48 h). The urinary lactulose levels and the urinary lactulose-mannitol ratios in the early group were significantly lower than in the delayed group as well as the levels of serum endotoxin and TNF-α. It was suggested that early enteral feeding may decrease intestinal permeability, preserve the intestinal mucosal barrier and have a beneficial effect on the reduction of enterogenic infection. A recent RCT from Slovenia in 52 patients with multiple injuries demonstrated that EN administered on admission, as compared to enteral feeding started after 24 h of admission, was associated with a lower incidence of upper intestinal intolerance and nosocomial pneumonia [82]. A meta-analysis by Marik and Zaloga demonstrated the benefits of early EN (started from 2 to 24 h after operation) versus delayed feeding in terms of reducing episodes of infection and length of hospital stay in patients after abdominal surgery [83].

However, the usefulness of early onset of enteral feeding has not been shown in some other studies. In 2004, Peck et al [84] reported the results of their RCT on 27 patients with burn injury. Study demonstrated that early EN (< 24 h of injury) had no beneficial effect on postburn hypermetabolism when compared with late (> 7 d) enteral feeding and also did not result in a reduction of mortality, infectious complications or hospital stay. In other trial, Dvorak et al [85] randomized 17 patients with acute spinal cord injury to early (initiated before 72 h after injury) or late (started more than 120 h after injury) enteral feeding. The RCT failed to detect any differences in the incidence of infection, nutritional status, feeding complications, or length of stay between studied groups. Unfortunately, both RCT were underpowered and thereby presented results should be interpreted with caution.

Considering the results from RCTs on this subject in patients with surgical conditions, it seems that there is a sufficient body of evidence to state the need for high quality RCT on the efficacy of early versus delayed enteral nutritional strategy in patients with severe acute pancreatitis.

Continuos vs Intermittent Enteral Nutrition

The impaired gastrointestinal motility is an important factor in the pathogenesis of complications of acute pancreatitis [14,15]. It may lead to proximal stagnation, gastric and small intestinal bacterial overgrowth with subsequent bacterial translocation and infection of pancreatic necrosis [16,17]. Thereby, a recent study questioned the rationale of fasting patients with acute pancreatitis prior to oral refeeding and advocated the early enteral feeding to prevent or attenuate ileus [86]. The logic behind early EN is that feeding may stimulate motor migrating complex which is responsible for coordinated propulsive activity of the gastrointestinal tract. At the same time, gut hormones may have an important role in regulating gastrointestinal motility.

In particular, high cholecystokinin level is known to cause delay in gastric empting, to regulate nutrient-induced jejuno-gastric feedback mechanism and, thereby, can have influence on the tolerance of enteral feeding [87]. Traditionally, continuous, as opposite to intermittent, EN has been recommended to increase the tolerance of nutrition. Nutritional diet is usually started at low rates (15 mL/h), with gradual advancement to ensure tolerance. However, this tactic has never been tested in RCTs. By contrast, it was reported in a RCT on continuous versus cyclic jejunal nutrition in patients undergoing pylorus-preserving pancreatoduodenectomy that patients on cyclic (discontinuing the nutrition during the night) EN had significantly lower levels of cholecystokinin during interruption of feeding [88]. Clinically this finding was associated with shorter length of hospital stay (p<0.05) and earlier resumption of oral diet (p<0.05) in the intermittent group. In accordance with these data, a recent RCT [89] on continuous versus intermittent gastric feeding in critically ill trauma patients showed that the intermittent regimen patients (100 ml of enteral feed during a 30- to 60-minute period of time every 8 h) reached the nutritional goal faster (p=0.01). However, there was no difference between group in terms of complications and mortality.

The data mentioned above suggest that a RCT on continuous versus intermittent enteral feeding may be of practical importance in patients with acute pancreatitis.

Conclusion

The strategy of nutritional management in acute pancreatitis has not simply undergone substantial changes over the past several decades but rather has tested a range of alternative approaches from famine to feast, from the conception of nil-per-os regimen and "pancreatic rest" through the advocating of nasojejunal and, subsequently, nasogastric tube feeding till the most recent successful reports of early oral feeding. Since acute pancreatitis induces intestinal bacterial overgrowth and secondary pancreatic infections are intestine-derived, the gut serves as the "motor" of pancreatic infection, systemic inflammatory response syndrome and organ failure. Enteral feeding as a treatment strategy targeting at protection of gut defence against bacterial translocation and its sequelae provides a range of clinical benefits. There is strong evidence of the advantages of enteral over parenteral feeding in patients with severe acute pancreatitis in terms of statistically significant reductions in the risk of infectious complications, hyperglycemia and mortality. Thereby, in the continuation of abovementioned "mechanical" allegory, enteral feeding may serve as a reliable "brake" of pancreatic sepsis and should be considered as a drug in patients with acute pancreatitis. The quest for optimal timing, content, rhythm and site of the enteral tube feeding may further amplify its usefulness in this clinical setting.

References

[1]   Lankisch PG. Natural course of chronic pancreatitis. *Pancreatology* 2001;1:3-14.
[2]   Moynihan B. Acute pancreatitis. *Ann Surg* 1925;81:132-42.
[3]   McKay CJ, Evans S, Sinclair M, Carter CR, Imrie CW. High early mortality rate from acute pancreatitis in Scotland, 1984–1995. *Br J Surg* 1999;86:1302–5.
[4]   Johnson CD, Abu-Hilal M. Persistent organ failure during the first week as a marker of fatal outcome in acute pancreatitis. *Gut* 2004;53:1340-4.
[5]   Blum T, Maisonneuve P, Lowenfels AB, Lankisch PG. Fatal outcome in acute pancreatitis: its occurrence and early prediction. *Pancreatology* 2001;1:237-41.
[6]   Baron TH, Morgan DE. Acute necrotizing pancreatitis. *N Engl J Med* 1999;340: 1412–7.

[7] Schmid SW, Uhl W, Friess H, Malfertheiner P, Buchler MW. The role of infection in acute pancreatitis. *Gut* 1999;45:311-6.

[8] Gloor B, Muller CA, Worni M, Martignoni ME, Uhl W, Buchler MW. Late mortality in patients with severe acute pancreatitis. *Br J Surg* 2001;88:975-9.

[9] Sackett DL. Clinical epidemiology. What, who, and whither. *J Clin Epidemiol* 2002;55:1161-6.

[10] van Nieuwenhoven CA, Buskens E, van Tiel FH, Bonten MJM. Relationship between methodological trial quality and the effects of selective digestive decontamination on pneumonia and mortality in critically ill patients. *JAMA* 2001;286:335-40.

[11] Cassim MM, Allardyce DB. Pancreatic secretion in response to jejunal feeding of elemental diet. *Ann Surg* 1974;180:228-31.

[12] Grant JP, James S, Grabowski V, Trexler KM. Total parenteral nutrition in pancreatic disease. *Ann Surg* 1984;200:627–31.

[13] Wicks C, Somasundaram S, Bjarnason I, Menzies IS, Routley D, Potter D, Tan KC, Williams R. Comparison of enteral feeding and total parenteral nutrition after liver transplantation. *Lancet* 1994;344:837–40.

[14] Swank GM, Deitch EA. Role of the gut in multiple organ failure: bacterial translocation and permeability changes. *World J Surg* 1996;20:411–7.

[15] Medich D, Lee T, Melhem M. Pathogenesis of pancreatic sepsis. *Am J Surg* 1993;165:46-50.

[16] Ammori BJ. Role of the gut in the course of severe acute pancreatitis. *Pancreas* 2003;26:122-9.

[17] Cicalese L, Sahai A, Sileri P. Acute pancreatitis and bacterial translocation. *Dig Dis Sci* 2001;46:1127–32.

[18] Kalfarentzos F, Kehagias J, Mead N, Kokkinis K, Gogos CA. Enteral nutrition is superior to parenteral nutrition in severe acute pancreatitis: results of a randomized prospective trial. *Br J Surg* 1997;84:1665-9.

[19] Paraskeva C, Smailis D, Priovolos A, Sofianou K, Lytras D, Avgerinos C, Rizos S, Karagiannis J, Dervenis C. Early enteral nutrition reduces the need for surgery in severe acute pancreatitis. *Pancreatology* 2001;1:372. [Abstract]

[20] Gupta R, Patel K, Calder PC, Yaqoob P, Primrose JN, Johnson CD. A randomised clinical trial to assess the effect of total enteral and total parenteral nutritional support on metabolic, inflammatory and oxidative markers in patients with predicted severe acute pancreatitis (APACHE II > or =6). *Pancreatology* 2003;3:406-13.

[21] Louie BE, Noseworthy T, Hailey D, Gramlich LM, Jacobs P, Warnock GL. 2004 MacLean-Mueller prize enteral or parenteral nutrition for severe pancreatitis: a randomized controlled trial and health technology assessment. *Can J Surg* 2005;48:298-306.

[22] Eckerwall GE, Axelsson JB, Andersson RG. Early nasogastric feeding in predicted severe acute pancreatitis: a clinical, randomized study. Ann Surg 2006;244:959-65.

[23] Petrov MS, Kukosh MV, Emelyanov NV. A randomized controlled trial of enteral versus parenteral feeding in patients with predicted severe acute pancreatitis shows a significant reduction in mortality and in infected pancreatic complications with total enteral nutrition. *Dig Surg* 2006;23:336-44.

[24] Casas M, Mora J, Fort E, Aracil C, Busquets D, Galter S, Jauregui CE, Ayala E, Cardona D, Gich I, Farre A. Total enteral nutrition vs. total parenteral nutrition in patients with severe acute pancreatitis. *Rev Esp Enferm Dig* 2007;99:264-9.

[25] Petrov MS, van Santvoort HC, Besselink MGH, van der Heijden GJMG, Windsor JA, Gooszen HG. Enteral nutrition reduced the risk of mortality and infectious complications in patients with severe acute pancreatitis: a meta-analysis comparing enteral and parenteral nutrition. *Arch Surg* 2008 [in press].

[26] Lehocky P, Sarr MG. Early enteral feeding in severe acute pancreatitis: can it prevent secondary pancreatic (super) infection? *Dig Surg* 2000;17:571-7.

[27] Dervenis C. Enteral nutrition in severe acute pancreatitis: future development. *JOP* 2004;5:60-63.

[28] Kotani J, Usami M, Nomura H, Iso A, Kasahara H, Kuroda Y, Oyanagi H, Saitoh Y. Enteral nutrition prevents bacterial translocation but does not improve survival during acute pancreatitis. *Arch Surg* 1999;134:287-92.

[29] Juvonen PO, Alhava EM, Takala JA. Gut permeability in patients with acute pancreatitis. *Scand J Gastroenterol* 2000;35:1314-8.

[30] Ammori BJ, Leeder PC, King RF, Barclay GR, Martin IG, Larvin M, McMahon MJ. Early increase in intestinal permeability in patients with severe acute pancreatitis: correlation with endotoxemia, organ failure, and mortality. *J Gastrointest Surg* 1999;3:252-62.

[31] Nagpal K, Minocha VR, Agrawal V, Kapur S. Evaluation of intestinal mucosal permeability function in patients with acute pancreatitis. *Am J Surg* 2006;192:24-8.

[32] Powell JJ, Murchison JT, Fearon KC, Ross JA, Siriwardena AK. Randomized controlled trial of the effect of early enteral nutrition on markers of the inflammatory response in predicted severe acute pancreatitis. *Br J Surg* 2000;87:1375-81.

[33] Windsor AC, Kanwar S, Li AG, Barnes E, Guthrie JA, Spark JI, Welsh F, Guillou PJ, Reynolds JV. Compared with parenteral nutrition, enteral feeding attenuates the acute phase response and improves disease severity in acute pancreatitis. *Gut* 1998;42:431-5.

[34] McCowen KC, Malhotra A, Bistrian BR. Stress-induced hyperglycemia. *Crit Care Clin* 2001;17:107-24.

[35] Petrov MS, Zagainov VE. Influence of enteral versus parenteral nutrition on blood glucose control in acute pancreatitis: a systematic review. *Clin Nutr* 2007;26:514-23.

[36] Van den Berghe G, Wouters P, Weekers F, Verwaest C, Bruyninckx F, Schetz M, Vlasselaers D, Ferdinande P, Lauwers P, Bouillon R. Intensive insulin therapy in critically ill patients. *N Engl J Med* 2001;345:1359-67.

[37] Suchner U, Senftleben U, Eckart T, Scholz MR, Beck K, Murr R, Enzenbach R, Peter K. Enteral versus parenteral nutrition: effects on gastrointestinal function and metabolism. *Nutrition* 1996;12:13-22.

[38] Moore FA, Moore EE, Jones TN, McCroskey BL, Peterson VM. TEN versus TPN following major abdominal trauma-reduced septic morbidity. *J Trauma* 1989;29:916-22.

[39] Bistrian BR, McCowen KC. Nutritional and metabolic support in the adult intensive care unit: Key controversies. *Crit Care Med* 2006;34:1525–31.

[40] McCowen KC, Maykel JA, Bistrian BR. Intensive insulin therapy in critically ill patients. *N Engl J Med* 2002;346:1586-8.

[41] Marik PE, Zaloga GP. Gastric versus post-pyloric feeding: a systematic review. Crit Care 2003;7:46-51.

[42] Vu MK, Van Der Veek P, Frolich M, Souverijn JH, Biemond I, Lamers CB, Masclee AA. Does jejunal feeding activate exocrine pancreatic secretion? *Eur J Clin Invest* 1999;29:1053-9.

[43] Kaushik N, Pietraszewski M, Holst JJ, O'Keefe SJ. Enteral feeding without pancreatic stimulation. *Pancreas* 2005;31:353-9.

[44] Eatock FC, Brombacher GD, Steven A, Imrie CW, McKay CJ, Carter R. Nasogastric feeding in severe acute pancreatitis may be practical and safe. *Int J Pancreatol* 2000;28:23-9.

[45] Eatock FC, Chong P, Menezes N, Murray L, McKay CJ, Carter CR, Imrie CW. A randomized study of early nasogastric versus nasojejunal feeding in severe acute pancreatitis. *Am J Gastroenterol* 2005;100:432-9.

[46] Kumar A, Singh N, Prakash S, Saraya A, Joshi YK. Early enteral nutrition in severe acute pancreatitis: a prospective randomized controlled trial comparing nasojejunal and nasogastric routes. *J Clin Gastroenterol* 2006;40:431-4.

[47] O'Keefe SJ, Lee RB, Li J, Zhou W, Stoll B, Dang Q. Trypsin and splanchnic protein turnover during feeding and fasting in human subjects. *Am J Physiol Gastrointest Liver Physiol* 2006;290:G213–21.

[48] O'Keefe SJ, Lee RB, Li J, Stevens S, Abou-Assi S, Zhou W. Trypsin secretion and turnover in patients with acute pancreatitis. *Am J Physiol Gastrointest Liver Physiol* 2005;289:G181-7.

[49] Bengmark S. Gut microenvironment and immune function. *Curr Opinion Clin Nutrit Metab Care* 1999;2:1-3.

[50] Phillips MC, Olson LR. The immunological role of the gastrointestinal tract. *Crit Care Nurs North Am* 1993;5:107–20.

[51] Schloerb PR. Immune-enhancing diets: products, components and their rationales. *JPEN J Parenter Enteral Nutr* 2001;25:S3–7.

[52] Grant J. Nutritional support in critically ill patients. *Ann Surg* 1994;220:610 –6.

[53] Foitzik T, Kruschewski M, Kroesen AJ, Hotz HG, Eibl G, Buhr HJ. Does glutamine reduce bacterial translocation? A study in two animal models with impaired gut barrier. *Int J Colorectal Dis* 1999;14:143-9.

[54] Foitzik T, Eibl G, Schneider P, Wenger FA, Jacobi CA, Buhr HJ. Omega-3 fatty acid supplementation increases anti-inflammatory cytokines and attenuates systemic disease sequelae in experimental pancreatitis. *JPEN J Parenter Enteral Nutr* 2002; 26:351-6.

[55] Beale RJ, Bryg DJ, Bihari DJ. Immunonutrition in the critically ill: a systematic review of clinical outcome. *Crit Care Med* 1999;27:2799-805.

[56] Heys SD, Walker LG, Smith I, Eremin O. Enteral nutritional supplementation with key nutrients in patients with critical illness and cancer: a meta-analysis of randomized controlled clinical trials. *Ann Surg* 1999; 229:467-77.

[57] Heyland D K, Novak F, Drover J W, Jain M, Su X, Suchner U. Should immunonutrition become routine in critically ill patients? A systematic review of the evidence. *JAMA* 2001;286:944-53.

[58] Hallay J, Kovacs G, Szatmari K. Early jejunal nutrition and changes in the immunological parameters of patients with acute pancreatitis. *Hepatogastroenterology* 2001;48:1488-92.

[59] Lasztity N, Hamvas J, Biro L, Németh E, Marosvölgyi T, Decsi T, Pap A, Antal M. Effect of enterally administered n-3 polyunsaturated fatty acids in acute pancreatitis - a prospective randomized clinical trial. *Clin Nutr* 2005;24:198-205.

[60] Pearce CB, Sadek SA, Walters AM, Goggin PM, Somers SS, Toh SK, Johns T, Duncan HD. A double-blind, randomised, controlled trial to study the effects of an enteral feed supplemented with glutamine, arginine, and omega-3 fatty acid in predicted acute severe pancreatitis. *JOP* 2006;7:361-71.

[61] Takama S, Kishino Y. Dietary effects on pancreatic lesions induced by excess arginine in rats. *Br J Nutr* 1985;54:37-42.

[62] Luiking YC, Deutz NE. Biomarkers of arginine and lysine excess. *J Nutr* 2007;137:S1662-8.

[63] Furst P, Kuhn KS. Fish oil emulsions: what benefit can they bring? *Clin Nutr* 2000;19:7–14.

[64] Bertolini G, Luciani D, Biolo G. Immunonutrition in septic patients: a philosophical view of the current situation. *Clin Nutr* 2007;26:25–29.

[65] Petrov MS, Zagainov VE. Advanced enteral therapy in acute pancreatitis: from immunonutrition to econutrition? [submitted].

[66] Bengmark S. Ecological control of the gastrointestinal tract. The role of probiotic flora. *Gut* 1998;42:2–7.

[67] Pezzilli R, Fantini L. Probiotics and severe acute pancreatitis. *JOP J Pancreas* (Online) 2006;7:92-93.

[68] Muftuoglu MA, Isikgor S, Tosun S, Saglam A. Effects of probiotics on the severity of experimental acute pancreatitis. *Eur J Clin Nutr* 2006;60:464-8.

[69] van Minnen LP, Timmerman HM, Lutgendorff F, Verheem A, Harmsen W, Konstantinov SR, Smidt H, Visser MR, Rijkers GT, Gooszen HG, Akkermans LM. Modification of intestinal flora with multispecies probiotics reduces bacterial translocation and improves clinical course in a rat model of acute pancreatitis. *Surgery* 2007;141:470-80.

[70] Besselink MG, Timmerman HM, Buskens E, Nieuwenhuijs VB, Akkermans LM, Gooszen HG. Dutch Acute Pancreatitis Study Group. Probiotic prophylaxis in patients with predicted severe acute pancreatitis (PROPATRIA): design and rationale of a double-blind, placebo-controlled randomised multicenter trial [ISRCTN38327949]. *BMC Surg* 2004; 4:12.

[71] Karakan T, Ergun M, Dogan I, Cindoruk M, Unal S. Comparison of early enteral nutrition in severe acute pancreatitis with prebiotic fiber supplementation versus standard enteral solution: a prospective randomized double-blind study. *World J Gastroenterol* 2007;13:2733-7.

[72] Olah A, Belagyi T, Issekutz A, Gamal ME, Bengmark S. Randomized clinical trial of specific lactobacillus and fibre supplement to early enteral nutrition in patients with acute pancreatitis. *Br J Surg* 2002;89:1103-7.

[73] Olah A, Belagyi T, Poto L, Romics L Jr, Bengmark S. Synbiotic control of inflammation and infection in severe acute pancreatitis: a prospective, randomized, double blind study. *Hepatogastroenterology* 2007;54:594-8.

[74] Wilson PG, Manji M, Neoptolemos JP. Acute pancreatitis as a model of sepsis. *J Antimicrob Chemother* 1998;41 Suppl A:51-63.

[75] Dervenis C, Smailis D, Hatzitheoklitos E. Bacterial translocation and its prevention in acute pancreatitis. *J Hepatobiliary Pancreat Surg* 2003;10:415-8.

[76] Nakad A, Piessevaux H, Marot JC, Hoang P, Geubel A, Van Steenbergen W, Reynaert M. Is early enteral nutrition in acute pancreatitis dangerous? About 20 patients fed by an endoscopically placed nasogastrojejunal tube. *Pancreas* 1998;17:187-93.

[77] Makola D, Krenitsky J, Parrish C, Dunston E, Shaffer HA, Yeaton P, Kahaleh M. Efficacy of enteral nutrition for the treatment of pancreatitis using standard enteral formula. *Am J Gastroenterol* 2006;101:2347-55.

[78] Tiengou LE, Gloro R, Pouzoulet J, Bouhier K, Read MH, Arnaud-Battandier F, Plaze JM, Blaizot X, Dao T, Piquet MA. Semi-elemental formula or polymeric formula: is there a better choice for enteral nutrition in acute pancreatitis? Randomized comparative study. *JPEN J Parenter Enteral Nutr* 2006;30:1-5.

[79] Chiarelli A, Enzi G, Casadei A, Baggio B, Valerio A, Mazzoleni F. Very early nutrition supplementation in burned patients. *Am J Clin Nutr* 1990;51:1035-9.

[80] Grahm TW, Zadrozny DB, Harrington T. The benefits of early jejunal hyperalimentation in the head-injured patient. *Neurosurgery* 1989;25:729-35.

[81] Peng YZ, Yuan ZQ, Xiao GX. Effects of early enteral feeding on the prevention of enterogenic infection in severely burned patients. *Burns* 2001;27:145-9.

[82] Kompan L, Kremzar B, Gadzijev E, Prosek M. Effects of early enteral nutrition on intestinal permeability and the development of multiple organ failure after multiple injury. *Intensive Care Med* 1999;25:157-61.

[83] Marik PE, Zaloga GP. Early enteral nutrition in acutely ill patients: a systematic review. *Crit Care Med* 2001;29:2264-70.

[84] Peck MD, Kessler M, Cairns BA, Chang YH, Ivanova A, Schooler W. Early enteral nutrition does not decrease hypermetabolism associated with burn injury. *J Trauma* 2004;57:1143-8.

[85] Dvorak MF, Noonan VK, Belanger L, Bruun B, Wing PC, Boyd MC, Fisher C. Early versus late enteral feeding in patients with acute cervical spinal cord injury: a pilot study. *Spine* 2004;29:175-80.

[86] Petrov MS, van Santvoort HC, Besselink MGH, Circel GA, Brink MA, Gooszen HG. Oral refeeding after onset of acute pancreatitis: a review of literature. *Am J Gastroenterol* 2007;102:2079-84.

[87] Kleibeuker JH, Beekhuis H, Jansen JB, Piers DA, Lamers CB. Cholecystokinin is a physiological hormonal mediator of fat-induced inhibition of gastric emptying in man. *Eur J Clin Invest* 1988;18:173-7.

[88] Van Berge Henegouwen MI, Akkermans LM, van Gulik TM, Masclee AA, Moojen TM, Obertop H, Gouma DJ. Prospective, randomized trial on the effect of cyclic versus continuous enteral nutrition on postoperative gastric function after pylorus-preserving pancreatoduodenectomy. *Ann Surg* 1997;226:677-85.

[89] MacLeod JB, Lefton J, Houghton D, Roland C, Doherty J, Cohn SM, Barquist ES. Prospective randomized control trial of intermittent versus continuous gastric feeds for critically ill trauma patients. *J Trauma* 2007;63:57-61.

Index

C

E

F

I

J

N

O

Q

R

S